Library of Congress Cataloging-in-Publication Data

Sharkey, Brian J.
  Fitness and health / Brian J. Sharkey, Steven E. Gaskill.-- 6th ed.
     p. cm.
  Includes bibliographical references and index.
  ISBN-13: 978-0-7360-5614-4 (soft cover)
  ISBN-10: 0-7360-5614-9 (soft cover)
  1. Physical fitness. 2. Health. I. Gaskill, Steven E., 1952- II. Title.
  RA781.S527 2007
  613.7--dc22

                              2006008698

ISBN-10: 0-7360-5614-9
ISBN-13: 978-0-7360-5614-4

Permission notices for material reprinted in this book from other sources can be found on page ix.

Acquisitions Editor: Michael S. Bahrke, PhD; **Developmental Editor:** Heather Healy; **Assistant Editors:** Mandy Maiden, Christine Horger; **Copyeditor:** Robert Replinger; **Proofreader:** Anne Rogers; **Indexer:** Bobbi Swanson; **Permission Manager:** Carly Breeding; **Graphic Designer:** Nancy Rasmus; **Graphic Artist:** Francine Hamerski; **Photo Manager:** Dan Wendt; **Cover Designer:** Keith Blomberg; **Photographer (cover):** © www.imagesource.com; **Photographer (interior):** Dan Wendt unless otherwise noted, Photos on pages 61, 81, 95, 143, 157 (fig. 9.1*b*), 181, 209, 265, 281, 297, 299, 332, 354, 365, and 373 © Human Kinetics; **Art Manager:** Kareema McLendon-Foster; **Illustrators:** Kareema McLendon-Foster, Mic Greenburg

Human Kinetics books are available at special discounts for bulk purchase. Special editions or book excerpts can also be created to specification. For details, contact the Special Sales Manager at Human Kinetics.

Printed in Hong Kong   10 9 8 7 6 5 4 3 2 1

Human Kinetics
Web site: www.HumanKinetics.com

United States: Human Kinetics
P.O. Box 5076
Champaign, IL 61825-5076
800-747-4457
e-mail: humank@hkusa.com

Canada: Human Kinetics
475 Devonshire Road Unit 100
Windsor, ON N8Y 2L5
800-465-7301 (in Canada only)
e-mail: orders@hkcanada.com

Europe: Human Kinetics
107 Bradford Road
Stanningley
Leeds LS28 6AT, United Kingdom
+44 (0) 113 255 5665
e-mail: hk@hkeurope.com

Australia: Human Kinetics
57A Price Avenue
Lower Mitcham, South Australia 5062
08 8277 1555
e-mail: liaw@hkaustralia.com

New Zealand: Human Kinetics
Division of Sports Distributors NZ Ltd.
P.O. Box 300 226 Albany
North Shore City
Auckland
0064 9 448 1207
e-mail: info@humankinetics.co.nz

Fitness & Health

Sixth Edition

Brian J. Sharkey, PhD

Steven E. Gaskill, PhD

University of Montana

049810

To Barbara and Kathy, perfect companions for the long run.

Contents

Preface

In 1968 Brian Sharkey began a manuscript that emerged as his first book. Refined by several years of classroom use, *Physiological Fitness and Weight Control* was published in 1974. It provided sound advice for exercise and weight control, advice that, according to the Centers for Disease Control (USDHHS 1996), could save over 250,000 lives annually, then and now! That information has been around for years, yet the population is far less active, and we now face an epidemic of overweight and obesity. All this has occurred in a period in which we have learned a great deal more about physical activity, fitness, and health. These exciting research developments led to a new title and expansion of the original version of the book in 1979, and then second and third editions in 1984 and 1990. The editions of that book, *Physiology of Fitness*, became a chronicle of new developments and the author's journey from fitness enthusiast to performance advocate and, finally, to campaigner for the benefits of the active life.

In 1997 the fourth edition was retitled *Fitness and Health*. Epidemiological studies demonstrated that people can achieve many health benefits with regular, moderate physical activity and can earn even greater rewards by improving their level of fitness. But the greatest gains, for personal and public health, come when people move from sedentary to active lifestyles. The new title affirms the importance of physical activity and fitness, highlighting one of the most exciting public health messages of our time. The fifth edition of the book was published in 2002.

After 30 years of solitary effort Brian decided that for this sixth edition, he would seek the assistance of a friend and colleague, Steve Gaskill. They met in 1980 when Steve was a coach and Brian was sport physiologist for the U.S. Nordic Ski Team. In the late 1980s their lives took separate directions, but they remained friends and kept in touch. In 1998, after completing his doctorate in exercise physiology, Steve applied for a position at the University of Montana, where Brian was retiring. Since then they have renewed their professional and personal association, conducting research and development activities in the Human Performance Laboratory and in the field. Steve brings new ideas and energy to the book. Together they plan to make this the best and most useful source available, one that will add purpose and meaning to involvement in regular, moderate physical activity.

Written for adults of all ages, this book is especially intended for the person who wants to develop a deeper understanding of fitness and health, for the enthusiast who wants to know why and how the body responds, for the newcomer who needs motivation, and for the skeptic who needs proof. The book has always sought to be the thinking person's fitness book; the authors hope you'll find that this edition meets that description.

Part I conveys the importance of regular, moderate physical activity. It describes how the active life contributes to physical and mental health as well as the quality of life. The added benefits associated with improved aerobic and muscular fitness are also discussed. Part II covers everything that you want to know about aerobic fitness, and part III provides information and guidelines for muscular fitness training. Part IV presents new information in the areas of nutrition and weight control, information that could reverse the current epidemic of obesity. Part V shows you how to improve your performance in sport and work and how to cope with the environment. Part VI includes an expanded look at the psychology of activity and a discussion of the role of activity in aging and longevity. The final chapter shows you how to improve your personal life, the lives of those in your family, and life in your community. It portrays the importance of the environment to health, fitness, and the quality of life, and enlists your aid in the struggle to preserve and expand opportunities for healthful, enjoyable physical activity.

Each chapter includes useful information in tables and figures, and some contain testing procedures and proven fitness programs. The special inserts (shaded boxes) provide additional background and details concerning fitness and health.

So join us as we enter a new era of physical activity and fitness, an era in which the benefits are great relative to the effort, enjoyment and satisfaction replace guilt and failure, and activity and fitness are recognized and practiced as vital contributors to health and the quality of life.

Credits

Figure in the Introduction "Activity Index"—Adapted from "The Effects of Exercise and Fitness on Serum Lipids in College Women," p. 46, by D. Kasari, 1976, unpublished master's thesis, University of Montana.

Figure 3.2—Source: American Heart Association. www.americanheart.org

Figure 3.4—Adapted, by permission, from K. Powel and R. Paffenbarger, 1985, "Workshop on epidemiologic and public health aspects of physical activity and exercise: A summary," *Public Health Reports* 100 (2):118-126.

Figures 4.2, 4.3, and 16.1—Adapted from B.J. Sharkey, 1997, *Fitness and work capacity*, 2nd ed. (Missoula, MT: USDA Forest Service).

Figures 5.5, 8.1, and 9.2—Adapted from B.J. Sharkey, 1975, *Physiology and physical activity* (New York: Harper and Row).

Figure 11.1—Adapted from B.J. Sharkey, 1984, *Training for cross-country ski racing* (Champaign, IL: Human Kinetics).

Figure 12.9—Recreated with permission from *Research Quarterly for Exercise and Sport*, Vol. 52, p. 382, Copyright 1981 by the American Alliance for Health, Physical Education, Recreation and Dance, 1900 Association Drive, Reston, VA 20191.

Figures 13.1 and 16.2—Reprinted, by permission, from B.J. Sharkey, 1974, *Physiological fitness and weight control* (Missoula, MT: Mountain Press), 92, 130.

Figure 16.3—Courtesy of the National Oceanic and Atmospheric Administration. www.noaa.gov

Figure 17.1—Adapted from *Vital Statistics of the United States*, 1977 (Volume II, Section 5), DHEW Publication PHS 80-1104, National Center for Health Statistics.

Tables 1.1, 1.3, 12.1, 12.2—Adapted, by permission, from B.J. Sharkey, 1974, *Physiological fitness and weight control* (Missoula, MT: Mountain Press), 11, 15, 22, 28.

Table 3.1—From www.nhlbi.nih.gov 2004.

Tables 3.2*a*–*e* and 3.4—Source: American Heart Association. www.americanheart.org

Table 6.2—G. Borg, 1998, *Borg's Perceived Exertion and Pain Scales* (Champaign, IL: Human Kinetics), 47. © Gunnar Borg, 1970, 1985, 1994, 1998.

Table 6.5—Adapted from B.J. Sharkey, 1997, *Fitness and work capacity*, 2nd ed. (Missoula, MT: USDA Forest Service).

Table 8.1—Reprinted from B.J. Sharkey, 2002, *Fitness and health*, 5th ed. (Champaign, IL: Human Kinetics).

Table 12.5—Reprinted with permission of the Metropolitan Life Insurance Company.

Table 17.1—Adapted, by permission, from J.F. Fries and L. Crapo, 1981, *Vitality and aging* (San Francisco: W.H. Freeman), 125.

Text, "Food Portions," pp. 224–226—Adapted from *Dietary guidelines for Americans 2005*, Department of Agriculture (USDA) and Department of Health and Human Services (HHS).

Text, "Training Principles," pp. 300–303—Adapted, by permission, from B.J. Sharkey and S. Gaskill, 2006, *Sport physiology for coaches* (Champaign, IL: Human Kinetics).

Photos on pp. 88 and 427—Courtesy of Steven Gaskill.

Photo on p. 157 (figure 9.1*a*)—Courtesy of www.vasatrainer.com

Photo on p. 16—Courtesy of Vascular Disease Foundation. www.vdf.org

Photo on p. 323—© Aurora Photos

Photos on pp. 1, 23, and 85—© Digital Vision Royalty Free

Photos on p. 170—© Jumpfoto

Photos on pp. 5, 7, 11, 75, 117, 130, 135, 137, 147, 151, 173, 207, 231, 267, 275, 294, and 305—© EyeWire/Photodisc/Getty Images

Photos on pp. 13, 28, 31, 36, 42, 45, 56, 69, 71, 78, 99, 105, 111, 115, 132, 141, 144, 218, 226, 254, 272, 279, 317, 327, 341, 345, 347, 350, 359, 379, 382, 384, and 388—© PhotoDisc Royalty Free

Introduction to the Active Life

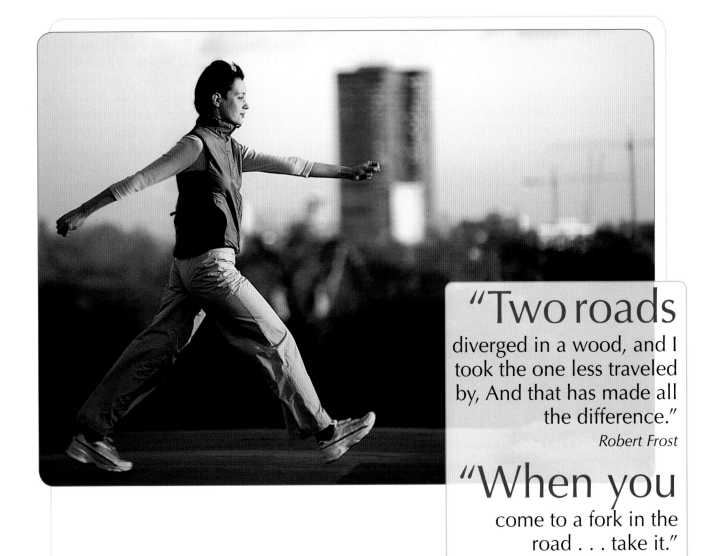

"Two roads diverged in a wood, and I took the one less traveled by, And that has made all the difference."
Robert Frost

"When you come to a fork in the road . . . take it."
Yogi Berra

You've come to a fork in the road. One path shows evidence of heavy traffic, whereas the other, the one less traveled, is faintly etched upon the land. One travels downhill, the route of least resistance, whereas the other rises slowly to distant heights. Will you be seduced by the easy route or motivated by the high road and the view from above? Sadly, many choose the easy route, and consequently we Americans have lost our identity as a vigorous, vital people. Along the way we have become the fattest nation in the world, beset with chronic fatigue, depression, and degenerative diseases of the heart and lungs, of cancer and diabetes. Our goal is to convince you to take the road less traveled, knowing that it will make all the difference in your life.

What is the road less traveled? Simply stated, it is the active life, a way of living based on regular physical activity and a cluster of related behaviors, including healthy food choices, weight control, stress management, abstinence from tobacco and drugs, moderate use of alcohol, attention to safety (wearing seat belts and helmets), and disease prevention. It is the path of individual responsibility that leads not only to health, vigor, and vitality but also to self-respect and control of your destiny. This family of health-related behaviors has proved to be a profound paradox for our society, simple to comprehend but difficult to adopt.

The active life is the one that people led before society achieved the benefits of industrial modernization—technological developments, the automobile, labor-saving devices, television, and computers. These marvels of ingenuity now make it possible to minimize daily energy expenditure by using buttons, keystrokes, and voice commands to meet survival, work, and entertainment needs. Parallel to the decline in the need for human energy expenditure has been an increase in the consumption of highly processed, calorie-rich, convenience, and fast foods. Calorie-rich refined sugars have replaced complex carbohydrates, such as corn, rice, beans, and whole-grained breads and pasta. Food chemists added hydrogen to vegetable oils (hydrogenated or trans-fatty acids) to prolong shelf life but not human life. Low-cost palm and coconut oils have replaced other ingredients to cater to our demand for tasty food—in a hurry. Restaurant and fast-food servings grew larger while physical activity declined. Individually, the decline in activity or the rise in food consumption may not have been such a problem. Coming together as they have in recent years, the potential exists for alarming growth in the epidemic of diseases caused by the way we live. Fortunately, we can change these behaviors.

This introduction will help you

- understand the dimensions of the active life,
- see how activity and other health behaviors interact,
- define the amount of activity needed for health, and
- compare your current level of activity with recommended values.

The Active Life

Our species, *Homo sapiens*, emerged in central Africa some 50,000 years ago. Genetic information indicates that our ancestors spread across the face of the earth as hunter–gatherers. Agriculture emerged some 10,000 years ago. Throughout this migration and until recently, by necessity we humans have lived an active life. But that has changed, slowly at first until the last few decades when we accelerated our transformation to sedentary ways. Now less than 30 percent of the U.S. population gets the minimum amount of exercise associated with health (30 minutes of moderate activity most days of the week) (Booth and Chakravarthy 2002). A small percentage (about 10 percent) engages in sufficient activity to improve fitness and achieve additional health benefits. Few of us understand and appreciate the pleasures and benefits of the active life.

Sports psychologist William Morgan (2001) suggests that part of the reason people don't start or drop out of exercise programs is that the physical activity presented to the population lacks purpose and the exercise prescription focuses on measuring heart rates and duration instead of enjoyment or accomplishment.

"Why do strong arms fatigue themselves with frivolous dumbbells?
To dig a vineyard is worthier exercise for men."

Marcus Valerius Martialis, A.D. 38–103

Morgan presents evidence of lifelong exercisers who (as do your authors) engage in meaningful activity, almost every day of their lives. Stone and Klein (2004) have found that long-term exercisers did so for fitness and health, but more important for the powerful feelings generated by their regular participation (e.g., energy, enjoyment). Their activity had purpose, and yours should too. Keep that in mind as we explore the active life.

Healthy Behaviors

The active life is at the core of a family of behaviors or habits that, viewed one at a time, seem too simplistic to be of much value. Yet collectively they are our greatest hope for personal health and vitality, and for the integrity of the nation's health care system. Many of the behaviors remind us of our mothers' admonitions.

Physical Activity

The U.S. Centers for Disease Control and Prevention (CDC) and the American College of Sports Medicine (ACSM) reported that as many as 250,000 lives are lost annually because of lack of regular, moderate physical activity (USDHHS 1996). Compare that number to the number of lives lost annually in the United States in automobile accidents (40,000), from unprotected sexual intercourse (30,000), or from drug overdoses (20,000). Lack of physical activity is now considered as much a contributor to heart disease as are high blood cholesterol, high blood pressure, and cigarette smoking, not because inactivity is more potent, but because so many of us are inactive or sedentary. Activity can reduce heart disease and control heart disease risk factors—elevated cholesterol, high blood pressure, diabetes, and obesity. Inactivity contributes to a substantial number of the deaths annually and costs $94 billion a year in medical expenses in the United States (Colditz 1999).

> As many as 250,000 lives are lost annually because of lack of regular, moderate physical activity.

Healthy Food Choices

Poor food choices contribute directly to overweight, obesity, heart disease, diabetes, and cancer, and indirectly to other problems such as depression. After years of health education, the average American still gets 30 to 40 percent of his or her daily calories from fat, and a substantial portion of the carbohydrate calories come from highly processed simple sugars instead of from fruits, vegetables, grains, and fiber.

The World Is Fatter, Not Better Fed

Just because people are gaining weight does not mean the world is better fed or healthier, says the environmental group Worldwatch Institute. For the first time in history the number of overweight people in the world is the same as the number of underfed people, about 1.1 billion of each. Being obese or underweight often results from the same problem—malnutrition. In the United States and other wealthy countries, the richer and the better educated people tend to eat right, whereas the poor often balloon from a diet of cheap and fatty fast foods. "Often, nations simply have traded hunger for obesity, and diseases of poverty for diseases of excess," said Worldwatch researchers. In the United States well over 60 percent of the population is overweight, with one in four adults considered obese (Associated Press, March 5, 2000).

Understanding the importance of nutrition and food choices becomes even more important as greater numbers of Americans enter the workforce; work longer hours; and rely more on convenience foods, take-home meals, and eating out. Along with healthy food choices, the modern urban warrior needs to develop eating survival techniques. Poor diet, coupled with lack of exercise, causes at least 300,000 deaths a year, mostly from heart disease, and contributes to an increased risk of diabetes, cancer, and other ills. We'll say much more about food and nutrition in part IV.

Weight Control

Dieting for weight loss is the most unsuccessful health intervention in all of medicine. Over 90 percent of people who have lost 25 pounds (11 kilograms) or more will return to their previous weight within the year. Worse yet, many weight-loss programs (diets) contribute to obesity. The truth that has emerged from the last decade of research is that diet alone won't help people achieve permanent weight loss. What will? The active life, combined with healthy food choices, and behavior therapy if necessary, is the answer to lifelong weight control. Activity maintains or builds the lean tissue (muscle) that has the capability to burn calories. Diet, by itself, leads to loss of muscle and a reduction in daily caloric expenditure, resulting in increased storage of fat.

> Dieting for weight loss is the most unsuccessful health intervention in all of medicine.

Stress Management

Stress is our emotional response to events in life. What one person perceives as stress may be stimulating to another. Stress management implies the learning of effective coping strategies, or ways to deal with the many sources of stress in modern life. Stress has been linked to heart disease, cancer, ulcers, immunosuppression, and other

Activity builds lean tissue and is a lifelong solution to weight control.

ills. The link is uncertain, however, because of the difficulty in measuring stress and because some ills have been found to have other causes (e.g., ulcers are caused by bacteria). What is certain is that people can learn to cope with minor irritations and most major threats. The best results come when a person combines learned behavior changes with an arsenal of coping skills. Regular, moderate activity is the ideal way to cope with stress because it is effective, long lasting, much less expensive than drugs, and provides other health benefits. As you'll see in chapter 2, activity can be psychologically therapeutic as well as preventive.

Other Healthy Behaviors

Another important aspect of the active life includes the elimination of negative behaviors, such as addiction to tobacco and other drugs, and moderation in the use of alcohol. According to the Public Health Service's Office for Disease Prevention and Health Promotion, tobacco causes over 400,000 deaths annually, including 30 percent of cancer deaths (85 percent of all lung cancer deaths) and 21 percent of cardiovascular deaths. Illegal drug deaths total 20,000 per year, including overdose, suicide, homicide, AIDS (HIV infection), and more. Alcohol misuse causes 100,000 deaths a year, including almost half of all deaths from motor vehicle accidents (U.S. Department of Health and Human Services, Public Health Service 1991). Yet one or two drinks of alcohol each day, whether wine, beer, or the hard stuff, are associated with reduced risk of heart disease. Who says disease prevention and health promotion have to be boring?

One of the enjoyable little moments that Brian experiences daily is sitting down to watch the evening news with a light beer and some low-fat pretzels. The beer provides a tasty way to relax, reduce stress, and lower heart disease risk. Likewise, Steve joins his wife for what she terms "booze and news" when they enjoy PBS news and a small glass of red wine.

Safety habits such as the use of seat belts and child restraints in automobiles contribute to health and longevity. Bicycle, motorcycle, and skiing helmets reduce the severity and cost of accidents. Those who refuse to use safety devices should consider the effect on family, friends, and themselves.

The final category of health behaviors that we want to mention is the habitual practice of preventive measures appropriate to your age, sex, medical condition, and family history. These measures include vaccinations and other preventive measures such as blood pressure and cholesterol checks and tests for glaucoma and prostate, breast, and skin cancer. The fact is that you, not your doctor, are responsible for your health. By combining personal responsibility with prevention and early detection tests, you have a cost-effective strategy for survival. The strategy is cost effective because prevention is always cheaper than treatment, because you use lower-cost health providers, and because you need to see physicians less frequently. If your employer has a comprehensive employee health or wellness program, use it. If not, create your own as you assume personal responsibility for your health.

> By combining personal responsibility with prevention and early detection tests, you have a cost-effective strategy for survival.

Integration

By now you've noticed how many facets of the active life interact in a reciprocal manner. Activity maintains muscle, which burns calories, helps maintain a healthy weight, and reduces the risk of heart disease, diabetes, and cancer, while also serving as the centerpiece of the stress management program. Of course, activity helps you look better, improves vitality, and reduces fatigue. Healthy food choices help you maintain or lose weight; lower cholesterol; reduce the risk of heart disease, cancer, and other ills; and make physical activity more enjoyable. The active life is not a hodgepodge of unrelated habits; it is a highly integrated family of behaviors that become more potent in combination than each is individually.

The Road Less Traveled

Some 28 percent of the U.S. population is completely sedentary, getting no physical activity, and another 42 percent does less than the minimum recommended activity (30 minutes of moderate activity most days of the week). Therefore, only 30 percent get the minimum recommended activity (Booth and Chakravarthy 2002), and probably about 10 percent achieve the Institute of Medicine recommendation (1 hour of moderate activity, most days) and are active enough to ensure the physical and mental benefits of regular physical activity. Most people deprive themselves of the joys and benefits of the active life and are likely to burden their families and the health care system. According to the CDC, sedentary habits vary by state, ranging from a low of 17 percent (Utah) to a high of 51 percent (Arizona). Activity differs by age, education, gender, and race (Macera et al. 2003, www.cdc.gov). Related data show that overweight and obesity increased from 55.9 to 64.5 percent in the last decade (Flegal et al. 2002). Indeed, the active life is the road less traveled. Isn't it time that you joined the ranks of the few, informed, resolute people who have the good sense and conviction needed to take the fork in the road, take personal responsibility, and embark on the active life?

Some view the active life and its associated behaviors as a medieval torture or religious rite, replete with fasting, denial, and mortification of the flesh. These folks are unwilling to give up the pleasures of rich (fatty) foods, unable to break addictions to tobacco, drugs, or alcohol. Because behaviors are often interrelated in a pattern of self-indulgence, these same people are likely to disdain the pleasures and rewards of the active life. Sadly, they do so at considerable cost to themselves and to society. Although few admit sorrow or repent their indulgences, they are destined to suffer a penance of fatigue, the purgatory of depression, and in time, frailty, disease, and early death. And the rest of us are expected to pay their bills and pick up the pieces of their lives.

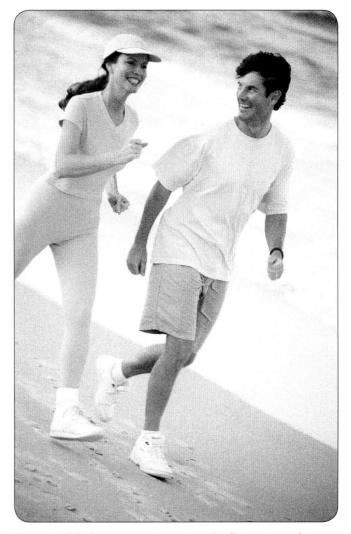

The active life does not require pain and suffering. Instead, it can be a joyful experience.

Zealous fitness instructors have been heard to say, "No pain, no gain," "Go for the burn," or "It has to hurt to be good." Of course, none of these statements is true for health and fitness. Any pain, burn, or hurt should be seen as an identifiable end point during exercise. The active life is not one of denial and deprivation, nor is it one of pain and suffering. It is a joyful experience, an affirmation of what we can be—physically, mentally, socially, and spiritually. The active life provides the energy to begin, the vigor to pursue, and the vitality to persist, to go the distance. It replaces overindulgence with moderation; substitutes positive addictions for negative ones; and yields health, energy, and the capacity to live.

How Much Is Enough?

The public and some fitness instructors are confused. For years they thought that exercise had to be intense if it was to yield desired benefits. For competitive performance and to achieve high levels of fitness, that recommendation still holds true. But what if your interest is in improving or maintaining health? In the summer of 1993, a group of world-renowned experts came together with the ACSM and the CDC to develop new recommendations for physical activity and health. They reviewed the latest scientific evidence and reached consensus on the following recommendation:

- Every American should accumulate 30 to 60 minutes of moderate-intensity physical activity on most days of the week.
- Because most adult Americans fail to meet this recommended level of moderate-intensity physical activity, almost all should strive to increase their participation in moderate or vigorous physical activity.

The recommendation suggests that a wide range of activities can contribute to the exercise total, including walking, gardening, and dancing. The 30 to 60 minutes of physical activity may come from planned exercise or recreation, such as brisk walking, jogging, cycling, or swimming. The recommendation notes that a specific way to meet the standard is to walk 2 miles (3.2 kilometers) briskly. The ACSM–CDC recommendation tells those who currently do not engage in regular activity to begin with a few minutes of daily activity and build gradually to 30 minutes (Pate et al. 1995).

These recommendations are based on research that shows that adults who engage in regular, moderate activity, enough to burn at least 200 calories a day (e.g., brisk 2-mile, or 3.2-kilometer, walk or jog), can expect many of the health benefits of exercise. From a public health perspective, we gain more if millions become active than we do if a few become superbly fit.

This CDC–ACSM recommendation was modified when scientists convened at the request of the Institute of Medicine (www.iom.edu). They increased the recommendation from a minimum of 30 minutes of regular, moderate activity to 60 minutes. They doubled the recommendation to increase caloric expenditure and slow the growing epidemic of obesity, an epidemic that has rapidly moved the proportion of overweight or obese people well beyond 64 percent (Brooks et al. 2004). So, you should view the 30-minute recommendation as the minimum, realizing that more health benefits are possible if you do more and add resistance training and flexibility exercises (Blair, LaMonte, and Nichaman 2004).

Activity Index

Before we move on, you may want to gauge your current level of activity using the following simple assessment tool. Developed in the 1970s, the index proved to be related to a laboratory test of aerobic fitness (maximal oxygen intake). As you increase the intensity, duration, and frequency of exercise, your index score and fitness both go up. How much activity do you need? You'll make that decision as you become better acquainted with the pleasures and benefits of activity. A score of 40 or more on the activity index is an indication that you are active enough to earn some of the health benefits associated with regular activity. By increasing the amount or intensity of exercise you will earn additional health benefits as you raise your aerobic fitness.

If your index score is below 40, you should begin today to increase your daily activity. Then, when we get into a discussion of the extra benefits associated with improved fitness (chapter 13), you will be ready to make a reasoned response to the question "Am I satisfied with my current level of activity and fitness, or do I feel the need to undertake a training program?"

Activity Index

Using your regular daily activity, calculate your activity index by multiplying your score for each category (score = intensity $\times$ duration $\times$ frequency).

	Score	Daily activity
Intensity	5	Sustained heavy breathing and perspiration
	4	Intermittent heavy breathing and perspiration—as in tennis, racquetball
	3	Moderately heavy—as in recreational sports and cycling
	2	Moderate—as in volleyball, softball
	1	Light—as in fishing, walking
Duration	4	More than 60 min
	3	30 min to 60 min
	2	20 to 30 min
	1	Less than 20 min
Frequency	5	Daily or almost daily
	4	3 to 5 times a week
	3	1 to 2 times a week
	2	Few times a month
	1	Less than once a month

Evaluation and Fitness Category

Score	Evaluation	Fitness category[*]
100	Very active lifestyle	High
80 to 100	Active and healthy	Very good
60 to 80	Active	Good
40 to 60	Acceptable (could be better)	Fair
20 to 40	Not good enough	Poor
Under 20	Sedentary	Very poor

[*]Index score is associated with aerobic fitness.

Adapted from Kasari, 1976.

Summary

This introduction began with a description of the active life as the road less traveled, described how the health behaviors of the active life interact, and finished with a simple assessment of your level of activity. Along the way we documented the fact that less than 15 percent of the population is active enough to get the physical and mental benefits of regular activity, and we defined the amount of activity needed to achieve health benefits. This question remains: How did Americans reach such a dramatic level of inactivity?

We began as a vigorous nation of farmers, miners, loggers, laborers, and merchants; survived a revolution, a civil war, and the industrial revolution; migrated across the continent; and continued to thrive in spite of two world wars, a depression, and current world conflicts. Yet today, we are gaining the reputation of being an overweight, lazy, complacent people, content to while away the hours with fast food, television, video games, and computer chat rooms. We have become the fattest nation in the world, with one-third of our adult citizens classified as obese. We're the only developed country that has ignored the need for universal health care, and many of us have lost a sense of responsibility for our acts, expecting others to bear the cost of our personal habits and mistakes.

Will the active life change all that? Probably not, but it is a positive way to begin exercising individual responsibility, to lighten our burden on society, and to lead family and friends along the road less traveled. With the active life you'll feel better, look better, and improve your physical and psychological health. Your energy level will increase, along with your productivity. You'll be more attractive, even sexier. And if you stick with the active life, you'll delay chronic illness and prolong the period of adult vigor. You'll be able to romp with your grandchildren and, years later, have the vitality to enjoy your great-grandchildren. You might as well make plans to live for 85 years, give or take a few. Adopt the active life and you could live with vigor and vitality until the end of your years.

"There is no path. You make the path when you walk."

Antonio Machado

Part I

Physical Activity, Fitness, and Health

Would you be upset to learn that far more than 250,000 lives are lost, every year, for failure to apply a medically proven therapy? It's true. Our high-cost health care system has ignored a simple, low-cost health treatment with the capacity to save hundreds of thousands of lives and billions of dollars. This miracle treatment goes unused in favor of expensive drugs, costly operations, even organ transplants. How could this happen? One reason is that physicians are compensated for performing procedures rather than providing the counseling that leads to improved health habits. With the development of penicillin and other wonder drugs, we patients have sought a quick fix for problems and have relinquished personal responsibility for our health. Hospitals, drug and insurance companies, and, yes, even lawyers have reaped enormous profits in this so-called health care system while simple, inexpensive health habits have gone unused.

Fortunately, the times are changing. As we work to rebuild our ailing health care system, we are searching for ways to reduce costs and the reliance on drugs and medical procedures.

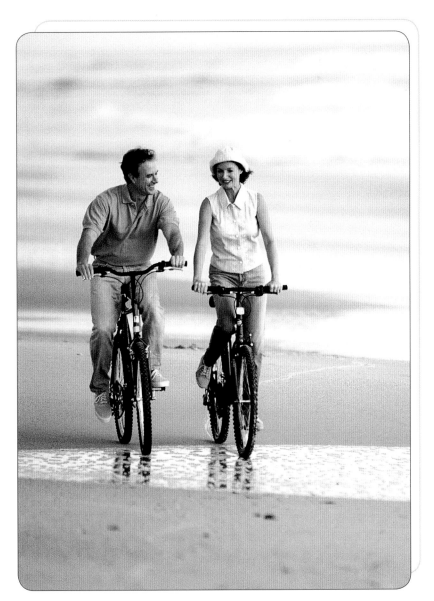

At the same time, researchers are questioning the value of operations and drugs and confirming the contributions of physical activity and related habits to health, longevity, and the quality of life. Finally, local, state, and federal organizations are moving to increase physical activity and curb the rise in sickness and death associated with inactivity. This section reviews studies that provide the modern foundation for the relationship of physical activity and fitness to physical and psychological health. It discusses the benefits and risks of activity, catalogs the extra benefits of fitness, and provides advice to help you begin your transformation to health, vitality, and the active life.

Health Benefits of Activity and Fitness

"Many of us spend half our time wishing for things we could have if we didn't spend half our time wishing."
Alexander Woollcott

The idea that physical activity is associated with good health is not new. The Chinese have long practiced tai chi and other forms of activity to prevent diseases associated with sedentary living. In Rome more than 1,500 years ago, the physician Galen prescribed exercise for health maintenance. References to the health values of exercise appear throughout recorded history, usually with little measurable effect on the populace. Why, then, do we invest time and energy to provide the latest evidence on the relationships between physical activity, physical fitness, and health? One reason is that we are devout optimists, the product of many years of professional experience and numerous heartwarming success stories. Another reason is that never before have so many studies said so many positive things about the health benefits of activity and fitness.

This chapter will help you

- understand the relationships among physical activity, fitness, and health;
- see how activity and fitness lower the risk of heart disease, hypertension, and stroke;
- appreciate how activity reduces the risk and severity of chronic diseases such as diabetes and some cancers;
- assess the role of activity in arthritis, osteoporosis, and low-back problems; and
- understand how regular, moderate physical activity contributes to the length and quality of life.

Active Living, Fitness, and Health

Epidemiology, the study of epidemics, is a fitting way to study the modern epidemic—diseases of lifestyle—that is responsible for more than half of all deaths in the United States. The epidemiologist studies populations to determine relationships between behaviors, such as physical activity, and the incidence of certain diseases. Researchers look at morbidity (sickness) and mortality (death). Studies can be retrospective, looking back at past behaviors; cross-sectional, looking at chronological slices of the population; or prospective, following a group into the future. Lack of solid information on activity, fitness, and other health habits often confound retrospective studies, whereas prospective studies face problems such as changing habits and participants who drop out. Issues of access to medical records (confidentiality) plague most studies, but the major problem is that of self-selection. Critics argue that subjects are active because they are well, not necessarily well because they are active.

Because self-selection confounds the results of retrospective and cross-sectional studies, only carefully controlled prospective studies, involving random assignment of participants to levels of activity (or inactivity), allow cause-and-effect conclusions. Because these studies are difficult to conduct and most likely unethical (inactivity is dangerous to health), we may never have absolute proof of the value of activity and fitness. But when the preponderance of studies support the health benefits of activity, and when the risks and costs are minimal, recommending a prudent, if not proved, course of action seems reasonable.

Risk Ratio

In a study of Harvard alumni, those with the least activity had 78.8 cardiovascular deaths per year per 10,000 study participants versus 43.0 for the most active, yielding a risk ratio of 54 percent (43.0 divided by 78.8 equals .54). Stated another way, the risk was 46 percent lower (100 minus 54 equals 46 percent) for the active alumni (Paffenbarger, Hyde, and Wing 1986).

Space does not permit a comprehensive review of the role of activity and fitness in health and disease, so we will review several classic studies and provide a summary of epidemiological findings. To avoid endless details, we will summarize the effects of activity and fitness with reference to the risk ratio (RR), the ratio of morbidity or mortality for the active members of the population to that for the inactive members. When possible we indicate plausible mechanisms or reasons that activity may have beneficial effects, and we conclude with a consideration of the risks and benefits of activity and recommendations for prudent behavior.

Activity Reduces the Risk of Coronary Artery Disease

In spite of tremendous progress in the past 30 years, heart disease, or, more specifically, coronary artery disease (CAD), remains the nation's number-one killer for men and women. Heart, stroke, and blood vessel diseases kill almost one million people in one year, far more than all the American lives lost in the four major wars of the last century (636,282). CAD is responsible for over half of those deaths, often in a sudden dramatic event called a heart attack. But this seemingly sudden event is actually the product of a process called atherosclerosis, a process that narrows the arteries and restricts the blood flow to the heart.

Atherosclerosis begins to develop during childhood, and the process is accelerated by a number of primary risk factors. In 1993, in recognition of the important role of activity, the American Heart Association (AHA) raised lack of physical activity to the level of the primary risk factors: cigarette smoking, elevated blood cholesterol, and high blood pressure (hypertension). Table 1.1 presents CAD risk factors and the possible influence of physical activity.

Atherosclerosis may be initiated by inflammation of the lining of the coronary artery, a protective response to injury or even an infection. Thereafter, high levels of circulating fats in the blood infiltrate the lining of the artery, aided perhaps by high blood pressure and chemicals, such as those in cigarette smoke. Cholesterol in low-density lipoprotein (LDL) becomes oxidized, leading to further damage to the artery. A scablike plaque forms and grows until it blocks the flow of blood or until a ruptured clot clogs the artery (see figure 1.1). C-reactive protein, a marker of inflammation from infection, is correlated to CAD risk. Some medical experts think that viruses may accelerate atherosclerosis or stimulate immune system responses that contribute to plaque formation and clotting. Gradual narrowing reduces blood flow (ischemia) and often leads to exertional pain (angina) experienced in the chest, left arm, or left shoulder.

Some plaque is hard and some is soft. The soft plaque has the potential to burst and cause a clot that can immediately interrupt blood flow and cause a heart attack

Table 1.1 CAD Risk Factors

Positively influenced by physical activity	May be influenced by physical activity	Not influenced by physical activity
Overweight and obesity	Electrocardiographic abnormalities	Family history of heart disease
Maintenance of blood glucose	Elevated uric acid and C-reactive protein	Gender (male has greater risk until age 55)
Elevated blood lipids	Pulmonary function (lung) abnormalities	Cigarette smoking
High blood pressure	Some cancers	Poor food choices
Physical inactivity	Personality or behavior pattern (hard driving, time conscious, aggressive, competitive, hostile)	
	Psychic reactivity (reaction to stress)	

Adapted from Sharkey, 1974.

Figure 1.1 Atherosclerosis plaque with recent bleeding into the center (arrow), making it more unstable and likely to cause a clot.

Courtesy of Vascular Disease Foundation

(myocardial infarct). Lack of blood and oxygen can damage heart muscle if it isn't treated quickly. This soft, or vulnerable, plaque may be the major cause of lethal heart attacks. The size, composition, and local inflammation processes may predispose a plaque to rupture. Biomechanical or hemodynamic forces, including increased blood pressure and heart rate, adrenalin, and even physical exertion sometimes trigger rupture and the onset of an acute heart attack. Ten percent of heart attacks are associated with physical activity; 90 percent are not. Inactive people are 56 times more likely to have a heart attack during exertion. In contrast, the risk for men who engage in habitual vigorous activity increases only 5 times during exercise. In addition, the overall risk for the active men was only 40 percent that of sedentary people (Siscovick et al. 1984).

Autopsy studies show that atherosclerosis is under way in some young adults, and recent surveys have confirmed the presence of CAD risk factors in children of all ages. When doctors examined teenage hearts donated after accidental deaths, they found that one in six already showed the blockage and plaque deposits characteristic of coronary artery disease (Tuzac 1999). Studies link atherosclerosis in youth to sedentary living and excess caloric consumption. Thus a program of risk factor identification and early intervention seems prudent, especially for those with a strong family history or multiple risk factors of heart disease. The active life can slow, stop, or reverse atherosclerosis. Indeed, a demanding intervention program consisting of activity, a low-fat diet, and medication, if needed, may halt and even reverse the process (Ornish 1993).

Inactivity and CAD

The famous London bus driver study published in 1954 (Morris and Raffle) focused world attention on inactivity as a factor in heart disease. The study compared the incidence of CAD between bus drivers and conductors. The more active conductors were found to have a rate 30 percent below that of the drivers. The disease appeared earlier in drivers, and their mortality rate was more than twice as high following the first heart attack. In spite of confounding factors (e.g., the stress of driving, drivers being more likely to be overweight), the study sparked interest in the role of activity.

SELF-EVALUATION FOR CAD

Do you have

- ❑ high blood pressure (greater than 130 millimeters of mercury)?
- ❑ elevated serum cholesterol (greater than 200 milligrams)?
- ❑ excess body weight? (See chapters 11 through 14.)

Are you

- ❑ a cigarette smoker?
- ❑ a bald male with a waist over 40 inches (102 centimeters)?
- ❑ physically inactive?

To determine your health risk, complete the health risk analysis at the end of chapter 3.

In a classic epidemiological study, Paffenbarger and associates (1986) studied thousands of Harvard alumni to determine the influence of activity, vigorous activity, and sports on cardiovascular illness and death. In comparison with less active subjects (those who engaged in less than 1,000 calories of activity per week, the equivalent of walking 30 minutes a day), those who participated in moderate and high levels of activity had mortality risk ratios of .71 and .54, respectively.

Less active	<1,000 calories per week	RR = 1.0
Moderate	1,000–2,500 calories per week	RR = .71
High activity	>2,500 calories per week	RR = .54

Moderate activity yielded a 29 percent reduction, and high levels of activity (2,500 calories per week is equivalent to 25 miles of jogging) yielded a 46 percent reduction in risk. Those who played light or moderately vigorous sports had mortality ratios of .79 and .63 when compared with those who played no sports. Risk ratios for mortality as well as first attacks of coronary artery disease were inversely related to physical activity, as indicated by calories of weekly exercise. The mortality ratio approached .5 when activity exceeded 2,500 calories per week, but when activity exceeded 3,500 calories per week, the contribution of activity seemed to diminish (see figure 1.2). The data of Paffenbarger and associates indicates that moderately vigorous activity and sport were more effective in reducing the risk of CAD. The risk for low-activity alumni who played no vigorous sports was 2.4 times that of active alumni who engaged in vigorous sports.

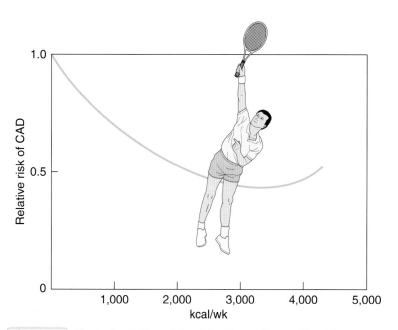

Figure 1.2 Physical activity and the risk of heart disease. The risk declines up to 3,500 calories per week and then begins to rise. This unexplained tendency for the risk to go back up may be the result of the small number of cases that report more than 3,500 calories per week.

Women's Risk

A study of 84,129 women participants in the Nurses' Health Study found that adherence to lifestyle guidelines involving diet, exercise, and abstinence from smoking is associated with a very low risk of CAD. Women in the low-risk category, defined as those who engaged in moderate to vigorous exercise for at least 30 minutes a day, did not currently smoke, had a favorable body mass index, consumed half a drink of alcohol daily, and scored in the top 40 percent on a diet high in fiber and low in saturated and trans-fatty acids and glycemic index, had a relative risk for CAD 17.8 percent below the population average (Stampfer et al. 2000).

Calories per Week

Throughout this book we will use the term *calorie* to refer to the kilocalorie, defined as the amount of heat required to raise 1 kilogram of water (1 liter) 1 degree centigrade. We use *calorie* because it is the common usage, the one that you see when you read food labels or diet books. By becoming familiar with the caloric cost of activities as well as the calories consumed in food, you will be an informed consumer of food and activity and will see how excess caloric intake requires an increase in caloric expenditure.

In general you burn about 100 calories when you jog 1 mile (or about 62.5 calories when you jog 1 kilometer). To burn 2,500 calories per week, you would need to jog 25 miles (40 kilometers). Alternatively, you could play singles tennis 3 hours each week (8 calories per minute times 50 minutes, with a 10-minute rest per hour, equals 400, times 3 hours equals 1,200 calories), walk briskly for 60 minutes (6 calories per minute times 60 minutes equals 360), and jog 3 miles (4.8 kilometers) three times (9 miles times 100 calories per mile, or 14.5 kilometers times 62.5 calories per kilometer, equals 900 calories), for a total of about 2,500 calories of vigorous activity per week.

Most other studies have shown similar results—that heart disease risk is inversely related to the amount of regular physical activity, be it occupational, leisure time, or vigorous sports. They show that the activity must be current or contemporaneous to be beneficial, that participation in high school or college sport did not confer protection later in life. In fact, regularly active adults maintain a lower risk of CAD whether or not they had been physically active during their youth. One study concludes that favorable long-term stabilization of most coronary risk factors is achievable with physical activity energy expenditure above 1,000 calories per week, and that 2,000 calories per week is associated with additional benefits, especially with favorable modification of HDL cholesterol and maintenance of weight (Drygas et al. 2000).

Autopsy studies conducted on American soldiers killed in the Korean conflict showed an alarming number (77 percent) with evidence of CAD, indicating that the pathology of atherosclerosis is developing by the age of 22 years (Enos, Beyer, and Holmes 1955). More alarming news comes from analysis of deceased teenage hearts. When doctors examined hearts donated after accidental deaths, they found that one in six already showed blockages and plaque deposits and concluded that heart disease, and therefore prevention, must begin much earlier than first believed (Tuzac 1999). Autopsies of older men (45 to 70 years) found that the incidence of scars, infarcts, and occlusions in the arteries were 30 percent less for those who had been moderately active and even lower for those who were heavily active (Morris and Crawford 1958).

Animal studies agree that moderate activity is beneficial but suggest that exhaustive or stressful effort may somehow accelerate the development of CAD. Exhaustion may be stressful for an animal, and stress provokes a hormonal response that suppresses the immune system and may accelerate the atherosclerotic process, in animals as well as in humans. No evidence exists that enormous amounts of activity, such as that performed by ultraendurance athletes, is detrimental to those athletes' health.

Physical Activity Versus Fitness

If activity and sport can lower the risk of CAD, what about improved fitness? Does one earn extra benefits by raising his or her level of fitness? Physical fitness, specifically aerobic fitness, has long been associated with better health. The issue was raised in 1988 at the annual meeting of the American College of Sports Medicine. Doctors Steven Blair and Harold Kohl reported on their study of more than 10,000 men. They analyzed all-cause death rates for sedentary and active men whose fitness had been assessed in a treadmill test. The surprising results have influenced the way we view activity, fitness, and the amount of exercise required to achieve public health benefits.

The all-cause death rate was almost three times higher for the sedentary men. And within the sedentary classification, aerobic fitness level made a difference only at the lowest level, where the least fit had twice the risk of other sedentary subjects (five times the risk for active men) (Blair and Kohl 1988). Among the active subjects, the death rates were not significantly different, regardless of the level of aerobic fitness! These findings suggested that, for the male subjects in this study, activity conferred most of the health benefits of exercise, and that higher levels of aerobic fitness didn't provide greater protection from all-cause mortality (heart disease contributes more than one-half of all-cause mortality) (see table 1.2).

Table 1.2   Physical Activity Versus Fitness

Fitness group	Lowest	2	3	4	Highest
Sedentary	74*	31	35	28	33
Active	13	8	14	16	13

*Age-adjusted death rate per 10,000; Blair and Kohl 1988.

Does this mean that physical fitness is not associated with better health? No, it does not. In fact, when the sedentary and active subjects are analyzed together, a trend toward a reduced death rate with increasing fitness is present (Blair et al. 1989).

Fitness level	Death rate*	Relative risk
1 Lowest	64.0	1.0
2	25.5	.40
3 Medium	27.1	.42
4	21.7	.34
5 Highest	18.6	.29

*All-cause deaths per 10,000.

Although higher levels of fitness are associated with only minor reductions in all-cause death rate, they are correlated with fewer risk factors and probably do provide added protection, especially for those with elevated risk (elevated cholesterol, triglycerides, hypertension, diabetes, obesity).

Are you wondering why some sedentary subjects are more fit than others? Physical fitness is a product of heredity and training. With good heredity a sedentary person could have a higher level of fitness than an active friend. The good news is that moving from sedentary to active living imparts a sizable drop in health risk and all-cause mortality. When an already active person improves his or her fitness, the decrease in risk is more subtle but still important, especially for someone with inherited risks.

In Review

Let us emphasize one of the most important public health messages of our time: Regular, moderate physical activity conveys many if not most of the important health benefits associated with exercise. From a public health standpoint, an increase in physical activity will provide millions of Americans with some level of protection from heart disease, hypertension, adult-onset diabetes, certain cancers, osteoporosis, depression, premature aging, and more. Improved aerobic fitness provides added benefits. Both the Blair and Lakka studies, however, showed that only moderate physical activity is necessary to achieve most of the gains, and that a large segment of the population can attain protection from many chronic diseases. Indeed, epidemiologist Dr. Steven Blair (2000) has called low fitness caused by sedentary habits our most important public health problem!

A study conducted in Finland offers further proof of the extra benefits of fitness. The authors concluded that higher levels of both leisure-time physical activity and fitness had a strong inverse relationship with the risk of heart attack. The study supports the conclusion that lower levels of physical activity and lower levels of fitness are independent risk factors for coronary artery disease in men (Lakka et al. 1994).

Cardioprotective Mechanisms

Numerous studies have shown that physical activity and fitness are associated with a lower risk of CAD. Yet because of self-selection, most of the studies do not allow cause-and-effect statements and the level of assurance desired in scientific and medical research. To conduct further investigations about the influence of activity on cardiovascular health, researchers have explored a number of hypotheses concerning cardioprotective mechanisms (see table 1.3).

Among the many possible ways in which activity may prevent or minimize the process of atherosclerosis, the major benefits are not directly related to the heart itself. But physical activity does improve the function of the heart through reduced workload, improved contractility of the cardiac muscle, increased blood volume, lower resting and exercise heart rates, and higher stroke volume. Other benefits of physical activity include slight increases in the concentration of aerobic enzymes, an increase in arterial diameters, an increase in the number of arterioles and capillaries, and a decrease in plaque formation. In our opinion, two of the major benefits of activity in reducing atherosclerosis are its ability to metabolize fat and lower circulating levels of fat in the blood (triglycerides and cholesterol) and its ability to maintain the elasticity of the major arteries. Let's explore some of these mechanisms to help explain why something as simple as regular, moderate activity is good for your health.

> The major benefits of activity are its ability to metabolize fat and lower circulating levels of fat in the blood and its ability to maintain the elasticity of the large arteries.

Effect of Activity on the Vascular System

Your vascular system, which delivers blood carrying oxygen, food, and hormones to the cells of your body, is the first line of defense against disease and removes waste products and heat. Physical activity provides beneficial changes in blood clotting, blood pressure, and blood distribution along with the specific benefits previously noted for your heart.

Table 1.3   Cardioprotective Mechanisms

EFFECTS OF PHYSICAL ACTIVITY	
Increase	**Decrease**
Oxidation of fat	Serum cholesterol and triglycerides
Number of coronary blood vessels	Glucose intolerance
Vessel size and arterial elasticity	Obesity, adiposity
Efficiency of heart	Platelet stickiness
Efficiency of peripheral blood distribution and return	Arterial blood pressure
Electron transport capacity	Heart rate (resting and active)
Fibrinolytic (clot-dissolving) capability	Vulnerability to heart rhythm problems
Arterial oxygen content	Overreaction to hormones
Red blood cells and blood volume	Psychic stress
Thyroid function	
Growth hormone production	
Tolerance to stress	
Prudent living habits	
Joy of living	

Adapted from Sharkey, 1974.

BLOOD CLOTTING   Blood is designed to form a clot and stem the flow of blood when we are injured. But a clot (called a thrombus) that forms within an uninjured vessel is dangerous, and a clot in a narrowed coronary artery could be disastrous. Clots form when the soluble protein fibrinogen is converted to insoluble threads of fibrin. Normally we are able to dissolve an unwanted thrombus by dissolving the fibrin (fibrinolysis). Exercise enhances this process, but the effect lasts only a day or two. The stress of exhaustive or highly competitive exercise seems to inhibit this system, allowing more rapid clotting time. Regular, moderate, or even vigorous, activity is the way to enhance the ability of the body to dissolve unwanted clots (Molz et al. 1993). Chronic aerobic exercise training may cause favorable adaptations that contribute to decreased risk for ischemic events (shortages of oxygen delivered to heart or skeletal muscle), both at rest and during exertion (Womack, Nagelkirk, and Coughlin 2003). In fact, a review of the literature concludes that regular exercise is the most practicable approach known to decrease plasma fibrinogen levels (Ernst 1993).

LARGE ARTERY ELASTICITY   Aging and sedentary living contribute to a loss of large artery compliance (elasticity). This loss of compliance increases systolic blood pressure and increases the risk of plaque rupture and heart attack. Recent research findings (Seals 2003) have shown that regular aerobic exercise may favorably attenuate age-associated decreases in arterial compliance. People who begin and maintain a moderate exercise program can improve arterial compliance and reduce their risk of myocardial infarction (heart attack). Regular exercisers, even those who show no improvement in fitness, have greater arterial compliance than sedentary people do (Ferreira et al. 2002).

BLOOD PRESSURE   High blood pressure, or hypertension, increases the workload of the heart by forcing it to contract against the greater resistance. Anything that lowers blood pressure also reduces the workload of the heart. Regular, moderate physical activity has been shown to reduce blood pressure in middle-aged or older people, especially those with elevated levels. Walking, but not weightlifting, has been shown to reduce systolic blood pressure in elderly people (Rejeski et al. 1995). Of course, changes in blood pressure could also be the consequence of weight loss or reduced stress, both known outcomes of regular activity.

BLOOD DISTRIBUTION   Regular physical activity teaches the body to distribute the blood to muscles better during exercise, further reducing the workload of the heart. Vessels leading to digestive and other organs learn to constrict, and dilating vessels that serve working muscles open to allow blood to flow where it is needed.

BLOOD VOLUME   The 10 to 15 percent increase in blood volume that comes with endurance training further enhances the performance of both the heart and skeletal muscles. These changes serve to lower the heart rate and blood pressure during physical activity. Because the oxygen needs of heart muscle are directly related to the product of heart rate and blood pressure, these improvements serve to reduce the likelihood that you'll exceed

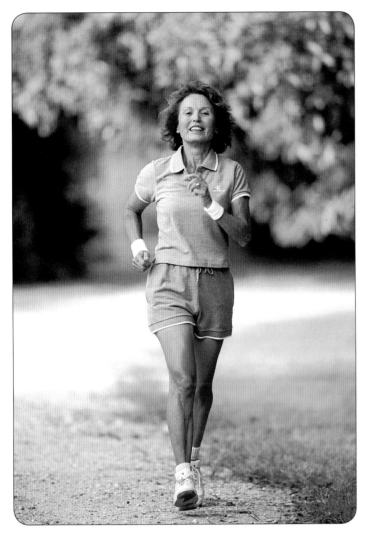

Regular, moderate exercise, such as walking, provides many benefits for the vascular system, including reduced blood pressure.

the ability to supply oxygen to cardiac muscle. As with most other effects of activity and training, the benefits depend on regular, not occasional, activity.

Metabolic Changes Due to Activity

The metabolic changes that result from activity may be the most important in the fight against CAD as well as several other disorders. The changes include increased fat mobilization and metabolism, reduced blood lipids, and changes in insulin sensitivity. The metabolic changes associated with physical activity contribute significantly to reductions in heart disease risk.

FAT METABOLISM   If you eat too much, you will gain weight in the form of stored fat. Excess fat is a health risk for heart disease, hypertension, diabetes, and some forms of cancer. You can diet (starve) to get rid of fat, but there is a hitch: The starving breaks down muscle tissue for energy, so you lose the only tissue that is capable of burning large amounts of fat. Muscular activity is the proved way to mobilize fat from adipose tissue storage and then to burn it for energy in skeletal muscles. Exercise burns fat and avoids loss of muscle protein. Regular activity can build additional muscle, thereby enhancing your ability to burn fat.

> The physically fit person is the owner of an efficient fat-burning furnace.

Regular activity burns calories, helping you maintain a desirable body weight and percent body fat and a leaner, healthier figure. Fitness training leads to enhanced ability to mobilize and metabolize fat. Training increases the proportion of energy derived from fat (versus carbohydrate) at rest and during moderate activity. The physically fit person is the owner of an efficient fat-burning furnace. This enhanced ability to use fat as an energy source leads to even greater benefits that are closely tied to reduced risk of atherosclerosis and CAD. Physical activity has even been found to decrease the risk of developing gallstones, independent of other risk factors such as obesity and recent rapid dietary weight loss (Leitzmann et al. 1999).

BLOOD LIPIDS   *Lipid* is another word for fat. The blood lipids include cholesterol and triglycerides, and each is related to the risk of heart disease. The level of cholesterol in the blood is an important predictor of the risk of heart disease. Total cholesterol includes low-density lipoprotein (LDL) cholesterol and high-density lipoprotein (HDL) cholesterol. Regular activity can lead to a modest decline in total cholesterol, but that is only part of the story. LDL is the dangerous subfraction of cholesterol found in the plaques that clog coronary arteries. Activity, diet, and weight loss all contribute to a drop in LDL. Regular activity, particularly prolonged or vigorous activity, and weight loss both contribute to a rise in HDL cholesterol, the beneficial subfraction that collects cholesterol from the arteries and transports it to the liver for removal from the body. So exercise reduces total cholesterol (especially the LDL portion), raises HDL, and greatly improves your total cholesterol to HDL ratio, one of the best predictors of heart disease risk.

Triglycerides, consisting of three fatty acids and a molecule of glycerol, constitute a transport and storage form of fat. High levels are associated with heart disease, obesity, and hypertension. Regular activity is a proved way to lower circulating levels of triglycerides. Levels decline after exercise, and the effect persists for 1 or 2 days. Several days of exercise lead to progressive reduction of triglyceride levels. The final plateau depends on diet, body weight, intensity and duration of exercise, and genetic tendencies. Clearly, regular, moderate activity leads to a significant reduction in triglycerides.

Aspirin

Studies have shown that one aspirin a day (or one every other day) reduces the risk of unwanted clots associated with heart disease and stroke. The aspirin reduces the stickiness of platelets, small particles in the blood that are caught in the fibrin threads of a developing clot. Most people tolerate one aspirin a day, taken with a meal. This practice is an inexpensive way to reduce the risk of CAD and stroke, and it may help reduce the risk of colon cancer. A small (81 milligrams) tablet may be adequate for most people, thereby reducing the risk of gastrointestinal problems. Some people, however, may require a higher dose (Kong 2004). Concurrent use of ibuprofen may decrease the heart benefit of aspirin (Gaziano and Gibson 2006), but a study of 3,859 patients found no increase in heart attacks among those who took aspirin and ibuprofen compared with those who took aspirin alone (Patel and Goldberg 2004). In either case, a coated aspirin may be a wise choice for long-term therapy.

Cholesterol to HDL Ratio

Before training and weight loss, Bill had a cholesterol level of 240 and an HDL of 40, for a ratio of 240 divided by 40, or 6, and a moderately high risk of CAD. Training and weight loss reduced the cholesterol to 200 and raised the HDL to 50, yielding a much improved ratio of 4. He could continue to improve his lipid profile and further reduce his risk of CAD by continuing training, maintaining or lowering his body weight, and reducing his consumption of total and saturated fat. Lowering cholesterol to 180 and raising HDL to 60 produces a favorable risk profile. We will say more about cholesterol in later chapters.

OTHER METABOLIC MECHANISMS A number of additional metabolic mechanisms support the value of activity as a cardioprotective therapy. Regular activity and training have been shown to increase insulin sensitivity and glucose tolerance. This effect of exercise is particularly important for people who are obese and those with adult-onset diabetes (also called type 2 diabetes or non-insulin-dependent diabetes mellitus—NIDDM). High levels of circulating fat inhibit the ability of insulin to transport glucose into muscles. Exercise enhances the transport of glucose into muscles, even in the absence of insulin. Thus, regular activity helps by reducing body weight and fat levels and by increasing insulin sensitivity and glucose transport. All these improvements reduce the risk of heart disease and NIDDM.

ELECTROLYTES Electrolytes, including potassium, sodium, and calcium, are essential to the function of muscles, including the heart. During exertion the untrained heart may experience diminished oxygen supply, which can trigger an imbalance of electrolytes, electrical instability, and disturbances in heart rhythms. Death can result from lethal rhythm disorders, such as tachycardia (rapid beating) or fibrillation (irregular, uncontrolled, unsynchronized beating). Fitness training minimizes this likelihood by reducing the workload of the heart, improving oxygen supply and efficiency, and correcting electrolyte imbalances.

Activity Reduces the Risk of Chronic Diseases

We have taken much time and space to establish the role of activity and fitness in reducing the risks of heart disease. Now we will briefly sketch how activity can protect you from a long list of chronic diseases and disorders.

Hypertension and Stroke

People with very high blood pressure (greater than 160/95) are three times more likely to experience CAD and four times more likely to get congestive heart failure than others. Resting blood pressure values above 130/85 are associated with an increased risk of CAD in middle-aged and older people, and the risk increases with age (Vasan et al. 2001). Hypertension also increases the risk of stroke and kidney failure. The causes of hypertension are still under investigation. But we do know that inactivity increases the risk of developing hypertension by 35 percent, and that unfit subjects have 52 percent greater risk than the fit. Regular endurance

Metabolic Syndrome

Defined as a clustering of metabolic abnormalities related to insulin, metabolic syndrome includes the following:

- Blood pressure greater than 130 millimeters of mercury
- Serum triglycerides greater than 150 milligrams
- HDL cholesterol less than 40 milligrams
- Fasting blood glucose greater than 110 milligrams per deciliter
- Central adiposity (waist circumference greater than 40 inches, or 102 centimeters)

Having three of these metabolic markers is associated with obesity, diabetes, and heart disease. Low levels of cardiorespiratory fitness are associated with increased clustering of the metabolic abnormalities of the syndrome in adult men and women (Whaley et al. 1999). A sedentary lifestyle and especially poor fitness are not only associated with metabolic syndrome but could be considered features of the syndrome. A low level of fitness may provide a means of identifying those who would benefit from interventions to prevent the syndrome and its dire consequences (Lakka et al. 2003). Excess central or abdominal fat, as indicated by waist circumference, is a predictor of the metabolic syndrome. High levels of visceral abdominal fat are also associated with measures of inflammation, which predict several chronic diseases, including heart disease (Despres 2004).

exercise lowers resting systolic and diastolic pressures by about 10 millimeters of mercury, with even greater benefits during activity. Active hypertensive patients have half the risk of death from all causes that inactive hypertensive patients do (Paffenbarger 1994).

A stroke, which is a clot or hemorrhage (bleeding) of a blood vessel in the brain, can result in loss of speech or muscle control or even death. The risk factors are similar to those for CAD. In most studies the risk of stroke decreases as activity increases. But with activity that is more vigorous and, possibly, with heavy lifting, the trend may reverse. Transient ischemic attacks (TIAs) are sudden, brief periods of weakness, vertigo, loss of vision, slurred speech, headache, or other symptoms that sometimes precede a stroke. Similar symptoms have been associated with heavy weightlifting exercises, especially in those with elevated blood pressure. Repeatedly, we find compelling arguments for moderation.

Cancer and Immunity

In recent years, evidence has been accumulating that an active lifestyle is associated with lower risk of certain types of cancers. Most often studied is the link between activity and lower risk of colon cancer. Some researchers hypothesize that regular activity shortens intestinal transit time for potential carcinogens in fecal material. If that is the mechanism, it is hard to understand why the incidence of rectal cancer isn't lower as well. But lack of physical activity is causally related to colon cancer; 12 to 14 percent of colon cancer can be attributed to lack of frequent involvement in vigorous physical activity (Slattery 2004). Some studies suggest that activity may help reduce the risk of prostate cancer. When activity was examined by intensity of effort, vigorous activity decreased prostate cancer risk by 30 percent (Friedenreich et al. 2004).

Women who were active in their youth have fewer cancers of the breast and the reproductive system (Frisch et al. 1985). These authors noted that body fat was lower in the previously active women. In fact, a study of more than 25,000 women found that the risk was lowest (RR, or risk ratio, was .28) in lean women who exercised at least 4 hours per week (Thune et al. 1997). A more recent study found that sustained activity throughout life, and particularly activity done later in life, may provide the greatest benefit in reducing the risk of breast cancer (Friedenreich, Courneya, and Bryant 2001). The role of dietary fat and obesity in the development of cancer continues to interest researchers. Increased body weight was associated with increased death rates for all cancers combined and for cancers and multiple specific sites (Calle et al. 2003).

A substance that causes genetic damage (e.g., carcinogens in meat or cigarette smoke) may initiate cancers. Promoters (such as estrogen in the case of breast cancer) then stimulate cell proliferation. A healthy immune system may play a role in the control of initiators or the suppression of transformed cells or their by-products. On the other hand, a compromised immune system may allow initiation and promotion to go unchecked. Regular, moderate physical activity enhances the function of the immune system, whereas high levels of stress or exhaustive exercise seem to suppress the system (Nieman 2003).

Diabetes and Obesity

Researchers have begun to suspect a link between NIDDM, CAD, and hypertension, specifically that all three share insulin resistance and that obesity and lack of activity are part of the problem. Insulin-resistant cells can't take in glucose, so glucose levels rise and the body secretes more insulin, which tends to increase blood pressure (through increased blood volume and vasoconstriction). Obesity and high levels of blood lipids seem to foster a resistance to insulin, whereas exercise increases insulin sensitivity and the movement of glucose into working muscles. Regular activity has returned to a place of prominence in the treatment of NIDDM, and for some it removes the need for insulin substitutes. In general, regularly active adults have a 42 percent lower risk of NIDDM (RR equals .58).

Arthritis, Osteoporosis, and Back Problems

This group of musculoskeletal problems accounts for significant pain and suffering, as well as massive sums of money for often unnecessary treatments. Activity can treat or prevent all these problems. Osteoarthritis, painful joint degeneration as in the knees, doesn't seem to be caused by exercise unless a previous injury has occurred. In addition, regular, moderate activity is an essential part of treatment for most forms of arthritis.

Osteoporosis is the progressive loss of bone mineral that occurs faster in women, especially after menopause. Cigarette smoking, low body weight—especially from dieting—and lack of activity accelerate its progress. With age, the condition can lead

Weight-bearing exercise helps maximize the bone density of the young, and it helps adults maintain their bone density.

to brittle bones, hip fractures, and the characteristic dowager's hump caused by the collapse of vertebrae in the neck. Adequate calcium intake can slow the loss of bone mineral. Weight-bearing exercise helps maximize bone mass during youth, maintain bone mass in middle age, and slow age-related losses in later years, and exercise helps older people avoid crippling falls (Beck and Snow 2003). Two years of intense exercise helped retain bone density in postmenopausal women (Kemmler et al. 2004). Weight-bearing exercises must serve upper- and lower-body sites. Running and calcium intake stimulated lower-body bone mass of women runners at the expense of bone mass from upper-body sites (Nevill et al. 2003). Continued participation in impact sports is also beneficial for the skeletal health of males, especially after the age of 40 years (VanLangendonck et al. 2003).

Back problems result from the acute or chronic assault to underused and under-trained bodies. Regular attention to abdominal exercises and flexibility of the back and hamstring muscles can minimize the risk or rehabilitate the back. Among the many therapies used on back problems, including surgery, manipulation, injections, and drugs, none has proved more effective than rapid return to physical activity. We will provide specific suggestions for back health in chapter 10.

Activity Increases Longevity

By decreasing the risk of CAD, cancer, and other diseases of lifestyle, regular activity extends the period of adult vigor and compresses the period of sickness that precedes death. In a real sense, activity adds life to your years, and evidence now indicates that it can also add years to your life. When Paffenbarger (1994) analyzed the effects of changing to more favorable health habits, moderate activity (1,500 calories per week) conferred an average of 1.57 years above less active living, and vigorous sports provided 1.54 years over no sports participation. Data on Harvard alumni indicated that vigorous activity (defined as more than 6.5 to 7.5 calories per minute, the equivalent of a brisk walk) was associated with reduced mortality. Mortality declined with increasing levels of vigorous activity up to about 3,500 calories per week, but not for nonvigorous activity (Lee, Hsieh, and Paffenbarger 1995).

A report from the Institute for Aerobics Research (Blair et al. 1995) confirmed that fit folks live longer. Data on 9,777 men aged 20 to 82 showed that those who were unfit when they entered the study were 44 percent less likely to die over the 18-year period of the study if they improved their fitness. Those who were fit at the start of the study and remained fit were 67 percent less likely to die than were those who remained unfit. The benefits were found across all age groups, and the most fit people had the lowest risk of premature death. We will say more about aging and how to live better and longer in chapter 17.

Summary

For over 50 years epidemiologists have studied the relationships of occupational and leisure-time activity with health, and an impressive list of benefits has emerged. The studies clearly show how activity enhances health while it reduces the risk of CAD, hypertension, and stroke as well as some cancers, diabetes, osteoporosis, obesity, and other chronic disorders. We've presented evidence of additional health benefits associated with vigorous activity and fitness and shown how regular, moderate physical activity extends the length and quality of life. Now we will turn our attention to the topic of psychological health, to see how the active life contributes to mental health and the joy of living.

Activity and Mental Health

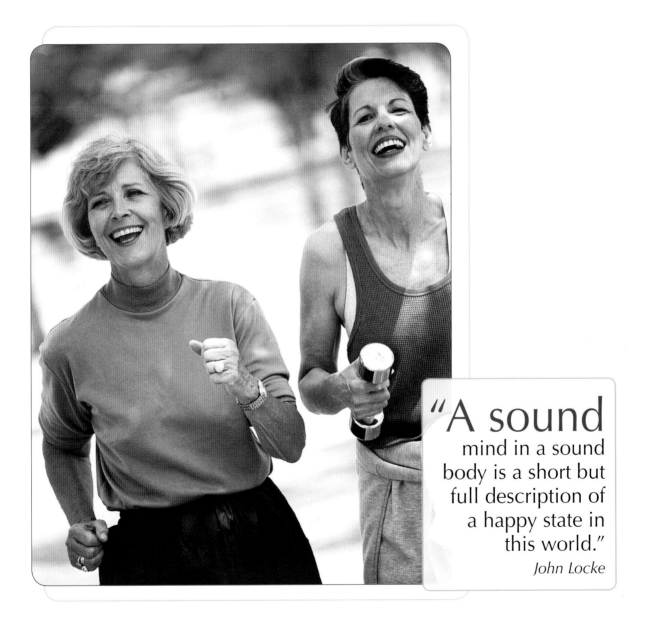

"A sound mind in a sound body is a short but full description of a happy state in this world."
John Locke

Everyone has heard of psychosomatic illness, a physical ailment caused or exacerbated by the state of mind. But few have heard the term *somatopsychic*, which suggests the effect of the body (soma) on the mind. This chapter describes how use of the body, specifically with regular, moderate physical activity, has a beneficial effect on the mind and mental health. Although the research in this area is still in its infancy and many questions remain, reviewing the case for what may be the most significant role for activity and fitness is important.

As with activity and physical health, we must wonder about self-selection: Does activity promote mental health, or does mental health promote activity? Do happy, less anxious, and nondepressed people have the interest, vigor, and energy to be active? Evidence from epidemiological studies indicates that the level of physical activity is positively associated with good mental health, when mental health is defined as positive mood, general well-being, and relatively infrequent symptoms of anxiety and depression (Stephens 1988). As you will see, in intervention studies, activity has been associated with reduced levels of anxiety and depression. If it is true, as some have estimated, that at any given time as many as 25 percent of the population suffer from mild to moderate anxiety, depression, and other emotional disorders, we should not ignore the potential of this safe, low-cost therapy.

This chapter will help you

- understand how activity reduces anxiety and depression,
- appreciate how activity helps us deal with stress, and
- recognize positive aspects of an addiction to activity.

Activity Reduces Anxiety and Depression

If activity were a drug and it could be proved effective in the prevention and treatment of anxiety and depression, it would be hailed as a modern miracle, worth billions to the company with legal rights to the formula. Well, activity isn't a drug, but rather a learned behavior that requires motivation to begin a program and persistence to adhere to it. This chapter deals with mental health problems, and chapter 18 provides the psychological support that you'll need to begin and continue the active life.

Anxiety

Anxiety has been defined as a diffuse apprehension of some vague threat, characterized by feelings of uncertainty and helplessness. Anxiety is more than ordinary worry in that a person can perceive it as a threat to his or her self-esteem. State anxiety is a transitory emotional response to a specific situation, characterized by feelings of tension, apprehension, and nervousness. Trait anxiety is a relatively stable level of anxiety proneness, a predisposition to respond to threats with elevated anxiety. Studies have investigated the effects of acute and chronic activity on state and trait anxiety.

Activity such as walking has been shown to reduce state anxiety, as have meditation, biofeedback, and some other forms of mental diversion (see table 2.1). So if you are tense and apprehensive about an upcoming responsibility, meeting, or presentation, go for a walk. Doing so certainly can't hurt, and it probably will help. A study showed that resistance training or aerobic exercise significantly reduced state anxiety. The effect was similar in both forms of effort, and the benefit remained throughout 8 weeks of training (Hale and Raglin 2002). If you become anxious about physical threats such as a steep ski slope or whitewater rapids, instruction, practice, and improved skill will help diminish future anxiety. Of greater importance is the question about whether regular (chronic) activity or training reduces trait anxiety.

Studies of police, firefighters, athletes, and even patients indicate that training and improved fitness are associated with reductions in trait anxiety. A comprehensive review of the research found that activity was statistically related to a reduction in state and trait anxiety as well as psycho-physiological measures of anxiety. The effects ranged from small to moderate (Landers and Petruzzello 1994). Studies show that moderate exercise is more effective than high-intensity exercise, that activity-induced reductions seem to persist for many weeks, and that reductions occur independently of age and health status (Weinberg and Gould 2003).

Table 2.1   Anxiety Exercise Prescription

Mode	Aerobic activities, such as walking.
Frequency	Regular (almost daily), especially when needed.
Intensity	Moderate.
Time	Not established, but 30 to 60 min should work.

Depression

Depression is characterized by sadness, low self-esteem, pessimism, hopelessness, and despair. Symptoms range from fatigue, irritability, lack of direction, and withdrawal to thoughts of suicide. Whereas mild depression may resolve without treatment and moderate depression may go away in 6 months, severe cases, in which suicide is a real risk, are usually treated with drugs. Most activity studies have been conducted on mild to moderate, nonclinical subjects.

A comprehensive statistical review of studies related to activity and depression concluded that activity significantly decreased depression for all age groups and fitness levels, and that larger decreases were associated with more sessions and longer exercise programs (North, McCullagh, and Tran 1990). A study evaluated the effects of treadmill exercise and found substantial rapid improvement in mood in patients with major depression (Bauer et al. 2001). Physical activity seems to work across all ages; more active children (Crews, Lochbaum, and Landers 2004) and teens are less depressed (Motl et al. 2004), and activity reduces the risk of subsequent depression in older adults (Strawbridge et al. 2002).

Although some researchers have hypothesized that exercise had to lead to improvements in aerobic fitness for it to decrease depression, results have not supported that theory. A study of women found that even low levels of activity (one or two times per week) have a positive effect on mental health (depressed feelings and psychological disorders) (Kull 2003). We may safely say that those with mild to moderate depression may experience at least as much relief from activity and training as they do from conventional forms of therapy (see table 2.2). Let's consider some reasons why this may be so.

Table 2.2   Depression Exercise Prescription

Mode	Aerobic exercise; some evidence supports light resistance exercise with multiple repetitions.
Frequency	Almost daily, with acute and long-term benefits.
Intensity	Light to moderate, with increased benefits associated with intensity, duration, and frequency.
Time	30 min or longer.

SELF-EVALUATION FOR DEPRESSION

The following statements, suggested by the National Institute of Mental Health, can help you determine whether you may be suffering from depression. Indicate whether you agree or disagree with the following:

- ❏ I feel downhearted, blue, and sad.
- ❏ I don't enjoy the things that I used to.
- ❏ I feel that others would be better off without me.
- ❏ I feel that I am not useful or needed.
- ❏ I notice that I am losing weight.
- ❏ I have trouble sleeping at night.
- ❏ I am restless and can't keep still.
- ❏ My mind isn't as clear as it used to be.
- ❏ I get tired for no reason.
- ❏ I feel hopeless about the future.

Total the number of statements with which you agreed. If you agreed with at least five, including one of the first two, and if you have had the symptoms for at least 2 weeks, you may need professional help. If you agreed with the third statement, seek help immediately.

How Activity Affects Anxiety and Depression

A number of hypotheses have been advanced to explain the effect of activity and training on mental health. They range from simple behavioral strategies to complex biochemical theories.

Coping Strategies

Regular activity serves as a positive coping strategy, a diversion, distraction, or time-out from the problems and stressors of everyday life. Activity occupies the mind, allowing the passage of time during difficult periods. It allows the substitution of good habits for bad ones, positive addictions for negative ones. Activity is a form of meditation, providing the benefits of other approaches along with improvement in health and fitness. It provides a sense of control over one's life and environment. People can be

> Regular physical activity is our primary coping mechanism.

separated into two groups—internals, who believe that they can control outcomes in their lives, and externals, who believe that chance or others control their lives. Internal controllers are more likely to adhere to healthy behaviors. Can a person change this locus of control? Can one become an internal and improve adherence to healthy behavior?

The perception of acquiring mastery in a particular area influences coping behavior. Perception of mastery also influences performance, and it is theorized that experience alters perception. Thus, successful experience may reinforce a coping behavior, thereby ensuring continuation of the behavior. Some have even suggested that this enhanced self-efficacy (defined as a sense of one's ability to organize and execute actions required to achieve designated outcomes) may generalize to other areas of performance. We have much to learn concerning these theories. We can say that regular activity provides a sense of control and mastery over one dimension of life, and it may improve control and mastery over others.

I Don't Do Lunch

Years ago Brian realized that midday was the best time for a personal exercise program. He enjoyed a noon-hour workout, with or without the company of friends, followed by a shower and a brown-bag lunch at his desk. Sometimes he set out with a problem and came back with a solution. Exercise before work was a struggle, and after work he was inclined to crash in front of the nightly news, with low-fat pretzels and a beer (for medicinal purposes of course). He looked forward to his daily activity and did all he could to keep the noon hour open. On weekends he started early for an extended workout, but during the week, noon hour was his time. In this era of power lunches you don't influence people or enhance your career when you announce, "I don't do lunch." Of course, you must make exceptions at times, but this resolve to keep the exercise time sacred is an indication of the importance of regular activity to physical and mental health. Regular physical activity is our primary coping mechanism.

Does activity measure up to other therapies? One study found that fitness training, embedded in a cognitive-behavioral program, was associated with positive changes in other relevant aspects of patient function, including coping strategies, sustained efforts to continue activities, and improved physical well-being. Other therapeutic efforts and drug therapy were associated with ambivalent patterns of positive as well as negative emotional and behavioral characteristics (VanderVliet et al. 2004).

Self-Esteem, Self-Concept, and Body Image

Can regular activity or improved fitness have a beneficial effect on self-esteem (self-approval) and self-concept, and could that reduce or prevent anxiety or depression? Self-concept is our knowledge, assumptions, and feelings about ourselves. A widely used test of self-concept employs 100 statements and a five-point answering scale to determine five components of self-concept: personal self, social self, family self, moral and ethical self, and physical self (body image). You might not expect activity and fitness to alter all the scales, but changes in physical and personal self seem possible.

An extensive review of research on children indicated that activity was associated with a positive self-concept, participation in activity programs contributed to self-esteem, and fitness activities were more effective than other components of the physical education program in developing self-concept (Gruber 1986). Research on

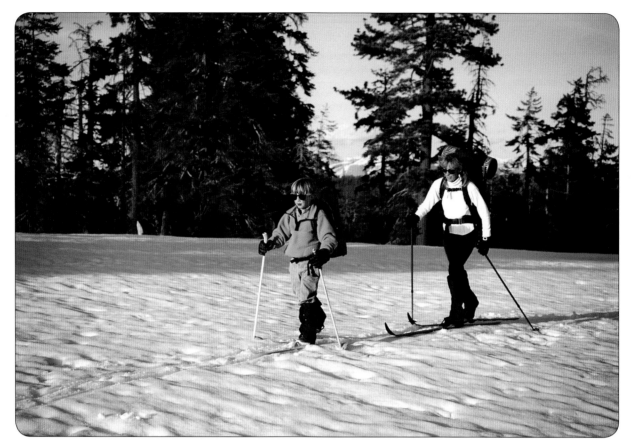

Activity has been shown to improve self-concept in children and adults.

adults agrees that activity and fitness improve self-concept. When you take control of your life, lose weight, improve strength and endurance, and enhance your appearance, you feel better about yourself and your body. This new confidence may alter your outlook on life, even your personality. As activity and fitness alter the self-image, this renewed confidence in the body can be an important step toward improved personal relations.

Self-esteem can be enhanced through participation in physical activity, perhaps by enhancing physical ability and self-estimation. Runners and other athletes identify with other participants. We define ourselves as runners, cyclists, swimmers, and so on and derive social acceptance from the group. One fear associated with injury is the loss of identity and social acceptance.

Biochemical Mechanisms

Activity and training can influence metabolism and a number of hormones. Regular participation provides biofeedback that leads to changes in heart rate, blood pressure, and other measures. Activity temporarily raises body temperature and induces relaxation and mild fatigue, factors related to the tranquilizing effect of exercise. A study by deVries and Adams (1972) showed that a single bout of exercise (walking) was as effective in reducing tension as a tranquilizer, and that the effect of the exercise lasted longer. Fitness training leads to profound metabolic effects that include increased efficiency and responsiveness to hormones, such as insulin. Training has a favorable influence on hormones and neurotransmitters associated with depression.

SELF-CONCEPT

Are you generally

__ relaxed or __ anxious?

__ in good shape or __ poor shape?

__ adventurous or __ conservative?

__ trim or __ overweight?

__ hardworking or __ lazy?

__ ambitious or __ aimless?

__ strong or __ weak?

__ physically attractive or __ unattractive?

__ persistent or __ not persistent?

__ extroverted or __ introverted?

__ self-confident or __ insecure?

__ a leader or __ a follower?

Do you want to improve some aspect of your self-concept? Select one or two attributes and find ways to make improvements.

Exercise also seems to enhance and protect brain function. Animals engaged in voluntary wheel running showed evidence of gene expression changes in the brain. Exercised animals showed an increase in a molecule (neurotrophic factor) that increases neuronal survival, enhances learning, and protects against cognitive decline (Cotman and Engesser-Cesar 2002). Researchers have also measured improved learning and delayed cognitive decline in active older adults. New research indicates that older people who exercise three or more times per week are less likely to develop Alzheimer's and other types of dementia. People who exercised regularly had a 30 to 40 percent lower risk of dementia. Even light activity such as walking helps to delay the onset of symptoms (Larson et al. 2006).

Some researchers also believe that activity increases levels of mood-altering substances called endorphins. Studies show that endorphins, morphinelike compounds produced in the brain, can reduce pain and induce a sense of euphoria. Runners whose levels of beta-endorphins in the blood increased after a marathon were quick to speculate that these opiates were responsible for the sensation known as the runner's high. Although blood endorphin levels increase during and after an endurance effort, studies have shown that the levels do not correspond with mood states (Markoff, Ryan, and Young 1982). But a lack of correlation between blood levels and moods should not be surprising because a barrier between the blood and brain prevents easy transport between the systemic circulation and the brain. Hence, blood levels of endorphins do not necessarily tell us what is happening to endorphin levels in the brain, where moods are formed. When rats were exercised daily for 1 hour on a treadmill, beta-endorphin levels in the brain (hypothalamus) were much higher than they were in control animals (Asahina et al. 2003). Increased levels in the blood are probably a reflection of the role of endorphins as a narcotic. Running feels easier after about 20 minutes, which is when researchers have detected increased levels of beta-endorphin. So if you have tried running and found it uncomfortable, try to continue beyond 20 minutes. You may find that it becomes easier with the help of your natural painkillers.

Clearly, activity and fitness have the potential to improve mild to moderate cases of anxiety and depression. But why wait until you are anxious or depressed to begin? Start now and you may be able to prevent or minimize assaults to your mental health.

Activity Minimizes Stress

Many believe that stress has become one of the major health problems of the modern age. Physiological responses necessary for the survival of primitive peoples may be unhealthy in highly complex societies. Stress, tension, and reactive behavior patterns have been associated with heart disease, hypertension, suppression of the immune system, and a variety of other ills. Structures in the brain, including the hypothalamus, mediate the emotional response to life events. When something excites or threatens us, the hypothalamus tells the anterior pituitary gland to secrete adrenocorticotropic hormone (ACTH), a chemical messenger that travels to the adrenal cortex and orders the release of hormones such as cortisol. These hormones are necessary for the body to respond to stressful situations. Stress has been defined as anything that increases the release of ACTH or cortisol.

Type A

The type A behavior pattern is characterized by extreme competitiveness, ambition, and a profound sense of time urgency. The type B personality, the opposite of type A, is relaxed, calm, and even phlegmatic. In studies by cardiologists Friedman and Rosenman (1973), type A subjects had higher cholesterol levels, faster blood-clotting times, higher adrenaline levels, more sudden deaths, and a sevenfold greater risk of heart disease. Subsequent studies, including the massive Framingham study, failed to find a link between the type A behavior pattern, stress, and heart disease. They did find a link between anger, repressed hostility, and heart disease risk (Wilson, Castelli, and Kannel 1987).

Although most of us intuitively accept stress as a risk factor for heart disease, the type A personality, in the absence of anger and hostility, does not seem to be a problem. Studies of corporate structure suggest that employees, not hard-driving executives, face the most stress. Executives live fast-paced lives but retain a sense of control. Employees often feel that they have no control over their lives, a circumstance that is stressful. A high level of anger in young men (concealed anger, griping, and irritability) is associated with increased risk of CAD and heart attacks (Chang et al. 2002).

Stressful situations also elicit a response in the sympathetic nervous system that leads to secretion of hormones from the adrenal medulla, including epinephrine (adrenaline) and norepinephrine. These hormones mobilize energy and support the cardiovascular response to the stressor. This aspect of the stress response is called the fight-or-flight mechanism. The hormones prepare the body to fight or run, but they have other effects that can be harmful to health. Epinephrine makes the blood clot faster and increases blood pressure, an advantage in a fight but a disadvantage in the workplace, where it can precipitate a heart attack or a stroke.

The stress response is necessary to prepare an athlete for maximal effort in a physical challenge, but it can be unhealthy if it occurs too often in the wrong setting. If you become stressed on the job, when a natural physical catharsis is impossible or improper, circulating hormones can be a problem. Recent research has suggested that some of us are hot reactors, exhibiting exaggerated blood pressure responses to everyday stressors. Hostile hot reactors become enraged when a driver cuts them off in traffic (road rage) or they experience other psychosocial stressors. This hostility elicits a flood of hormones designed for combat. Blood pressure and heart rate increase, arteries constrict, clotting time shortens, and blood flow to the heart drops off, contributing to increased risk of a heart attack. Hot reactors stew in their own juices, setting the stage for immediate or future health problems. Although occasional stress is not a threat, prolonged exposure to stress hormones eventually suppresses the immune system and reduces resistance to infection.

Some early animal studies suggested that exercise itself was a stressor (Selye 1956). Those results make sense when you realize that the researchers forced the animals to run on a treadmill and shocked them when they tried to rest, or forced them to swim to exhaustion in a deep tank with a weight tied around the tail. Electroshock and fear of drowning are stressful for most of us. For humans, exercise is stressful when it is highly competitive, exhausting, or threatening. Rock climbing, for example, is stressful for the neophyte but relaxing and exhilarating for the veteran. Stress is in the eye of the beholder.

Ulcers?

Years ago, ulcers were thought to be a product of stress, which led to increases in stomach acid, which then eroded a hole in the stomach (gastric ulcer). Today we know that *Helicobactor pylori*, an acid-resistant organism that survives in the stomach, causes many ulcers. Eliminating the bacterium with antibiotics cures the ulcer (Sachs et al. 2003).

Regular, moderate activity minimizes the effects of stress. It is relaxing and tranquilizing and counters the tendency to form blood clots, lowers blood pressure, and reduces epinephrine and cortisol. Regular activity enhances the function of the immune system, whereas the exhaustion of running a marathon is immunosuppressive. Occasional exposure to stressful activity is fine if one has trained for the event. Regular, moderate activity and fitness contribute to health, in part by reducing the diastolic blood pressure response to stress (Hendrix and Hughes 1997). Highly fit people experienced lower cardiovascular responses to stress than less fit people did, even though the groups did not differ in hostility (Alderman and Landers 2004). Another recent study correlated subclinical coronary artery disease, as measured by electron beam computed tomography, to depression, anxiety, hostility, and stress. This study of 630 active-duty military personnel found no correlation between CAD and any of the psychological factors, including stress (O'Malley et al. 2000). Perhaps the soldiers used activity to minimize their stress.

We know that regular activity is a coping mechanism that serves to improve tolerance to psychological stress. Although meditation and other forms of stress management are useful, regular, moderate activity is the best form of stress management, because it provides the benefits of meditation and relaxation while delivering added health benefits, including weight loss; reduced risk of CAD, hypertension, cancer, diabetes, and other ills; control of anxiety and depression; and improved appearance, vitality, and even longevity. Aerobic training is more effective than stress management in lowering heart rate and blood pressure during psychological stress (Spalding, Lyon, and Hatfield 2004).

STRESS TEST

Certain life events, both positive and negative, have been identified as stressful. A score of over 300 points in the past year has been associated with a serious illness within 2 years. Here are some of the events and their relative stressfulness (Roth and Holmes 1985).

Death of spouse	100 points
Divorce	73
Separation	65
Jail term	63
Death of family member	63
Personal injury or illness	53
Marriage	50
Fired from job	47
Retirement	45
Marital reconciliation	45
Pregnancy	40
Death of friend	37
Mortgage	31
Personal achievement	28
Spouse starts or stops work	26
Trouble with boss	23
Change of residence	20
Vacation	13

If life is getting too stressful, slow the pace of change.

Psychoneuroimmunology (PNI) studies the links between the brain, the nervous system, and the immune system. PNI focuses on how thoughts, emotions, and personality traits interact with the immune system and become manifest in sickness or health. Thoughts or emotions can enhance or suppress the immune system through neurotransmitters secreted by the sympathetic nervous system, or through hormones released by command of the brain (e.g., ACTH). The immune system is immensely complicated, consisting of lymphocytes, T cells, natural killer cells, antibodies, immunoglobulins, and more. The immune system serves to protect the body from foreign assaults. When exposed to prolonged stress, however, the system tends to break down, allowing invading microorganisms to proliferate. PNI suggests that by altering your perception of the supposed threat, by reprogramming your thinking and your outlook on life, you can reduce exposure to stress and spare the immune system.

Another way to bolster the immune system is by participating in regular activity. Studies confirm the beneficial effect of activity and training on components of the immune system. The studies agree that regular, moderate activity and training contribute to a healthy immune system (Mackinnon 1992; Nieman and Pedersen 1999). Intensity, duration, or frequency of training larger than a person is accustomed to increases the risk of overtraining, a condition characterized by fatigue, poor performance, and suppression of the immune system. On the other hand, well-trained athletes and workers are able to complete full days of physically challenging work with no decline in immune function. Studies of wildland firefighters showed that the firefighters could sustain up to 14 hours of hard work without adverse effects on immune function (Ruby et al. 2002). Activity, relaxation, imagery, and other coping strategies help you deal in a rational way with difficult problems, freeing the immune system to function on your behalf.

> If life is getting too stressful, slow the pace of change.

Physically active individuals tend to deal well with stress, have fewer upper respiratory tract infections (colds and sore throats), miss fewer work days because of illness, and are able to perform on the job or athletic field day after day. These health improvements appear related to improved immune function. In an ongoing study at the University of Montana, daily habitual activity levels appear to be inversely linked to levels of C-reactive protein, an inflammatory marker in the blood linked to increased risk for heart disease. In many ways, direct and indirect, the active life seems to reduce illness and increase vitality.

Activity and Addiction

Substance abuse with nicotine, alcohol, or prescription or recreational drugs presents a health and social dilemma that threatens to tear society apart. Each of these substances presents a staggering cost in health care, rehabilitation, and social services, not to mention loss of human potential. We don't pretend to have answers to this problem, but we do have some suggestions for prevention and individual responsibility.

In his book *Positive Addiction*, Dr. William Glasser contrasts positive and negative addictions (1976). Negative addictions such as drugs or alcohol relieve the pain of failure and provide temporary pleasure but at a terrible cost in terms of family, social, and professional life. Positive addictions, such as physical activity, lead to psychological strength, imagination, and creativity. Dr. Glasser suggests that as a person participates in meditation, yoga, or running, he or she eventually achieves a state of positive addiction. When the person reaches this state, the mind is free to become more imaginative or creative. The mind conceives more options in solving difficult or frustrating problems; it has more strength. Proof of addiction comes when guilt and anxiety accompany the early stages of withdrawal after a person is forced to abandon a habit.

Dr. Glasser suggested that positive addiction can be achieved from almost any activity you choose, as long as it meets the following criteria:

- The activity is not competitive.
- You do it for approximately 1 hour daily.
- The activity is easy to do and doesn't take much mental effort.
- You can do it alone or occasionally with others, but you don't rely on others to do it.
- You believe that it has some physical, mental, or spiritual value.
- You believe that if you persist you will improve.
- You can do it without criticizing yourself.

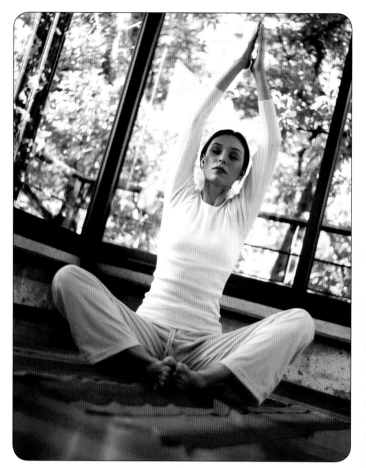

A positive addiction to meditation or activity can improve your creativity and help you deal with difficult problems.

In the chapter titled "Running—the Hardest But Surest Way," Dr. Glasser suggests that running, perhaps because it is our most basic solitary survival activity, produces the non-self-critical state more effectively than any other practice. He recommends running to everyone, from the weakest to the strongest. He feels that when a person can run an hour without fatigue, he or she will almost certainly achieve the positive addiction state on a regular basis. If the runner avoids competition and runs alone in a pleasant setting, addiction should occur within the year.

We knew that we were addicted to running long before Dr. Glasser wrote his book; we needed far less than an hour per day of running or a year to achieve it. Over the years the addiction to running has evolved to an addiction to activity. Addiction works with hiking, cycling, cross-country skiing, swimming, and even weight training as long as we keep it non-competitive and uncritical. As interests change or injuries occur, we've been able to transfer the addiction to new activities. The addiction ensures that we will remain active for the rest of our lives.

Is it possible to be too dedicated to activity, fitness, or training—to be negatively addicted or dependent? Probably. An old friend, the eminent and venerable sport psychologist Dr. William Morgan, first called attention to the possibility, noting runners who were so addicted that they neglected family and work. Some continued to train in spite of an illness or injury (Morgan 1979). We, too, have seen runners with an obsessive compulsion for their sport. Closer inspection revealed that some lives seemed confounded with other problems and that these people had turned to running as therapy. Several studies have linked compulsive running with the eating disorder anorexia nervosa. Others, however, found that addicted runners fell within the normal range of behavior whereas those with anorexia nervosa did not.

For our part we prefer a compulsion to running over a negative addiction to alcohol or drugs. The compulsive activity may alter family relationships and work performance, but it won't destroy the body and the mind. The obsession with running may serve as therapy, just as activity serves to reduce anxiety and depression. Dr. Glasser suggests that people can use positive addictions as replacements for negative ones. Imagine the health benefits of replacing smoking, alcohol, or drug use with daily activity! Although this replacement model clearly works for some people, the sizable dropout rates common in exercise programs and programs aimed at cessation of smoking, alcohol use, and drug use will limit its application.

Summary

Health has been called the first of all liberties. What some call optimal health or wellness implies a vitality and zest for living that is much more than the absence of disease. Our definition of health also embraces psychological, emotional, or mental health. Thus, healthy people are free from disease, anxiety, and depression. Their physical condition, nutritional state, and emotional outlook enable them to carry out daily tasks with vigor and alertness, without undue fatigue, and with ample energy to enjoy leisure-time pursuits and meet unforeseen emergencies.

The International Society of Sport Psychology (Tenenbaum and Singer 1992) believes that the benefits of regular vigorous activity include

- reduced state anxiety,
- decreased level of mild to moderate depression,
- reductions in neuroticism and anxiety,
- an adjunct to professional treatment of severe depression,
- reduction of stress indices, and
- beneficial emotional effects for all ages and both sexes.

We have seen how regular, moderate activity serves to enhance both physical and mental health. Now let's explore the role of health care in the active life.

Activity and Personal Health

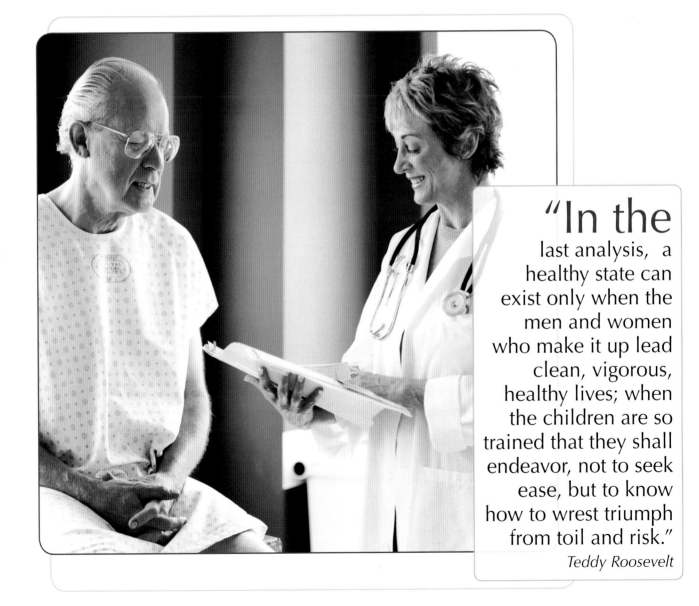

"In the last analysis, a healthy state can exist only when the men and women who make it up lead clean, vigorous, healthy lives; when the children are so trained that they shall endeavor, not to seek ease, but to know how to wrest triumph from toil and risk."

Teddy Roosevelt

The so-called American health care system is not about health, nor is it a system. Instead it is a chaotic mixture of doctors, hospitals, drug and insurance companies, lawyers, and—oh, yes—patients, held together by market factors, mutual dependence, and self-interest. The arrangement does not focus on prevention or health but on the treatment of illness, disease, and disabling injury. It isn't a system because it wasn't planned; it just grew. It defies economic theory. If demand goes down, prices go up (by 22 percent in 2003). Worst of all, it has fostered an unhealthy attitude: If we ignore commonsense health habits and become sick or injured, the health care system will perform a miracle cure and insurance will pay most of the enormous cost.

We're Number . . . 37!

The World Health Organization's year 2000 ranking of national health care systems found that the United States spends a large amount of money on health care per person ($3,724 in 2000 and $4,600 in 2004 according to newer WHO data), more than two times the average for other industrialized nations, yet ranks 37th in overall health care quality. Why? One reason is that the United States fails to insure 44 million citizens amid a patchwork of private insurance and government programs. Americans spend billions on diagnostics, drugs, and procedures but little on prevention. Japan, which spends less than $2,000 per person per year, beat the United States by 4 1/2 years in the category of how long people live in good health, not just how long they live.

Many Americans have come to rely on their doctors to take care of their health. Of course, that approach doesn't work. Your doctor can't make you stop smoking, lose weight, eat less fat, fasten your seat belt, or get regular exercise. These simple habits have more to do with health and disease than all the influences of medicine. More than half of all disease and death can be attributed to lifestyle. Granted, medical tests and treatments that prevent or minimize disease and disability are available, but not all the procedures require a physician.

This chapter will help you

- recognize the values and limitations of both health screening and early detection,
- develop a schedule for periodic medical examinations,
- determine the need for a preexercise medical exam, and
- understand the risks and benefits of regular, moderate physical activity.

Health Screening

One of us (Brian) has had the pleasure of working in two bureaucracies—a university and a federal agency. Although they are different in many respects, they share an interest in the health of their employees: Both have employee health or wellness programs. Most wellness programs use a computerized health risk analysis as the start of a comprehensive health-screening program. The analysis uses answers to questions about health habits and some basic information (age, sex, weight, blood pressure, and cholesterol) to calculate health risks and compute one's risk age. An overweight smoker with a family history of heart disease may have a risk age years above his or her chronological age. The health risk analysis is a simple, low-cost way to focus future health habits. A health risk analysis and longevity estimate are included in figure 3.6 (pages 64 through 68) at the end of this chapter.

Results from a cholesterol test could lead to a class on healthy food choices, an activity program, or even a doctor's visit and a prescription for cholesterol-lowering medication. The principle is simple: Use low-cost approaches to identify health habits and risks, apply more expensive tests but only for those at risk, and reserve high-cost tests and treatments for those in real need. Years ago, testing advocates promoted broad application of health-screening tests. Now we realize that many tests should be reserved for those who, by virtue of age, risk factors, family history, symptoms, or exposure, are most in need of the procedure. Generalized testing is costly, wastes the time and effort of medical personnel, and risks false positive results (indication of a problem when none exists).

Age, sex, health risks, family history, and occupation determine the need for health screening. Young, apparently healthy people do well with infrequent tests, unless, of course, they have a family history, symptoms, or exposure, or they change habits. Regrettably, age alone increases the need for certain onerous tests, such as a colonoscopy (for colon cancer) and digital prostate examination. A family history of glaucoma raises the need for a regular glaucoma test, and occupational exposure to noise or toxic chemicals calls for evaluation of hearing or lung function, respectively. A comprehensive worksite wellness program provides a wide range of health-screening procedures (see figure 3.1), along with appropriate immunizations (e.g., flu shots for retired employees) and booster shots.

Early Detection

For a time there was great interest in the development of tests to detect problems such as cancer. The idea was that early detection would improve the prognosis for recovery. Indeed, some studies showed that early detection was associated with extended survival. This notion is fine, as long as the extension of life exceeds the improvement in detection time. Early detection is meaningless, however, if no effective treatment for the disease is available. Of course, if the disease can be transmitted (e.g., AIDS) and its spread can be limited, early detection makes sense from a public health standpoint.

> Early detection is meaningless if no effective treatment for the disease is available.

In recent years medical opinion has changed concerning the course of treatment for several medical problems. For example, in older men, aggressive treatment of prostate cancer (surgery, radiation) is not necessarily superior to watching and waiting. Survival time doesn't always improve with aggressive treatment, and quality of life is often impaired (incontinence, impotency). Back operations and heart surgery, even for patients with obvious symptoms, have been performed more often than necessary, leading one to question the accuracy of detection and diagnosis. But many tests are warranted, especially when they lead to changes in behavior. Low-cost blood pressure and cholesterol tests can identify problems while time is still available to slow, stop, or even reverse the disease process. So if your age, sex, race, family history, health habits, or exposure puts you at risk for a disease, use an early detection test, as long as the proposed test meets the following criteria:

- The disease has a significant effect on the quality of life.
- Acceptable methods of treatment are available.

Figure 3.1 Adult preventive care timeline: recommendations of major authorities.

- Treatment during the asymptomatic (no symptom) period significantly reduces disability or death.
- Early treatment yields a superior result.
- Detection tests are available at reasonable cost.
- The incidence of the disease in the population is sufficient to justify the cost of screening.

Few tests meet these criteria; blood pressure tests, breast examinations, and Pap smears do, whereas exercise stress tests, diabetes screening, and X rays for lung cancer do not. Surprisingly, the routine (annual) medical examination also fails to meet the criteria.

Blood Pressure

High blood pressure, or hypertension, a silent killer with no obvious symptoms, is easy and inexpensive to test. Moreover, several acceptable methods of treatment are available, and successful control extends the quantity and quality of life. Systolic pressure is the pressure exerted against arterial walls when the heart contracts to send blood into the system. Diastolic pressure is the pressure against arterial walls between beats, when the heart is relaxed. Both measures contribute to the mean arterial pressure, and both have consequences for health. Use the information in table 3.1 to evaluate your blood pressure.

Table 3.1 Blood Pressure Evaluation

	Systolic BP (mm Hg)	Diastolic BP (mm Hg)	Action
Normal BP	<120	<80	Retest annually.
Prehypertension	120–130	80–85	Retest in 6 mo.[*]
Hypertension	≥130	≥85	See physician.[**]

[*]Change diet, weight loss, physical activity, stress reduction.
[**]Possible medication.

From www.nhlbi.nih.gov 2004.

Borderline cases often respond to diet, weight loss, and exercise. Cases that remain elevated with diet, weight loss, exercise, and stress reduction require medication. Studies clearly show the value of controlling blood pressure. Aerobic exercise combined with weight loss is recommended for the management of elevated blood pressure in sedentary, overweight individuals (Blumenthal et al. 2000). High blood pressure can damage arterial walls and contribute to atherosclerosis, and excess pressure increases the risk of stroke. Although salt intake, being overweight, and stress may exacerbate the problem, the cause is poorly understood, and more than 90 percent of all cases are of unknown origin. Modern molecular biology will someday unlock the cause of these constricted arteries, but you can't wait for someday. Check your pressure regularly and never rely on a single measure. If the pressure is elevated in several checks, restrict salt and fat, lose weight, engage in regular, moderate activity, and learn how to manage stress. If all that isn't enough, or if the pressure is above 160, see your physician. New medications provide control of blood pressure with fewer side effects. But don't rely on medications for control; continue with diet, exercise, weight loss, and stress management.

Annual Medical Examination

The typical medical examination includes a history, physical examination, and tests dictated by the patient's age, gender, and the findings of the exam. In the past, we all assumed that the annual medical examination would help us stay healthy and reduce the likelihood of illness or premature death. But when researchers compared those who had annual exams with those who did not, they found an equal number of chronic diseases and deaths in the two groups. Today many doctors agree that for persons with no symptoms or chronic disease, the annual medical exam is a waste of time and money. A past president of the American Medical Association has said that he hasn't had a routine physical since he joined the army decades ago, and he asks patients who request a checkup, "What do you want one for?" Let's consider a typical scenario to see why the annual medical exam pays off for the doctor and the laboratory but not for the patient.

Joe is a typical patient; he is 45, somewhat overweight and out of shape, smokes a pack a day, and indulges his love for meat and potatoes. His company pays for his annual medical exam, so the physician schedules a battery of tests, including a blood lipid panel, chest X ray, electrocardiogram (ECG), pulmonary function tests, and other procedures. Aside from somewhat elevated blood pressure and cholesterol and a low level of HDL cholesterol, Joe's ECG and other tests appear normal. So Joe goes out and celebrates his clean bill of health with a prime rib; baked potato with butter, sour cream, and bacon bits; a salad with lots of dressing; and a slice of cheesecake. The next morning he experiences a crushing pain in his chest and is rushed to the hospital with a heart attack.

This all-too-common scenario illustrates the fact that many tests lack the sensitivity to provide early detection. A resting ECG seldom predicts an impending myocardial infarction (heart attack). An exercise electrocardiogram (stress test) may have had a better chance of identifying Joe's problem, but the exercise test occasionally suggests heart disease when none is present. Pulmonary function tests and chest X rays seldom detect lung cancer early enough to improve the prognosis (the X ray actually increases the risk of cancer). And some tests increase the likelihood of surgery when it may not be needed. If Joe had complained of a back problem and the doctor had ordered an MRI (magnetic resonance imaging) that revealed a bulging disk, he might have been scheduled for an operation that could make things worse (Jensen et al. 1994). Does this mean that all tests and medical exams are a waste of time? Of course not; many valid reasons point to the need for a medical examination.

If you have symptoms or are in doubt about the condition of your health, see your physician. If you or a member of your family has a history of hypertension, check your pressure regularly. Buy a stethoscope and a blood pressure cuff (sphygmomanometer) and do it at home, at the drugstore, or at your worksite wellness program. Check elevated cholesterol regularly at worksite screenings, health fairs, or walk-in clinics. Check your kids to see whether they need to use diet and exercise to minimize a family problem. Use screening programs to check blood sugar, and if problems arise see your physician. Of course, women should have regular checkups throughout pregnancy. Studies fail to provide convincing evidence of the value of periodic medical examinations, let alone annual exams (Gordon, Senf, and Campos-Outcalt 1999). A reasonable frequency of examination includes the following:

> If you have symptoms or are in doubt about the condition of your health, by all means see your physician.

- At around 18 and 25 years of age
- Every 5 years between ages 35 and 65
- Every 2 years after age 65 (Gordon, Senf, and Campos-Outcalt 1999)

In our view, this schedule could be too intensive for the apparently healthy adult who is willing to take charge of his or her health. We use the physician when necessary, but we employ other ways to get answers to medical issues, such as the *Merck Manual*, the book that doctors use when they are stumped (www.merckmanual.com). We have a wellness program blood panel each year to keep track of blood lipids (e.g., cholesterol), and we take advantage of other worksite wellness and community health-screening programs that fit our needs. We see the dentist often enough and have periodic eye exams to adjust prescriptions and test for glaucoma. Otherwise, our visits to the doctor's office are for specifics, such as a trip to the dermatologist to check on a suspicious growth, or to the orthopedic surgeon for a major injury (we self-treat minor injuries or seek a friendly athletic trainer for advice). But, as we said, if you have symptoms or are in doubt about the condition of your health, see your physician.

Cholesterol Screening

Cholesterol is a serious heart disease risk factor. Although the risk rises with the level of cholesterol, some people with relatively low values experience problems with atherosclerosis (see tables 3.2, *a-e*). Cholesterol is a fatlike substance found in all human and animal tissues but not in plants. We ingest cholesterol in foods from animals (e.g., meat, eggs, fish, poultry, and dairy products), or we can synthesize it in the body. If you don't eat much cholesterol, the body will make all it needs from other fats. The blood transports cholesterol in low- or high-density lipoprotein packages.

The ideal total cholesterol level is below 150 milligrams. Values from 150 to 200 should respond to a moderate reduction of saturated and hydrogenated fats in the diet. Levels from 200 to 240 call for a concentrated effort to reduce these atherogenic fats and take additional dietary measures, including increasing intake of bran and other natural foods to reduce cholesterol. Cholesterol levels that remain above 240 after dietary, exercise, and weight-loss interventions may require drug therapy, especially if other risk factors are present. Fortunately, cholesterol drugs have been

Table 3.2*a*   Total Cholesterol and CAD Risk

Cholesterol (mg/100 ml)	Category
<200	Desirable
200–239	Borderline high risk
240 or over	High risk

Source: American Heart Association.

Table 3.2*b*   LDL Cholesterol and CAD Risk

LDL (mg/dl)	Category
<100	Optimal
100–129	Near optimal
130–159	Borderline high
160–189	High
>190	Very high

Source: American Heart Association.

Table 3.2*c*   HDL Cholesterol and CAD Risk

HDL (mg/dl)	Category
>60	Desirable
45 (men), 55 (women)	Average
<40	High risk

Source: American Heart Association.

Table 3.2*d*   Total Cholesterol to HDL Ratio and CAD Risk

Ratio (chol/HDL)	Category
<3.5	Desirable
3.5–5	Average
>5	High risk

Source: American Heart Association.

Table 3.2*e*   Triglycerides and CAD Risk

Triglycerides (mg/dl)	Category
<150	Normal
150–199	Borderline high
200–499	High
>500	Very high

Source: American Heart Association.

proved successful at lowering levels and the incidence of heart disease. Consult your physician for details.

Low-density lipoprotein cholesterol (LDL) is the dangerous version that finds its way into the lining of the coronary arteries. It can combine with oxygen and enhance the development of plaques in arteries. High-density lipoprotein cholesterol (HDL) acts like a transport system that picks up excess cholesterol and delivers it to the liver for reprocessing or removal. Thus, higher HDL levels are protective, with a one-milligram increase associated with a 2 to 3 percent reduction in CAD. Conversely, low values are an independent risk factor. So you can have a low total cholesterol level and still have some risk if your HDL is low. You should know all three numbers (total cholesterol, LDL, and HDL), as well as your cholesterol to HDL ratio. Table 3.2c shows the risk associated with blood lipids and displays how the risk declines as HDL levels rise.

Another way to assess your risk is to calculate your total cholesterol to HDL ratio. A ratio under 4 (e.g., 200 divided by 50) is associated with a low risk of heart disease, whereas a ratio over 6 (e.g., 240 divided by 40) is not. All adults should be tested every 5 years unless values are borderline or high, a circumstance that calls for annual testing and treatment.

Recent research has identified two additional tests to help determine one's risk of heart disease:

- Homocysteine is often elevated in the blood of those at high risk for heart problems. A blood test will show if a problem exists. If it does, the solution is simple: an increase in foods containing the B vitamin folate (or a folate supplement). Folate is also important for pregnant women or those planning to become pregnant.

- C-reactive protein (C-RP) is a sign of inflammatory activity that is associated with an increased risk of a heart attack (Ridker et al. 2000). C-RP may influence apoptosis or fragmentation of human coronary vascular smooth muscle cells, a key event in the development of atherosclerotic lesions and the vulnerability of plaque to rupture (Blaschke et al. 2004). But because C-RP is also associated with chronic infections and arthritis, it is viewed as a relatively moderate predictor of CAD (Danesh et al. 2004). Recent studies indicate that cholesterol-lowering statin drugs may also lower C-RP, and that those with lower C-RP levels have a greater reduction in coronary risk (Nissen et al. 2005). A blood test can determine the level. Efforts to reduce the risk may include daily intake of an aspirin, vitamin E, an alcoholic beverage, weight loss, statin therapy, and, of course, physical activity (see table 3.3).

In case you were wondering about triglyceride levels, some say that they do not provide clinically relevant information about CAD risk beyond that obtained with measures of cholesterol, LDL, and HDL (Avins and Neuhaus 2000). But elevated triglycerides may be a risk factor for CAD when cholesterol levels are low (see table

Table 3.3   Prescription for Elevated Cholesterol

Exercise	Thirty minutes of moderate daily aerobic activity will lower LDL a modest amount; higher intensity or duration exercise (e.g., jogging) will further reduce LDL and improve HDL cholesterol.
Diet	Reduce animal and hydrogenated fat intake, increase fiber by eating bran and whole-grained products, increase vitamin C and E intake, and consume some alcohol (one or two drinks a day).

3.2*e*). High triglycerides are often associated with low HDL and blood clotting, and may lead to enlargement of the liver. Normal fasted levels should be below 150 milligrams per 100 milliliters. We'll say more about the blood lipids, cholesterol, and triglycerides in later chapters.

If your risk of heart disease is high, you should know that new information is available that you can use to improve your health. The National Cholesterol Education Program has formulated new guidelines for LDL cholesterol. High-risk persons (based on risk factors) should aim to get LDL cholesterol below 70, well below the previous goal of 100 milligrams per deciliter. Studies indicate that the lower the LDL cholesterol level, the better. Achieving this level will probably require use of prescription drugs (Grundy et al. 2004).

Preexercise Medical Examination

Should you see your doctor before you embark on an increase in your physical activity? Here is the opinion of the eminent Swedish physician and exercise scientist Dr. Per Olaf Åstrand (Åstrand and Rodahl 1970, 608):

As a general rule, moderate activity is less harmful to the health than inactivity. You could also put it this way: A medical examination is more urgent for those who plan to remain inactive than for those who intend to get into good physical shape!

The active life is certain to enhance—not threaten—your health if you are free of symptoms, if you make a gradual transition to a more active life, and if you follow a sensible program. On the other hand, you should consider a preparticipation medical examination if you have been sedentary, if you are concerned about your health, if you have one or several primary heart disease risk factors (hypertension, elevated cholesterol, cigarette smoking, or inactivity), or if you are over 45 years of age (55 for women) and plan to engage in a vigorous exercise program. The American Heart Association (AHA) and the American College of Sports Medicine (ACSM) recommend a preparticipation medical exam including a progressive, ECG-monitored exercise test (stress test) for everyone with known cardiac, pulmonary, or metabolic disease, and for patients with symptoms and those over 45 (55 for women) before participation in vigorous exercise (Balady et al. 1998).

> A medical examination is more urgent for those who plan to remain inactive than for those who intend to get into good physical shape!

Health-Screening Questionnaire

For apparently healthy individuals under 45 years of age, the risk of participation in activity and fitness programs can be substantially reduced with inexpensive preparticipation health screening. Canadian researchers have developed the Physical Activity Readiness Questionnaire (PAR-Q) to identify the small number of adults for whom physical activity might be inappropriate or those who should have medical advice before participation (www.csep.com). The authors use a more comprehensive questionnaire (see figure 3.2). The questionnaire was adapted from the American Heart Association (www.americanheart.org) and the American College of Sports Medicine form that provides simple, self-administered preparticipation questions that identify heart disease risk factors and some other health issues.

Figure 3.2   Preexercise Screening Questionnaire

HISTORY

Have you had any of the following?

__ Heart attack

__ Heart surgery

__ Cardiac catheterization

__ Coronary angioplasty (PTCA)

__ Pacemaker or implantable cardiac defibrillator or rhythm disturbance

__ Heart valve disease

__ Heart failure

__ Heart transplantation

__ Congenital heart disease

If you marked any of the statements in this section, consult your health care provider before engaging in exercise. You may need to use a facility with a medically qualified staff.

CARDIOVASCULAR AND OTHER RISK FACTORS

__ You are a man older than 45 years.

__ You are a woman older than 55 years or you have had a hysterectomy or you are postmenopausal.

__ You smoke.

__ Your blood pressure is greater than 140/90.

__ You don't know your blood pressure.

__ You take blood pressure medication.

__ Your blood cholesterol level is greater than 240 mg/dl.

__ You don't know your cholesterol level.

__ You have a close blood relative who had a heart attack before age 55 (father or

    brother) or age 65 (mother or sister).

__ You have diabetes or take medicine to control your blood sugar.

__ You are physically inactive (i.e., you get less than 30 minutes of physical activity on at least 3 days per week).

__ You are more than 20 pounds (9 kilograms) overweight.

__ You have chest pain brought on by physical activity.

__ You developed chest pain in the past month.

__ You take heart medications.

__ You have musculoskeletal problems.

__ You have concerns about the safety of exercise.

__ You take prescription medications.

__ You are pregnant.

If you marked two or more of the statements in this section, consult your health care provider before engaging in exercise. You might benefit by using a facility with a professionally qualified exercise staff to guide your exercise program.

If none of the above are true you should be able to exercise safely without consulting your health care provider in almost any facility that meets your exercise program needs.

Note: If you have a temporary illness, such as a common cold, or are not feeling well at this time, postpone.

Source: American Heart Association www.americanheart.org.

Exercise Stress Test

Severe chest pain (angina pectoris) or even a heart attack can sometimes be the first sign of coronary artery problems. A gradually increased exercise challenge known as a stress test can detect indications of previously undiagnosed heart disease. Narrowed coronary arteries may be able to supply the blood that you need for sedentary pursuits, but during exercise the oxygen needs of heart muscle go up, and electrocardiographic abnormalities or physical symptoms may indicate a problem.

Maximal or near-maximal workloads may be needed to elicit the symptoms of previously undiagnosed heart disease. Many physicians choose to terminate the stress test when the heart rate reaches some percentage of the age-adjusted maximal heart rate, reasoning that it is unnecessary to risk a maximal test. Unfortunately, wide variability in maximal heart rates means that the test may be too strenuous for some and too easy for others (see table 3.4).

A physician uses a progressive ECG-monitored exercise test as a diagnostic tool to identify the presence of heart disease, as a preexercise test to reduce risks or set limits, as a postcoronary test to indicate the extent of damage and subsequent progress in therapeutic programs, or after a coronary bypass or angioplasty procedure to establish extent of recovery as well as work and activity limits. Although most stress tests are conducted on the treadmill, arm testing (cranking) may be required for individuals returning to jobs that require strenuous use of the upper body.

One reason for maximal testing is to evaluate individuals' functional capacity, their maximal attainable workload. The stress test can be used to clear a patient for hard work and to establish his or her work capacity. When treadmill tests are used to predict aerobic fitness, the subject should not support his or her weight by holding the railing of the

Table 3.4 Age and Maximal Heart Rates

Age	Average fitness
20	201
30	193
40	186
50	179
60	172
70	165

Maximal heart rate declines with age. The decline is slower among active and fit people (170 at 70 years). The decline is more rapid for those below average fitness (147 at 70 years). This measure has considerable variability.

Source: American Heart Association.

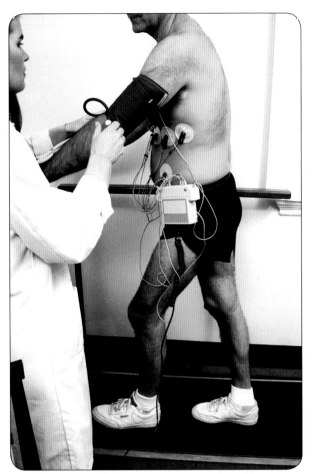

An ECG-monitored treadmill test can help reduce exercise risks.

treadmill. This practice lowers the actual work load and invalidates the prediction of fitness and work capacity.

The stress test should end when the subject cannot continue or has symptoms of exertional intolerance (chest pain, intolerable fatigue) or distress (staggering, dizziness, confusion, pallor, labored breathing, or nausea), when significant electrocardiographic changes occur, or when blood pressure drops in spite of increasing workload. Termination of the test at some predetermined percentage of the assumed maximal heart rate, on the other hand, risks missing important signs or symptoms. As we have noted, maximal heart rate is highly variable. Using an age-related maximal heart rate (e.g., 220 beats per minute minus age equals the predicted maximal heart rate) can lead to substantial errors. For example, the maximal heart rate for 40-year-old patients may average 180 beats per minute (220 minus 40 equals 180), but the range goes from below 144 to above 216. So a test terminated at 85 percent of the predicted maximal heart rate (.85 times 180 equals 153 beats per minute) may be too strenuous for a few and much too easy for others. For these reasons, we suggest continuing the stress test until the subject reaches fatigue or the termination criteria mentioned earlier.

Maximal Heart Rate

The variability in maximal heart rate, as defined by a statistic called the standard deviation (SD), is plus or minus 12 beats per minute: 68 percent of all cases fall within plus or minus one SD, 95 percent within plus or minus two SD, and 99 percent within plus or minus three SD. So, for our example, it is likely that one in a hundred 40-year-olds will have a maximal heart rate below 144 or above 216. Incidentally, as you'll see in chapter 4, this variability in maximal heart rate complicates the use of the heart rate for the prescription of exercise. And to make matters more confusing, the standard deviation for maximal heart rate goes up to 15 beats per minute for older people.

Exercise Electrocardiogram

The electrocardiogram (ECG) is a strip of paper with a record of the heart's electrical activity. Each complete ECG cycle (see figure 3.3) represents one beat of the heart. The P wave shows the electrical activity that immediately precedes the contraction of the upper chambers, or atria. The QRS complex represents the electrical discharge of the lower chambers, or ventricles, and the T wave results when the depolarized ventricles are recharged. Because the ECG paper moves at a specified speed (usually 25 millimeters per second), the timing and width of the waves can provide information

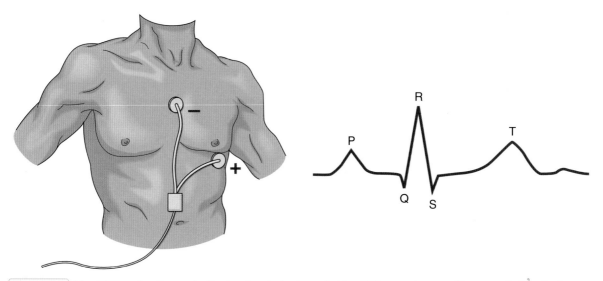

Figure 3.3 The ECG cycle. P wave indicates depolarization of atria. QRS wave is caused by spread of excitation through ventricles. T wave indicates repolarization of ventricles.

about the rate of electrical conduction. For example, if conduction is slow or blocked, the base of the QRS will be broad. The physician, nurse, or exercise test technologist administering a stress test pays careful attention to the ECG waveform and knows how to identify changes that suggest heart disease or other problems.

Conduction disturbances occasionally occur during stress tests, so emergency equipment and trained personnel should be available during evaluation of high-risk patients. Fortunately, most patients recover and are able to return to supervised activity after defibrillation. Tests conducted on apparently healthy individuals are not considered unsafe, but test administrators should know how to perform cardiopulmonary resuscitation (CPR) and other emergency techniques.

Test Results

When the exercise stress test results suggest heart problems (e.g., ECG abnormalities, chest pain, or abnormal blood pressure response) the test is called positive. Stress test findings are verified when they are confirmed with cardiac catheterization, an invasive imaging technique. In this procedure a catheter is inserted into a blood vessel in the leg and worked into position in the aorta. Injection of an opaque dye into each coronary artery allows X-ray detection of narrowing because of atherosclerosis. When narrowed arteries are found after a normal, or negative, stress test, the test is called a false negative. Results of a positive stress test are considered false when the catheter test reveals normal coronary arteries (i.e., a false positive stress test).

When cardiologists identify a positive test showing narrowed coronary arteries, the medical intervention is often a coronary bypass or angioplasty operation to repair one or more of the narrowed coronary arteries of the body. In a bypass surgery, the surgeon takes a small blood vessel from the leg or chest and uses it to bypass the section of severely narrowed coronary artery. Coronary angioplasty involves insertion of a catheter tipped with a balloon into the narrowed artery. Inflation of the balloon opens the artery, and the surgeon inserts a wire mesh stent to maintain blood flow. Both operations are expensive and may have complications. Before you get to the point where you require one of the invasive procedures, prevention seems prudent.

Nonsurgical Alternative

The United States has just 5 percent of the world's population but performs nearly half of the angioplasties and bypass surgeries worldwide. Some think that a quarter to a third of all cardiac procedures are unnecessary and that many people do as well with nonsurgical approaches. How do you know if you need the procedure that your doctor recommends? Dr. Thomas Graboys, a cardiologist at Harvard Medical School, employs three criteria to determine who can follow the nonsurgical route: the condition of the pump (a good heart muscle will do well); the electrical stability of the heart, especially under stress (treadmill); and the absence of symptoms. Those who meet these criteria may want to consider a nonsurgical approach involving drugs and lifestyle changes (Griffin 2004).

False negative results are disturbing because they indicate a failure to diagnose the presence of existing coronary artery disease. A small number of patients who undergo exercise stress tests fall into this category, and most of them do not go on for further evaluation. In such cases the first indication of a problem may be the last, a myocardial infarction or heart attack. Because of this, the physician cannot rely on the stress test alone but must employ clinical judgment, the patient's medical history, and other diagnostic tools. For example, patient reports of indigestion or chest pain during exertion may be useful, because the gradual warm-up of the stress test may allow patients with narrowed arteries to adjust to the increased workload, thus disguising the problem. Recent research shows that partially occluded vessels, which may not produce symptoms during a stress test, contain unstable plaque, which may rupture and cause a heart attack with no warning.

False positive tests are also disturbing because they may cause otherwise healthy individuals to become cardiac neurotics, morbidly obsessed with a heart condition that may not exist. Estimates of the frequency of false positive results range from as little as 10 percent to more than 30 percent, depending on the group studied (ACSM 1999). False positive results are more prevalent in highly active subjects and women (who may be more likely to hyperventilate during the test). Endurance athletes often exhibit ECG abnormalities during the stress test, and experienced doctors have learned to disregard the findings in the absence of other signs or symptoms. But what about the active nonathlete who receives word that the stress test indicates possible coronary artery disease? What does he or she do next?

In the past the coronary angiogram was the only way to confirm or deny the existence of coronary artery disease. If the stress test indicated possible disease, the patient had two choices: have the invasive catheter test or ignore the findings and fret about the possibilities, even giving up an active lifestyle for a heart condition that might not exist. Today the patient has other choices. Myocardial scintigraphy involves a less invasive assessment of myocardial blood flow during rest and exercise. In this procedure, radioactive thallium is injected into the circulation, and its uptake in cardiac muscle is observed with a scintillation camera. Cold spots indicate areas where blood flow is inadequate during exercise, allowing confirmation of stress test results (Froelicher 1984). Recently, drugs have been used to stress the heart and simulate the stress test, and computerized tomography (CT) scans are being used successfully to detect plaques in coronary arteries. The ideal will be a simple, noninvasive, low-cost alternative, such as a comparison of blood pressure readings taken from the arm and leg. A difference between the two readings may indicate the presence of circulatory problems or atherosclerosis. These developments may someday make the stress test obsolete as a test for heart disease.

Some experts think that false positive tests occur infrequently. They reason that a coronary artery spasm may occur during the vigorous effort of the stress test. Because the catheterization test is routinely performed at rest, the spasm may not show up. The thallium scan mentioned earlier helps solve this problem, and drugs can indicate the tendency for spasms during catheterization. For more on exercise testing, visit the Web pages for the American Heart Association (www.americanheart.org) and the American College of Sports Medicine (www.acsm.org).

Risk of Activity

Anecdotal notes on the dangers of exercise appear often in exercise literature, leading many people to have concerns about the safety of physical activity. Research has confirmed that activity greatly reduces but doesn't eliminate the risks associated with inherited or lifestyle diseases. When inactive people engage in vigorous exercise, their risk rises 56 times above resting levels when they first start an activity program, but the risk drops rapidly as the program progresses and overall risk during nonexercise periods also drops dramatically. The habitually active person has a 60 percent lower risk of heart attack than his or her sedentary counterpart does. The risk for the active person rises only 5 times during vigorous exercise, to a level slightly above the risk of sedentary living (Siscovick, LaPorte, and Newman 1985). The bottom line: Start an exercise program gradually, keep it going, and enjoy the lowered risk of heart disease and the improved quality of life for many years to come.

The risks of activity and fitness range from minor musculoskeletal problems to major coronary events. The risks are low for low-intensity and moderate-duration activity. Overuse injuries are more common when a person rapidly increases distance, with more miles (kilometers) per week, with high-intensity training (e.g., interval training), and with eccentric exercise (e.g., downhill running). The risk of a coronary event is low for an asymptomatic adult, in either training or testing, and the exerciser can cut the risk in half by taking the preexercise screening questionnaire (see figure 3.2).

When patients take a stress test in a medical setting, the risk is one cardiac episode per 187,000 person-hours of testing. The average test lasts 15 minutes, so the odds of an event are 1 in 788,000, or about 1/100 of the chance of being in a major automobile accident per hour of driving. But when presumably healthy (asymptomatic) individuals are tested, the risks are much lower. The incident of sudden cardiac death during vigorous exertion in healthy adults is only one death per year in every 15,000 to 18,000 people (ACSM 2005). For patients in a medically supervised cardiac rehabilitation program, the risk of death is one per every 60,000 person-hours of participation. Clearly, the health benefits of physical activity outweigh the risks (Morrey and Hensrud 1999).

Figure 3.4 provides a graphic view of the relationships between the benefits and risks of activity. The figure indicates

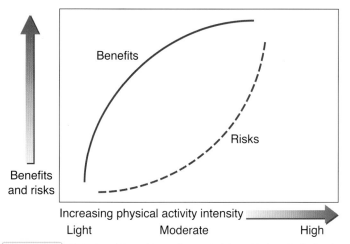

Figure 3.4   Relationships of benefits and risks with level of physical activity.

Adapted from Powel and Paffenbarger, 1985.

that benefits increase rapidly at first but eventually reach a plateau, with little additional reward at higher levels of activity. Risks, on the other hand, rise slowly at first and then more rapidly at higher levels of activity. The prudent approach to maximizing benefits and minimizing risks is to engage in a level of activity associated with enhanced health—regular, moderate activity.

As you engage in physical activity, be aware of these warning signs.

Stop Signs

If any of these occur, even once, stop exercising and consult your physician before resuming.

- Abnormal heart action: irregular pulse; fluttering, pumping, or palpitations in the chest or throat; a sudden burst of rapid heartbeats; or a very slow pulse that a moment earlier had been beating at a moderate rate (may occur either during or after exercise).

- Pain or pressure in the middle of the chest or in the arm or throat during or after exercise.

- Dizziness, lightheadedness, sudden loss of coordination, confusion, cold sweat, glassy stare, pallor, blueness, or fainting. In this case, stop the exercise—don't try to cool down—and lie with your feet elevated or sit and put your head down between your legs until the symptoms pass.

Yield Signs

Try the suggested remedy; if no relief occurs, consult a doctor.

- Persistent rapid heart action. Heart rate increases with exercise intensity. High heart rate values may occur when you are exercising vigorously and for 5 to 10 minutes thereafter. To correct the problem, lower exercise intensity (heart rate) to a comfortable level and increase it slowly over a period of weeks. Consult a physician if the action is persistent.

- Flare-up of bone or joint conditions. Rest and resume exercise when the condition subsides. If you have no relief with the usual remedies, see your doctor.

Caution Signs

You can usually remedy these signs without medical consultation, although you may wish to report them to your doctor.

- Nausea or vomiting after exercise. Wait at least 2 to 3 hours after eating before you exercise, avoid extreme heat, exercise less vigorously, and take a longer cool-down period.

- Extreme breathlessness lasting more than 10 minutes after stopping exercise. Exercise less vigorously, at a level at which you can hold a conversation (talk test). If breathlessness persists, see your doctor.

- Prolonged fatigue. If you remain tired 24 or more hours after exercising or have insomnia related to physical activity, lower your intensity and increase it gradually over a period of weeks.

- Side stitch. Lean forward while sitting and attempt to push the abdominal organs up against the diaphragm.

Special Considerations for Exercise

This section provides a brief summary for those with special exercise needs or limitations. Consult references, the Internet, community services, or your physician for additional information.

OLDER ADULTS   With age comes increasing need for muscular fitness. Seniors should undertake exercises to develop and maintain muscular strength and endurance. A wise approach is to increase strength to required levels before loss of strength limits self-sufficiency. Chapter 17 explores issues of age, activity, and vitality.

WOMEN   The exercise advice and prescriptions in this book work for both men and women, but women should consider some specific issues. Young women need to know that high-volume vigorous prepubertal training may delay the onset of the menstrual cycle. On the positive side, that delay is associated with lower risk of cancers of the breast and the reproductive system. Long delays in the onset of menstruation or the onset of amenorrhea because of excess endurance training in young women can reduce bone mineral content, cause stress fractures, and pose future bone problems (osteoporosis). Conversely, strength training strengthens bones and increases strength and muscle mass.

Pregnant women may continue their exercise habits with physician approval. Most doctors recommend eliminating high-impact aerobics, keeping the exercise heart rate below 140 beats per minute, and avoiding prolonged exposure to high temperature during activity.

Postmenopausal women should participate in activities that put a moderate degree of stress on the muscles and bones of the upper body as well as the legs, to minimize the progress of osteoporosis. And women of all ages need to be aware of their special nutritional needs (e.g., calcium and iron).

A disability needn't stop participation or competition.

CHILDREN   Children are not miniature adults; their bones are still forming, and their capacity for exercise in certain circumstances is different from that of adults. Moreover, the value of early (prepubertal) strength or endurance training is still far from established. Therefore, moderation is the best approach. Children should avoid heavy training, prolonged hard work in the heat, and excess competition (if only to prevent later burnout). Give children the freedom to develop their own games, to play, to explore, and to be kids. Don't impose an adult model or adult goals on children, but do encourage an active lifestyle that will last a lifetime.

PEOPLE WITH DISABILITIES   Each disability carries its own restrictions, but each has potential as well. People with disabilities participate and compete all the way up to international competitions, but only after establishing control over their conditions. They have learned to ski, to kayak, to do just about anything, and more opportunities are becoming available. Wheelchair athletes compete in marathons, play basketball, and fish at special access sites. People with multiple sclerosis respond better to moderate activity, such as swimming. For more information contact your recreation department, community service organizations, or the National Center on Physical Activity and Disability, which maintains a wonderful free electronic newsletter and Web site (www.ncpad.org).

RACIAL CONSIDERATIONS   We've long known about the greater prevalence of hypertension among African Americans (Lubell 1988). One in every three African American adults has hypertension, compared with one in four non-African Americans, and African Americans are three times more likely to have severe hypertension than whites. All people benefit from aerobic and moderate lifting activities. Those with hypertension may want to avoid extremely heavy lifting or exercises with an isometric (static) component, because straining against a heavy load can elevate blood pressure dramatically. Moderate aerobic exercise and weight loss will help lower blood pressure, but people with hypertension should undergo a preexercise medical examination, follow dietary recommendations, and take prescribed medications.

Health and Wellness

In the past health was defined as the absence of disease, and that is how many people still think of the term. In the 1980s the definition of health was expanded to include a state of complete physical, mental, and emotional well-being, not merely the absence of disease or infirmity. In that context the relationship of activity to health becomes clearer. The relationship of health and wellness is equally clear. Ardell (1984) defined wellness as "a conscious and deliberate approach to an advanced state of physical and psychological/spiritual health." So wellness defines movement toward an advanced state of health, also called optimal or high-level health (figure 3.5).

The old view of health placed illness on one side of a line and health on the other, with doctors and the treatment-oriented health care system defending the line. We now view wellness as a dynamic process in which you, the individual, are responsible for your health. The health care system is treatment oriented. Workers in the system focus on correcting problems brought on by illness, disease, injury, or disability. Wellness involves disease prevention and promotion of behaviors that lower the risk of illness or injury. The treatment system employs an army of high-priced professionals and costs billions. Wellness relies on individual responsibility, low-cost helpers, and reduced reliance on costly specialists and procedures. The active life is the keystone of health and wellness.

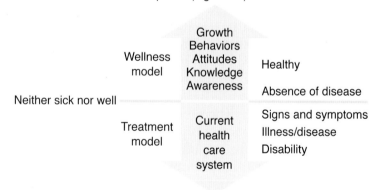

Figure 3.5   The health continuum.

Health Risk Analysis

Use the health risk analysis in figure 3.6 as a learning tool to identify positive and negative aspects of your health behavior. Although many of the effects are based on real findings from large epidemiological investigations, the estimates are generalized and you should not take them too literally. Accurately predicting how long you will live or when you will die is impossible.

Plus one (+1) represents a positive effect that could add a year to your life or life to your years, and minus one (–1) indicates a loss in the quantity or quality of life. Complete each section and record the totals in section VIII of figure 3.6 on page 68.

What Can You Do?

If you find that your risk of heart disease is high, you can take a number of steps to lower the risk, including the following:

- Engage in regular, moderate physical activity, 30 minutes on most days.
- Eat less saturated and trans fat and more fresh fruits and vegetables.
- Eat soy protein and olive oil.
- Keep your body mass index below 25 (see page 242).
- Take a low-dose coated aspirin daily or every other day.
- Have one alcoholic drink (red wine or beer) daily or every other day.

In subsequent chapters we will tell you reasons why you should consider these and other possible steps, such as vitamins.

Summary

Until recently the medical community has been cautious concerning exercise, suggesting a visit to the physician and even a stress test before participation. This approach is understandable given that few medical schools offer more than a few lectures on exercise physiology. Unless your doctor is active or has special training in physiology or sports medicine, he or she may know little about the benefits of activity and how to prescribe exercise to achieve those benefits. But as the benefits and risks become better understood, physicians are turning to exercise physiologists to design and conduct preventive and rehabilitative exercise programs.

Of course, you don't have to see your physician to participate in moderate activity such as walking. If you feel good and answer no to all the questions in the health-screening questionnaire (page 54), you don't have to spend large sums to confirm what you already know. Start slowly, increase intensity and duration gradually, and read the next section of this book. Use health screening, early detection, and periodic medical examinations to help you maintain your health.

Figure 3.6   Section I: Coronary Heart Disease (CHD) Risk Factors

Cholesterol or total cholesterol to HDL ratio					Score:
	<160	160–200	200–240	240–280	>280
	<3	3–4	4–5	5–6	>6
Score:	+2	+1	–1	–2	–4

Blood pressure (choose your highest number for either value)					Score:
	<110	110–120	120–150	150–170	170
	60–80	60–80	80–90	90–100	>100
	+1	0	–1	–2	–4

Smoking					Score:
	Never	Quit	Smoke cigar or pipe or close family member smokes	One pack of cigarettes daily	Two or more packs daily
	+1	0	–1	–3	–5

Heredity					Score:
	No family history of CHD	One close relative over 60 with CHD	Two close relatives over 60 with CHD	One close relative under 60 with CHD	Two or more close relatives under 60 with CHD
	+2	0	–1	–2	–4

Body mass index (BMI, use table on page 242)					Score:
	19–25	<19	26–30	31–40*	>40*
	+2	0	–1	–3	–5

*If waist is under 40 in. (102 cm) subtract one less (e.g., –2 or –4)

Gender					Score:
	Female under 55 years	Female over 55 years	Male	Stocky male	Bald, stocky male
	0	–1	–1	–2	–4

Stress					Score:
	Phlegmatic, unhurried, generally happy	Ambitious but generally relaxed	Sometimes hard-driving, time-consious, competitive	Hard-driving, time-conscious, competitive (type A)	Type A with repressed hostility
	+1	0	0	–1	–3

Physical activity					Score:
	High intensity, 60 min most days	Moderate, 30 min most days	Moderate, 20–30 min, 3–5 times per week	Light, 10–20 min,1–2 times per week	Little or none
	+3	**+2**	**+1**	**–1**	**–3**

Total: CHD risk factors: _____

Enter in section VIII

Section II: Health Habits (Related to Good Health and Longevity)

Breakfast				Score:
Daily	Sometimes	None	Coffee	Coffee and doughnut
+1	0	−1	−2	−3

Regular meals				Score:
Three or more	Two daily	Not regular	Fad diets	Starve and stuff
+1	0	−1	−2	−3

Sleep				Score:
7–8 hr	8–9 hr	6–7 hr	9 hr	6 hr
+1	0	0	−1	−2

Alcohol				Score:
None	Women 3/wk	Men 1–2 daily	3–6 daily	>6 daily
+1	+1	+1	−2	−4

Total: Health habits _____

Enter in section VIII

Section III: Medical Factors

Medical exam and screening tests (blood pressure, diabetes, glaucoma)				Score:
Regular tests, see doctor when necessary	Periodic medical exam and selected tests	Periodic medical exam	Sometimes get tests	No tests or medical exams
+1	+1	0	0	−1

Heart				Score:
No history of problems, self or family	Some history	Rheumatic fever as child, no murmur now	Rheumatic fever as a child, have murmur	Have ECG abnormality or angina pectoris
+2	0	−1	−2	−3

Lung (including pneumonia and tuberculosis)				Score:
No problem	Some past problem	Mild asthma or bronchitis	Emphysema, severe asthma, or bronchitis	Severe lung problems
+1	0	−1	−1	−3

Digestive tract				Score:
No problem	Occasional diarrhea, loss of appetite	Frequent diarrhea or stomach upset	Ulcers, colitis, gall bladder, or liver problems	Severe gastrointestinal disorders
+1	0	−1	−2	−3

Diabetes				Score:
No problem or family history	Controlled hypoglycemia (low blood sugar)	Hypoglycemia and family history	Mild diabetes (diet and exercise)	Diabetes (insulin)
+1	0	−1	−2	−4

Drugs				Score:
Seldom take	Minimal but regular use of aspirin or other drugs	Heavy use of aspirin or other drugs	Regular use of mood-altering or psychogenic drugs	Heavy use of mood-altering or psychogenic drugs
+1	0	−1	−2	−3

Total: Medical factors_____

Enter in section VIII

(continued)

Section IV: Safety Factors

Driving in car				Score:
<7,000 mi (11,000 km) per year, mostly local	7,000–10,000 mi (11,000–16,000 km) per year, local and some highway	10,000–15,000 mi (16,000–24,000 km) per year, local and highway	>15,000 mi (24,000 km) per year, high-way and some local	>15,000 mi (24,000 km) per year, mostly highway
+1	0	0	–1	–2

Using seat belts				Score:
Always	Most of time (>75%)	On highway only	Seldom (<25%)	Never
+1	0	–1	–2	–4

Risk-taking behavior (Motorcycle, skydive, mountain climb, fly small plane, etc.)				Score:
Some with careful preparation	Never	Occasional	Often	Try anything for thrills
+1	0	–1	–1	–2

Total: Safety factors _____
Enter in section VIII

Section V: Personal Factors

Diet				Score:
*Low fat, low calories	Balanced complex carbohydrate	High protein, limited fat	Extra calories, low carbohydrate	Fad diets and fat
+2	+1	unknown?	–1	–2
*See chapter 13				

Longevity				Score:
Grandparents lived past 90, parents past 80	Grandparents lived past 80, parents past 70	Grandparents lived past 70, parents past 60	Few relatives lived past 60	Few relatives lived past 50
+2	+1	0	–1	–3

Love and marriage				Score:
Happily married	Married	Unmarried	Divorced	Extramarital relationship(s)
+2	+1	0	–1	–3

Education				Score:
Postgraduate or master craftsman	College graduate or skilled craftsman	Some college or trade school	High school graduate	Grade school graduate
+1	+1	0	–1	–2

Job satisfaction				Score:
Enjoy job, see results, room for advancement	Enjoy job, see some results, able to advance	Job OK, no results, nowhere to go	Dislike job	Hate job
+1	+1	0	–1	–2

Social				Score:
Have some close friends	Have some friends	Have no good friends	Stuck with people I don't enjoy	Have no friends at all
+1	0	–1	–2	–3

Race				Score:
White or Asian	Black or Hispanic	American Indian		
0	–1	–2		

Total: Personal factors_____
Enter in section VIII

Section VI: Psychological Factors

Outlook				**Score:**
Feel good about present and future	Satisfied	Unsure about present or future	Unhappy in present, don't look forward to future	Miserable, rather not get out of bed
+1	0	–1	–2	–3
Depression				**Score:**
No family history of depression	Some family history, feel OK	Family history and mildly depressed	Sometimes feel life isn't worth living	Thoughts of suicide
+1	0	–1	–2	–3
Anxiety				**Score:**
Seldom anxious	Occasionally anxious	Often anxious	Always anxious	Panic attacks
+1	0	–1	–2	–3
Relaxation				**Score:**
Relax meditate daily	Relax often	Seldom relax	Usually tense	Always tense
+1	0	–1	–2	–3

Total: Psychological factors_____
Enter in section VIII

Section VII: For Women Only

Health care				**Score:**
Regular breast and Pap tests	Occasional breast and Pap tests	Never have exams	Treated disorder	Untreated cancer
+1	0	–1	–2	–4
Birth control pill				**Score:**
Never used	Quit 5 years ago	Still use, under 30 years	Use pill and smoke	Use pill, smoke, over 35
+1	0	0	–2	–3

Total: For women only _____
Enter in section VIII

(continued)

Section VIII: Summary

You can now estimate your longevity. Add your total score from the previous sections to your normal life expectancy (from the chart below) to find your longevity estimate. If you would like to improve your longevity estimate, go back and decide on some lifestyle areas you would like to improve.

Category	Score (+ or – from previous sections)
I. CHD risk factors	_____
II. Health habits	_____
III. Medical factors	_____
IV. Safety factors	_____
V. Personal factors	_____
VI. Psychological factors	_____
VII. For women only	_____

Total   _____ + _____ = _____

Totals from   Life expectancy   Your longevity
sections I-VII   for your age from   estimate
              table below

Life expectancy[*]		
	Expectancy (all races)	
Nearest age	**Male**	**Female**
30	75.9	80.6
35	76.3	80.8
40	76.7	81.0
45	77.2	81.3
50	77.9	81.8
55	78.8	82.4
60	79.9	83.1
65	81.3	84.2
70	83.0	85.5

[*]From CDC, *National Vital Statistics Reports*, December 2002 (www.cdc.gov).

Part II

Aerobic Fitness

Somewhere above the pace of your normal daily activities but well below maximal effort, you will find aerobic exercise. If you do aerobic exercise often enough you will improve your aerobic fitness, and as fitness improves you'll further enhance your health, appearance, vitality, and quality of life. Aerobic fitness describes how well you are able to take oxygen from the atmosphere into the lungs and then into the blood and pump it through the heart and circulatory system to working muscles, where it is used to oxidize carbohydrate and fat to produce energy. No other measure says more about the health and capacity of your lungs, heart, circulatory system, and, most important, your skeletal muscles.

Rhythmic large-muscle activities such as brisk walking, jogging, cycling, swimming, cross-country skiing, and rowing are aerobic exercises. They demand sustained increases in respiration, circulation, and muscle metabolism and lead to adaptations in the systems and muscles involved. Aerobic exercise is associated

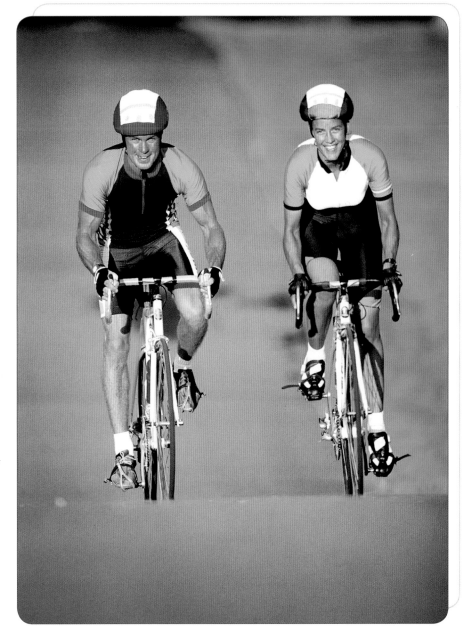

with health and longevity, regular participation in aerobic exercise improves aerobic fitness, and improved fitness further enhances health. In many physical, psychological, and social ways, aerobic fitness is good for health and the quality of life. It improves appearance, boosts self-confidence and body image, and opens the door to a challenging new world filled with new experiences and interesting people. Let's see how you can integrate fitness into your busy schedule so that you can reap the many extra benefits.

4

Understanding Aerobic Fitness

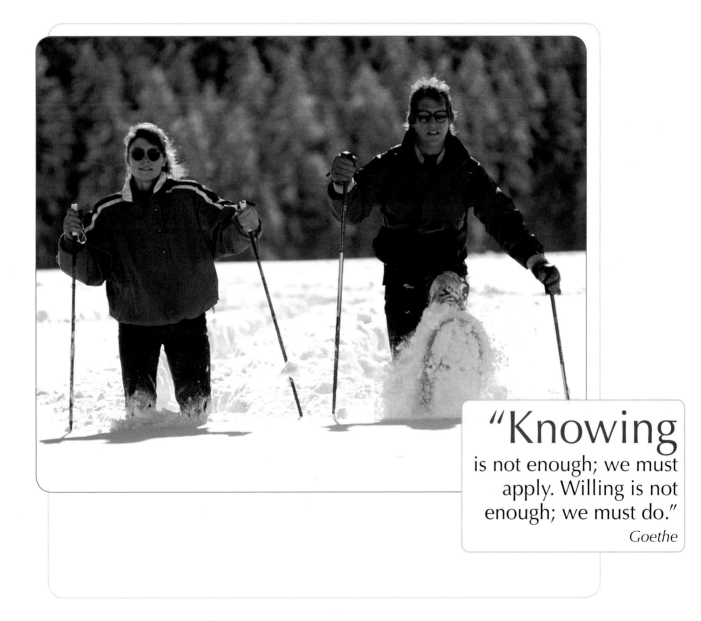

> ## "Knowing
> is not enough; we must apply. Willing is not enough; we must do."
> *Goethe*

Aerobic fitness is synonymous with endurance or stamina. It describes the ability, part inherited and part trained, to persevere or persist in prolonged endeavors. Those who pursue fitness earn far more than enhanced health and performance. For many, the process becomes more important than the goal, providing discipline, challenge, and time for reflection. For the moment we'll consider the physiology of fitness; later we'll ponder its other dimensions.

This chapter will help you

- understand the terms *aerobic* and *anaerobic*,
- determine the meaning of aerobic exercise and aerobic fitness,
- experience the concept of exercise intensity and the lactate thresholds, and
- understand the factors that influence aerobic fitness.

Aerobic Exercise

To learn about aerobic exercise, dress for exercise, warm up, and head out at a walking pace. Increase the pace a little as each minute passes, going from a slow walk to a fast walk. As you approach 5 miles (8 kilometers) per hour (12 minutes per mile, or 7 minutes 30 seconds per kilometer), you'll feel the need to jog. Continue to increase your speed gradually until the effort becomes uncomfortable, breathing becomes labored, and you doubt your ability to continue. As you increase your intensity from easy to hard you have moved from aerobic exercise, which means exercise in the presence of oxygen, to exercise that relies increasingly on anaerobic, or nonoxidative, energy production. During aerobic exercise, energy comes from the oxidation of fat and carbohydrate. If you continue to increase the intensity of exercise, the muscles gradually make a transition to anaerobic energy production, which involves intense effort of necessarily short duration and accumulation of lactic acid in the muscles and blood.

Lactic acid is both an energy carrier and a metabolic by-product of intense effort. Its accumulation is a sign that you are using energy faster than your body can produce it aerobically. Too much lactic acid interferes with the contractile and metabolic capabilities of the muscles. Lactic acid and the high levels of carbon dioxide produced in vigorous effort are associated with labored breathing, fatigue, and discomfort. Aerobic exercise can be defined as exercise below the point at which blood lactic acid levels rise—the lactate threshold (see figure 4.1). In simple terms, aerobic exercise includes all large-muscle activities that you can comfortably sustain for 15 minutes or more.

> The oxidation of abundant fat reserves during aerobic exercise ensures an adequate supply of energy for extended periods of effort.

Aerobic metabolism is far more efficient than anaerobic metabolism, yielding 38 molecules of adenosine triphosphate (ATP), the high-energy compound that fuels muscular contractions, per molecule of glucose, versus only 2 molecules of ATP through anaerobic metabolism. Because it produces little lactic acid, aerobic exercise is relatively pleasant and relaxing and not painful. The oxidation of abundant fat reserves during aerobic exercise ensures an adequate supply of energy for extended periods of effort. You can sustain aerobic exercise for several minutes to many hours, and you can carry on a conversation during moderate aerobic exercise.

Stored fats (triglycerides) and carbohydrate are the fuels for aerobic exercise. As exercise intensity increases we move from reliance on fats during low-intensity exercise to increasing use of carbohydrate at higher intensities of effort. Carbohydrate produces 50 percent of ATP during easy effort. At the first lactate threshold, carbohydrate produces 75 percent of ATP, and at the second lactate threshold, 100 percent of ATP comes from carbohydrate oxidation (see figure 4.1).

Aerobic and anaerobic exercises differ in intensity; light to moderate activity is aerobic, whereas extremely vigorous or intense effort is anaerobic. Table 4.1 illustrates how heart rate and breathing increase with exercise intensity, and how we switch from burning fat to carbohydrate as exercise becomes more vigorous. The table also shows how the nervous system recruits different muscle fiber types as the effort becomes more intense.

Figure 4.1 Lactate thresholds. As exercise intensity (percent $\dot{V}O_2$max) increases we continually recruit additional SO fibers, FOG fibers, and finally FG fibers. The first lactate threshold (LT1) occurs as muscles produce more lactic acid than can be cleared from the blood. This generally occurs at a moderate intensity and represents long-duration sustainable capacity. The second lactate threshold (LT2) occurs when blood lactate accumulates rapidly and breathing becomes labored. Exercise over LT2 cannot be long sustained. Above LT1, and especially above LT2, more blood lactate accumulates because FG fibers produce more lactic acid and because most muscle fibers are active and therefore unable to remove (take up) lactate.

Table 4.1   Levels of Exercise Intensity

	EXERCISE INTENSITY		
	Light	**Moderate**	**Intense**
Example exercise	Walking	Jogging	Running
Metabolism*	Aerobic	Aerobic	Aerobic and anaerobic
Energy source*	Fat > CHO	CHO > fat	Mostly CHO
Heart rate**	<120	120–150	>150
Breathing*	Easy	Can talk easily	Hard to talk
Muscle fiber recruited	SO	FOG	FG

CHO = carbohydrate
*Depends on fitness
**Depends on age and fitness

Endurance

A biologist friend who has studied locomotion throughout the animal kingdom has noted that when it comes to running short distances, humans are inferior to other species. Cheetahs, gazelles, antelopes, horses, camels, and even grizzly bears are much faster than humans. But as the distance increases, the human becomes more competitive, and at long distances, human endurance qualities stand out. Unfortunately, this superiority emerges only at distances few are willing to negotiate. When a proud Montana horseman bragged about the endurance and speed of his Arabian, a local physician wagered that he could outrun the horse over a mountainous marathon course (26.2 miles, or 42.2 kilometers). Perhaps the distance wasn't long enough, because the horse finished 16 minutes ahead of the physician. Another factor may have been that the fit but 49-year-old physician was slightly past his prime, whereas the horse was not.

We have ample evidence that humans are able to run extremely long distances. The Tarahumara Indians of Mexico run more than 100 miles (161 kilometers) while kicking a small ball, and runners throughout the world do 100-mile footraces, sometimes over difficult mountain terrain. Early in the 20th century, crowds flocked to big cities to watch 6-day races in which athletes attempted to run as far as possible. Today the 6-day record is well over 635 miles (1,022 kilometers), for an average of 106 miles (171 kilometers) per day! In spite of the publicity given short races and sports that emphasize bursts of speed, the human body has evolved with the capacity to accomplish prodigious feats of endurance.

Humans have three main types of muscle fibers: slow-twitch (slow oxidative, or SO) fibers that are efficient in the use of oxygen; a faster-contracting type that can work with oxygen or without (fast oxidative glycolytic, or FOG); and a fast-twitch fiber that uses muscle glycogen for short, intense contractions (fast glycolytic, or FG) without oxygen. As we go from a walk to a jog to a run we sequentially recruit SO, FOG, and then FG fibers to help us go faster. If we recruit too many FG fibers, the effort becomes anaerobic. The fibers produce lactic acid, and we are forced to slow down or stop.

Aerobic Fitness

Aerobic fitness, defined as the maximal capacity to take in, transport, and use oxygen, is best measured in a laboratory test called the maximal oxygen intake (or $\dot{V}O_2max$) test. The test, which defines the highest intensity of effort, requires a treadmill or other exercise device (e.g., bicycle ergometer); a metabolic measurement system to measure oxygen, carbon dioxide, and the volume of expired air; and a computer to do the calculations. After a health risk assessment, the person being tested signs an informed consent form and is fitted with ECG electrodes to monitor the heart and measure heart rate.

After a brief warm-up, the person begins the test wearing a mask or mouthpiece to direct the expired air into the analyzer. The test involves increasing intensity of exercise, starting at an easy rate and grade, with increases every minute or two. Oxygen intake is computed each minute as the test proceeds toward maximal effort. The test ends when oxygen intake levels off in spite of increased treadmill rate or grade, or when the person can no longer keep up with the treadmill. The highest level of oxygen used is called the maximal oxygen intake ($\dot{V}O_2max$), or peak aerobic fitness.

The $\dot{V}O_2$max test signifies the maximum volume (V) of oxygen (O_2) used. The test takes from 8 to 12 minutes and uses either metabolic measurements to measure oxygen intake or a table to estimate the value. The protocol should allow the test to be tailored to the subject's level of fitness and previous training. The test should be specific to the person's activity—a treadmill for runners and a bicycle ergometer for cyclists. The test can be conducted on any mode of aerobic exercise. Our example focuses on the treadmill.

Measure oxygen intake or use the final rate and grade on the treadmill to estimate $\dot{V}O_2$max (see table 4.2). For example, if the last minute of the test was at 6 miles (9.7 kilometers) per hour and 10 percent grade, the aerobic fitness estimate is 50 milliliters of oxygen per kilogram of body weight per minute. The person being tested should not hold on to the railing of the treadmill if the intention is to estimate the maximal value. Holding on to the railing reduces the workload and overestimates the estimation of oxygen uptake.

The $\dot{V}O_2$max test measures the maximal capacity to take in, transport, and use oxygen.

Table 4.2   Estimating $\dot{V}O_2$max From Treadmill Test: Approximate Oxygen Intake Required for Final Rate and Grade Combinations*

Miles (km) per hour	GRADE				
	8%	10%	12%	14%	15%
WALK					
3.0 (4.8 km)	22	26	30	34	37
3.5 (5.6 km)	24	29	34	39	43
4.0 (6.4 km)	26	32	38	44	48
RUN					
6.0 (9.7 km)	47	50	53	56	59
7.0 (11.3 km)	54	58	61	65	69
8.0 (12.9 km)	62	66	70	74	78

*ml · kg^{-1} · min^{-1}, varies with efficiency

Scores in the range of 3 to 4 liters of oxygen per minute are typical, and values of 5 to 6 liters have been reported for endurance athletes. When reported in liters per minute (called aerobic capacity), the score provides information about the total capacity of the cardiorespiratory systems and is a predictor of endurance performance in non-weight-bearing sports (e.g., cycling, rowing). But because this value is related to body size, larger people tend to have higher scores.

To eliminate the influence of body size, the maximal oxygen intake score in liters (1 liter equals 1,000 milliliters) is divided by the body weight in kilograms (1 kilogram equals 2.2 pounds). In this example, maximal oxygen intake score is 3 liters (3,000 milliliters), and body weight is 60 kilograms (132 pounds):

$$3 \text{ L/min} \div 60 \text{ kg} = 50 \text{ ml} \cdot \text{kg}^{-1} \cdot \text{min}^{-1}$$

The resulting value allows direct comparison of individuals regardless of body size. This measure, also known as aerobic power, is more related to endurance performance in running and other weight-bearing sports, and it is the preferred way to express maximal aerobic fitness. If two people have the same score in liters, which one is more fit, the one who weighs 60 kilograms (132 pounds) or the other who weighs 100 kilograms (220 pounds)? Divide the score for the latter by the respective body weight:

$$3 \text{ L/min} \div 100 \text{ kg} = 30 \text{ ml} \cdot \text{kg}^{-1} \cdot \text{min}^{-1}$$

In a footrace, the one with a score of 50 would be better able to take in, transport, and use oxygen in the working muscles than the one with the score of 30. The average young male (18 to 25 years old) scores 42 to 45 milliliters per kilogram of body weight per minute, and the average young female scores 39 to 41. Active men score in the 50s and 60s, and similarly active women in the 40s and 50s. Male endurance athletes achieve measurements in the 80s, and top female athletes are not far behind with scores in the 70s (see table 4.3). Although average values decline with age, as much as 8 to 10 percent per decade in sedentary populations, regular activity cuts the rate of decline in half (4 to 5 percent per decade), and aerobic training can cut that rate in half again (2 to 3 percent per decade).

Until recently, the aerobic fitness score ($\dot{V}O_2$max) was viewed as the best measure of fitness and was believed to be correlated to health and related to performance in work and sport. During the last 10 to 15 years, other ways to measure fitness have emerged, and some are better correlated to endurance and to performance in sport. The maximal oxygen intake test, or $\dot{V}O_2$max test, which uses the highest score attained, is a test of exercise intensity, best correlated to events lasting 5 to 15 minutes.

Table 4.3   Aerobic Fitness Comparison

Subjects	Age	Men (ml · kg⁻¹ · min⁻¹)	Women (ml · kg⁻¹ · min⁻¹)
Untrained	18–22	43	38
Active	18–22	50	43
Trained	18–22	57	53
Elite	18–22	70	63
World class	18–22	≥80	≥70
Untrained	40–50	36	27
Active	40–50	46	39
Trained	40–50	52	44
Elite	40–50	≥60	≥50

As exercise intensity increases from easy to moderately hard, aerobic metabolism shifts from using primarily fat to a greater reliance on carbohydrate to provide the energy for metabolism. The first lactate threshold (LT1) is defined as the intensity of aerobic exercise at which blood lactate begins to increase. The intensity at which this occurs is generally defined as moderate, and is associated with the highest intensity that a person can comfortably sustain for an hour or more. This threshold defines the point at which lactic acid begins to accumulate in the blood more rapidly than it can be removed. The first lactate threshold is an excellent indicator of performance in aerobic events lasting more than 3 hours. This threshold also defines what we call sustainable aerobic fitness—the intensity that people can sustain for long periods. The first lactate threshold is an important measure of aerobic fitness (see figure 4.1).

Laboratory tests can identify LT1 by drawing blood samples during each stage of an incremental exercise test and then analyzing the blood for lactate levels. During easy to moderate intensities, blood lactate will remain level as the blood clears the lactate as quickly as it is produced. After LT1 is reached, blood lactate concentrations begin to increase gradually until the second lactate threshold is reached, where blood lactate increases more rapidly. Ventilatory measurements during the exercise test permit a less invasive measure of LT1. Several methods can be used to select LT1 through respiratory measurements. Most exercise laboratories or clinical centers are able to perform these measurements.

The second lactate threshold can also be estimated using respiratory data. The respiratory compensation point, defined as the point at which ventilation (liters of air per minute) rises disproportionably to increasing work, corresponds to LT2. This point is also referred to as breakaway ventilation. This rapid rise in ventilation (respiratory rate and depth) provides a perceptible signal indicating that the person is flirting with excess anaerobic effort and exhaustion, and should ease off. Perceptive people learn to listen to the information that their bodies provide during exertion.

The second lactate threshold is a better indicator of endurance performance than aerobic fitness ($\dot{V}O_2max$) in events such as a 10-kilometer road race. The threshold indicates the oxygen-using capabilities of the muscles. In chapter 6 we'll show you how to use the thresholds in an aerobic training program, and in chapter 15 we'll show you how to use the thresholds in training for competition.

Dimensions of Aerobic Fitness

Aerobic fitness has three important dimensions. Each has its own value, and a single treadmill test can determine all of them (see table 4.4).

The first lactate threshold defines the level of effort that a person can sustain for prolonged periods. Expressed as a percentage of $\dot{V}O_2max$, it may be low or high, depending on the person's level of activity and training. People can increase all dimensions of aerobic fitness by training according to the principles presented in chapters 6 and 15.

Table 4.4   Dimensions of Aerobic Fitness

Test	Measures	Best related to
$\dot{V}O_2max$	Intensity	Events lasting 5 to 15 min (1 to 3 mi, or 1.6 to 4.8 km)
Second lactate threshold	Duration	30 min to 3 hr (10K to marathon)
First lactate threshold*	Long duration	Prolonged work or sport (up to 8 hr or longer)

*Also called sustainable fitness, it is defined as the first rise, or breakpoint, in the lactate or ventilatory response to increasing rate or grade of exercise (see figure 4.1).

Factors Influencing Aerobic Fitness

Is a high aerobic fitness score the product of heredity or training? How much can training influence fitness? How do other factors such as gender, age, and body fat influence your attainable level of fitness?

Heredity

Achieving high-level endurance performances requires tremendous natural endowment and years of systematic training. Researchers have studied differences in aerobic fitness among fraternal (dizygotic) and identical (monozygotic) twins and found that intrapair differences were far greater among fraternal twins than among identical twins. The largest difference between identical twins was smaller than the smallest difference between fraternal pairs (Klissouras 1976). Bouchard et al. (1999) estimated that heredity accounts for 47 percent or more of the variance in $\dot{V}O_2$max values, and Sundet, Magnus, and Tambs (1994) contend that more than half of the variance in maximal aerobic power is due to genotypic differences, with the remainder accounted for by environmental factors (nutrition, training). This finding supports the notion that the way to become a world-class endurance athlete is to pick your parents carefully, especially your mother, because maternal transmission accounts for almost 60 percent of the inherited component (Bouchard et al. 1999)!

> The way to become a world-class endurance athlete is to pick your parents carefully.

Picking your parents well may help you achieve elite athlete status, but training will dictate how close you get to your potential. In a training study, 80 percent of the improvements in ventilatory threshold (LT1) were due to training, with the remaining

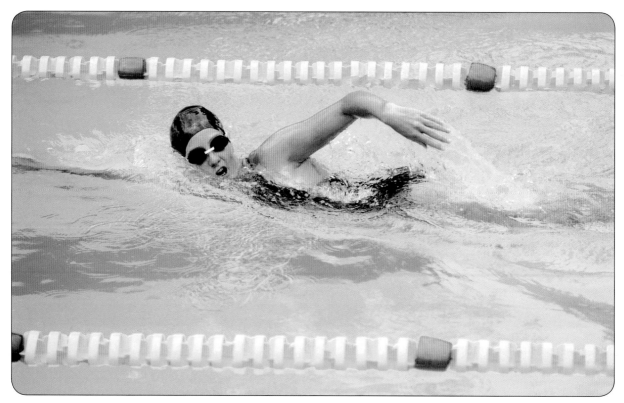

Although heredity influences aerobic fitness, training can help you reach your potential.

20 percent related to familial or genetic influences (Gaskill et al. 2001). Genes play an important role in how sustainable fitness responds to training, but the majority of the effects are due to training.

We inherit many factors that are important to aerobic fitness, including the capacity of the respiratory and cardiovascular systems, the size of the heart, the number of red blood cells and hemoglobin, and the percentage of oxidative (slow oxidative and fast oxidative glycolytic) muscle fibers. Mitochondria, the energy-producing units of muscle and other cells, are inherited from the maternal side. Studies indicate that the capacity of muscle to respond to training is also inherited, with improvements in aerobic fitness ranging from 5 percent to over 30 percent (Bouchard et al. 1988). Other inherited factors such as physique and body composition also influence the potential to perform at a high level.

Training

The potential to improve aerobic fitness ($\dot{V}O_2$max) with training is limited. Although most studies confirm the potential to improve 20 to 25 percent (more with loss of body fat), only adolescents can hope to improve much more than 30 percent. Consider two people, one with an untrained $\dot{V}O_2$max of 40 milliliters per kilogram per minute and the other with a score of 60. Let us assume that heredity accounts for the difference in scores. What happens if each trains and gains a 25 percent improvement in $\dot{V}O_2$max?

a. $40 \text{ ml} \cdot \text{kg}^{-1} \cdot \text{min}^{-1}$ increased 25% = 40 + 10 = $50 \text{ ml} \cdot \text{kg}^{-1} \cdot \text{min}^{-1}$

b. $60 \text{ ml} \cdot \text{kg}^{-1} \cdot \text{min}^{-1}$ increased 25% = 60 + 15 = $75 \text{ ml} \cdot \text{kg}^{-1} \cdot \text{min}^{-1}$

Training raises the first person above the average for young men, whereas the second person rises to the level of elite endurance athletes. Even in an untrained state, the second person has a higher $\dot{V}O_2$max than the first person does when trained. Whoever said that life was fair?

Training improves the function and capacity of the respiratory and cardiovascular systems and boosts blood volume, but the most important changes take place in the muscle fibers used in the training. Aerobic training improves the ability of the muscles to produce energy aerobically and metabolize fat. Training makes muscle an efficient furnace for the combustion of fat, producing perhaps the single most important health benefit of regular exercise. Burning fat reduces fat storage, blood fat levels, and cardiovascular risk, and it improves insulin sensitivity and reduces the risk of diabetes. This fat metabolism may also contribute to a lower risk of some cancers. Of course, training enhances the ability to perform, but the improvement is limited to the activity used in training. Long-duration training will increase LT1, and higher-intensity effort will raise LT2. We'll say more about the specificity of training in later chapters.

> Training makes muscle an efficient furnace for the combustion of fat, producing perhaps the single most important health benefit of regular exercise.

Gender

Before puberty, boys and girls differ little in aerobic fitness, but from then on girls fall behind. Young women average 10 to 20 percent less in aerobic fitness compared with young men, depending on their level of activity. But highly trained young female endurance athletes are only 10 percent below elite males in $\dot{V}O_2$max and performance times. One reason for the difference between genders may be hemoglobin, the oxygen-carrying compound found in red blood cells. Men average about 2 grams more hemoglobin per 100 milliliters of blood (15 grams versus 13 grams per deciliter), and total hemoglobin is correlated to $\dot{V}O_2$max and endurance. On the other hand, some women have higher values than male endurance athletes do (Sharkey 1986).

Other reasons may be that women are smaller and have less muscle mass, or that women have more body fat than men on average (25 to 30 percent versus 12.5 to 17.5 percent for college-age women and men, respectively). Because aerobic fitness is usually reported per unit of body weight, those with more fat and less lean tissue (muscle) will have some disadvantage. Of course, a portion of the difference is sex-specific fat that is essential for reproductive function and health. For those and other reasons (e.g., osteoporosis), women shouldn't try to become too thin. We raise the issue only to explain why the average male has some advantage over the average female in aerobic fitness.

Until the 1970s women were discouraged or even banned from competing in races longer than .5 mile (.8 kilometer). Overprotective or prejudiced officials worried that frail females couldn't stand the strain. Today women run marathons and 100-mile (160-kilometer) races; compete in the Ironman triathlon; and swim, ski, and cycle prodigious distances. A woman led much of the 1994 high-altitude Leadville 100-Mile Trail Run until a male Tarahumara Indian from Mexico passed her. We've learned that women are well suited for fat-burning endurance events and that some tolerate heat, cold, and other indignities as well as or better than men. Yet at the highest level, women's endurance performances remain about 10 percent behind those of the best males.

Age

Earlier we alluded to the effects of age on aerobic fitness, with a decline approaching 8 to 10 percent per decade for inactive people, regardless of their initial level of fitness (see figure 4.2). Those who decide to remain active can cut the decline in half (4 to 5 percent per decade), and those who engage in fitness training can cut that rate in half again (2 to 3 percent per decade).

A friend who served as a subject in many of our studies had a $\dot{V}O_2$max of 46 milliliters per kilogram per minute when he started aerobic training at age 30. His score

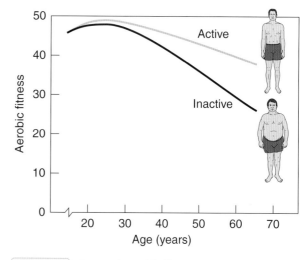

Figure 4.2   Age and aerobic fitness.
Adapted from Sharkey, 1997.

rose to 54 in a few months and then declined slowly for 3 decades as he continued his active lifestyle. When retirement allowed him time for even more activity, his fitness score was 52, well above his starting point at age 30. Although trainability may decline somewhat with age, exercise gerontologist Dr. Herb deVries has shown that people can improve their fitness even after age 70 (deVries and Housh 1994). It is never too late to start. At age 81 Eula Weaver had a heart attack to add to her problems of congestive heart failure and poor circulation. Unable to walk even 100 feet (30 meters) at first, she worked up to jogging a mile (1.6 kilometers) each day and riding her stationary bicycle for several more. She even lifted weights several days a week. At age 85 she won the gold medal for the mile run in her age group at the Senior Olympics. We'll say more about age and performance in chapter 17.

Body Fat

Remember that fitness is calculated per unit of body weight, so if fat increases, aerobic fitness declines. About half the decline in fitness with age can be attributed to an increase in body fat. So the easiest way to maintain or even improve fitness is to get rid of excess fat. For example, if Bob, at 100 kilograms, or 220 pounds, and 20 percent fat, loses 10 kilograms (22 pounds), or half his body fat, his aerobic fitness score will go from

$$4 \text{ L} / 100 \text{ kg} = 40 \text{ ml} \cdot \text{kg}^{-1} \cdot \text{min}^{-1}$$

to

$$4 \text{ L} / 90 \text{ kg} = 44.4 \text{ ml} \cdot \text{kg}^{-1} \cdot \text{min}^{-1}$$

Without any exercise, just weight loss, his fitness, both maximal and submaximal, has improved 10 percent! Now, if he earns an additional 20 percent improvement from training, his fitness could rise above 53 milliliters per kilogram per minute (44.4 times 20 percent equals 8.88 milliliters per kilogram per minute, plus 44.4 equals 53.3). Unlikely? Not at all. Our old friend Ernie smoked two packs a day, weighed over 250 pounds (113 kilograms), and bragged about his sedentary lifestyle. When he took a fitness test it was all he could do to finish with a score in the low 30s. Ernie got the message. He stopped smoking, started training, and paid attention to his diet. Now, years later, you wouldn't recognize him. Under the fat he discovered a trim, handsome body. He weighs around 170 pounds (77 kilograms), his fitness score is 58, and he thoroughly enjoys the active life.

Activity

Finally, let us comment on the most obvious influence on fitness: your regular level of activity. What you do, day by day, year after year,

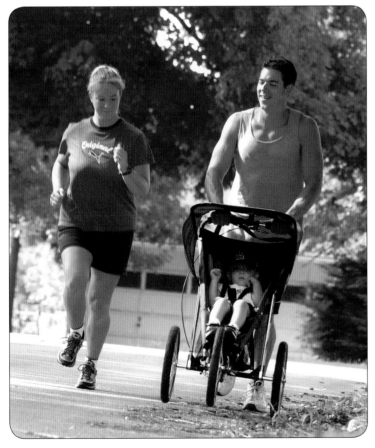

What you do day after day shapes your health and vitality.

shapes your health, vitality, and quality of life. You can lose the effect of years of training in a mere 12 weeks with the cessation of activity (Coyle, Hemmert, and Coggan 1986). Three weeks of complete bed rest, for example, may cause a fitness decline of 29 percent, or almost 10 percent per week, but you can easily restore the loss with regular activity (Saltin et al. 1968). Moderate activity leads to improved fitness and substantial health benefits; training leads to a higher level of fitness and extra health benefits; and prolonged, systematic training helps you achieve your potential. The choice is yours, but remember: Health has more to do with regular, moderate activity than with your level of fitness.

Relative Fitness

Aerobic training is the process of doing the best we can with what we are given. One way to monitor progress is to use a concept called relative fitness—the percentage of maximal aerobic capacity that you can sustain. As people become more fit, they can sustain a higher percentage of their maximal capacity. Relative fitness shows what percentage of $\dot{V}O_2$max people can sustain for events of different duration. This can be defined using either LT1 or LT2 in comparison with $\dot{V}O_2$max. As you train, both $\dot{V}O_2$max and your thresholds tend to increase. As your training program continues past several months, $\dot{V}O_2$max will plateau while improvements in submaximal fitness (LT1 and LT2) will continue. The closer your threshold values are to your maximal value, the more effective your training has been. Table 4.5 shows typical values for relative fitness. Over the course of training, the intensity gradually increased from 50 percent to 85 percent of $\dot{V}O_2$max.

Relative Fitness Comparison

A surprising finding in a large study of sedentary people was that many of the older participants had high relative fitness values, whereas some of the younger participants, including a number with $\dot{V}O_2$max values greater than 50 milliliters per kilogram per minute, had low relative fitness (Gaskill et al. 2001). Because all these people were sedentary they had similar relative fitness scores because of their low levels of activity. Relative fitness is calculated by dividing $\dot{V}O_2$ at the first lactate threshold by $\dot{V}O_2$max. For example, a genetically gifted but sedentary 21-year-old male with a $\dot{V}O_2$max of 54.5 milliliters per kilogram per minute and LT1 of 19.8 milliliters per kilogram per minute has a low relative fitness of 36 percent, whereas a 60-year-old sedentary female with a $\dot{V}O_2$max of 25.8 milliliters per kilogram per minute and a LT1 of 18.6 milliliters per kilogram per minute has a high relative fitness of 72 percent.

Relative fitness tells us what percentage of maximal capacity we can sustain. Because sedentary people require about 18 milliliters per kilogram per minute of oxygen to do tasks of daily living, they are essentially training at that level. By performing tasks of daily living, the older woman maintains her sustainable fitness at a relatively high percentage of her maximal capacity, whereas the young man is using but a low percentage of his capacity. Training will help these people increase both $\dot{V}O_2$max and sustainable fitness (LT1). Of course, the young male has much more room for improvement.

Table 4.5   Relative Fitness

Relative fitness level	LT1 as a % of $\dot{V}O_2$max	LT2 as a % of $\dot{V}O_2$max
Low	35–50%	45–60%
Medium	50–60%	60–70%
High	60–70%	70–80%
Very high	70–80%	80–90%

Training and genetics influence $\dot{V}O_2$max. Submaximal fitness seems to be related to what we do with our potential. Of course, to be successful at the elite level an athlete must have both high maximal capacity and high relative fitness.

Aerobic Fitness Field Tests

Another way to estimate your aerobic fitness is with a simple, inexpensive field test. If you are a walker, use the 1-mile (1.6-kilometer) walking test to estimate your $\dot{V}O_2$max. If you are a runner, you can use the 1.5-mile (2.4-kilometer) run test. Be sure to take the health-screening questionnaire (figure 3.2, page 54) before engaging in either test.

Walking Test

The Rockport Walking Test uses the time for a 1-mile (1.6-kilometer) walk and some personal information to estimate the $\dot{V}O_2$max. Walk the measured course as quickly as possible and then substitute the time (to the nearest hundredth of a minute), posttest heart rate, and other information in the following equation.

$$\dot{V}O_2\text{max} = 132.853 - (0.0769 \times \text{weight in lb } [0.03488 \times \text{weight in kg}]) -$$
$$(0.3877 \times \text{age in yr}) + (6.315 \times \text{gender } [0 \text{ for female, } 1 \text{ for male}]) -$$
$$(3.2649 \times \text{time } [\text{min to the nearest 100th}]) - (0.1565 \times \text{HR at end of test})$$

The result in milliliters per kilogram per minute is highly correlated to a laboratory measure of aerobic fitness (Kline et al. 1987).

Running Test

The 1.5-mile (2.4-kilometer) running test requires a near-maximal effort. If you've been inactive, precede training with an adjustment to activity (walking), and then begin 6 to 8 weeks of training for the test. People over the age of 45 should consider a medical examination, especially if you have two or more cardiovascular risk factors. Be sure to warm up and stretch before the test. The time for the 1.5-mile (2.4-kilometer) run is used to predict aerobic fitness and is based on the oxygen cost of running (see figure 4.3).

Figure 4.3 1.5-mile (2.4-kilometer) aerobic fitness test.
Note: Subtract altitude adjustment from 1.5-mile (2.4-kilometer) run time. Then use the graph to find your score.
Adapted from Sharkey, 1997.
Sources: Balke 1963; Cooper 1968; Sharkey 1997b; Daniels 1977, personal communication.

Summary

Aerobic fitness, defined as the ability to take in, transport, and use oxygen, is a measure of exercise intensity. The second lactate threshold, which defines the upper limit of sustainable aerobic exercise, is a measure of exercise duration and an excellent predictor of endurance performance in events lasting from 30 minutes to several hours. The first lactate threshold defines the level of work or sport that you can sustain for prolonged periods. Heredity and training as well as other factors such as age, gender, and body fat influence all the dimensions of aerobic fitness. Factors such as your current health, diet, hydration, level of rest, and acclimatization to heat and altitude will also influence your ability to perform an endurance event. Few of us ever reach our potential for fitness and endurance, and no laboratory test exists to pinpoint this potential. World-class athletes train daily for years to be the best that they can be. Most of us must be content to do the best we can within the time constraints imposed by family, profession, community, and other responsibilities. The best time to start training is as you approach puberty. The second best time to start is today. Chapter 6 provides a prescription to get you started, and chapter 15 provides additional guidance to help you reach your potential.

5

Aerobic Training Effect

"Nothing in the world can take the place of persistence."
Calvin Coolidge

Fifty years ago, the term *cardiovascular* was used to define fitness. Next came the term *cardiorespiratory*, and today we speak of *aerobic fitness*. The changes in terminology reflect insights derived from decades of research, based on a clearer view of the effects of training. We used *cardiovascular* when the best-documented effects of training were about the heart and circulation, measures of transport. *Cardiorespiratory* became popular when we began to understand the importance of oxygen intake as well as transport. And *aerobic* was adopted to indicate that oxygen intake, transport, and utilization all improved with training. Since 1967, when research first documented the effects of endurance training on the ability of the muscles to use oxygen, we have become increasingly aware that some of the most important effects of training involve skeletal muscles and their ability to carry out oxidative, or aerobic, energy production. To emphasize that point, we like to say that skeletal muscle is the target of aerobic training.

You've heard that fitness is good for the heart and the lungs, and that is true. But training requires the use of muscles, and major changes take place in the muscles that are used in training. Of course, important secondary adaptations take place in the cardiovascular, respiratory, and neuroendocrine systems and other tissues (fat, bone, ligaments, tendons). But it is impossible to improve the health or function of organs such as the heart without involving the skeletal muscles. All the beneficial changes begin with muscular activity. If you train the muscles properly, the secondary benefits follow; if you fail to train the muscles, the other changes are unlikely to occur.

This chapter will help you

- understand how systematic exercise (training) stimulates changes in
  - muscle fibers;
  - respiration and oxygen transport;
  - blood volume;
  - the heart and circulation;
  - the endocrine system;
  - fat metabolism and body composition; and
  - bones, ligaments, and tendons; and
- understand the specificity of training and its importance for the design of effective programs.

Training Effect

When you engage in an exercise such as walking or jogging at a level above your normal daily activity (load), you overload the muscles and their support systems, including the heart and lungs. If you repeat the exercise regularly (e.g., every other day) your body begins to adapt to the overload imposed by the exercise. We call the many adaptations the training effect. The exercise somehow signals muscle fibers and support systems to undergo changes that will permit more exercise in the future. How does it work? Let's look at a muscle fiber.

Figure 5.1 illustrates the basic structure of a muscle fiber. Something associated with training (metabolic by-products, chemical messenger, hormone) tells the deoxyribonucleic acid (DNA) in the nuclei of the muscle fiber to produce specific messengers in the form of ribonucleic acid (RNA). The messenger RNA (mRNA) travels to structures within the fiber called ribosomes to direct the synthesis of specific proteins, like aerobic enzymes. Transfer RNA (tRNA) reads the mRNA blueprint and then captures appropriate amino acids for use in the synthesis of the desired protein. Endurance training leads to an increase in the concentration of oxidative enzymes and to a rise in the size and number of mitochondria, the cellular power plants where all oxidative metabolism takes place (Hood et al. 2000). These particular adaptations are specific to endurance training, and they take place only in the muscles used in training.

Figure 5.1 Basic structures in a muscle fiber.

The effects of training have been determined in experimental studies. A typical study involves pretesting of volunteer subjects for aerobic fitness, lactate thresholds, and other measures; random assignment to experimental or control groups; weeks or even months of systematic and progressive training; and posttesting to measure the adaptations resulting from training. Studies have ranged from low to high intensity, using low- to high-fit subjects. We'll review the effects of aerobic training and then differentiate specific effects of long-duration, low-intensity training versus high-intensity training.

A variation of the training study involves detraining already fit subjects. Researchers convince habitual exercisers to forgo training for a period while they observe the decline of important measures and performance. Although this approach has limits, it eliminates the need for prolonged training. We'll look at both types of studies as well as animal research to help you understand the training effect.

Muscle: Target of Training

Muscle, the motive force and source of many of the benefits associated with exercise, is the primary target of training. The effects of aerobic training on muscle relate to the utilization of oxygen. Oxidative metabolism, the enzymatic breakdown of carbohydrate and fat to produce energy for muscular contractions, takes place in cellular powerhouses called mitochondria (Coggan and Williams 1995). Long, slow training improves the oxidative capabilities of slow oxidative fibers, whereas high-intensity training enhances the capabilities of fast oxidative glycolytic fibers. Aerobic training has the following effects on muscle:

> The effects of aerobic training on muscle relate to the utilization of oxygen.

- Increases the concentration of aerobic enzymes (protein compounds that catalyze metabolic reactions) needed for the metabolic breakdown of carbohydrate and fat to produce energy in the form of ATP (adenosine triphosphate, the cellular energy supply)

- Increases the size and number (volume) of mitochondria, which produce energy aerobically (with oxygen)

- Increases the ability of the muscle to use fat as a source of energy

- Increases the size of the fibers used in training

- Long-slow training improves the oxidative capabilities of slow oxidative fibers

Cellular Effects

Before 1967, research had failed to demonstrate the effects of training on muscle fibers. Dr. John Holloszy reasoned that previous studies failed to overload aerobic pathways, so he subjected laboratory rats to a strenuous treadmill program. Trained rats eventually were able to continue exercise for 4 to 8 hours, whereas untrained animals were exhausted within 30 minutes. Following the 12-week program, the animals were sacrificed to allow study of the muscle tissue. Holloszy found a 50 to 60 percent increase in mitochondrial protein, a twofold rise in the oxygen consumption of trained muscle, and enhanced ability to use (oxidize) carbohydrate and fat (1967). Other researchers have replicated these findings and confirmed them in humans, using a muscle biopsy technique.

Courtesy of Steven Gaskill.

Muscle biopsy technique: A hollow needle is inserted though an incision in the skin and fascia into the muscle. By removing a small piece of muscle about the size of a popcorn kernel, it is possible to measure aerobic and anaerobic enzymes, muscle glycogen stores, and gene expression as well as the study of an ever increasing list of muscle functions.

Today we know that the increase in mitochondrial mass is due to branching of existing mitochondria, and that the increase provides greater capacity for oxidation of energy sources, especially our abundant supply of fat (we store 50 times more fat energy than we do carbohydrate energy, and training makes that supply more available).

- High-intensity training enhances the capabilities of fast oxidative glycolytic fibers
- Increases the storage of muscle glycogen
- Increases the supply of intramuscular fat
- Increases the myoglobin (a compound that carries oxygen from the cell membrane to the mitochondria) in muscle fibers
- Increases the number of capillaries serving muscle fibers

Training Supply and Support Systems

The respiratory, circulatory, nervous, endocrine, and other systems supply and support the activities of muscles. How does aerobic training affect them? Aerobic training

- increases the efficiency of respiration and the endurance of respiratory muscles;
- improves blood volume, distribution, and delivery to working muscles;
- improves cardiovascular efficiency (increases stroke volume and cardiac output while decreasing resting and exercise heart rates); and
- fine-tunes nervous and hormonal control mechanisms.

Respiration and Oxygen Transport

Aerobic training doesn't alter the size of the lungs, but it does improve the endurance and efficiency of breathing muscles, allowing greater use of inherited capacity (see figure 5.2). Training reduces the residual volume, the portion of lung capacity that goes unused. Residual volume increases with age and inactivity, and this decline of lung volume eventually compromises exercise capacity. The human respiratory system is overbuilt for its task, however, so people don't notice the gradual decline at first. Aerobic training slows the decline, ensuring adequate respiratory capacity throughout life.

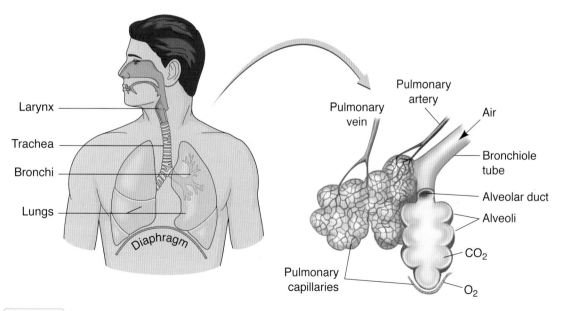

Figure 5.2 Respiratory system.

Training also enhances the efficiency of respiration, so the trained person needs fewer breaths to move the same volume of air. Ventilation is the amount of air moving in or out of the lungs. It is the product of respiratory rate (or frequency) times the volume of air in each breath (tidal volume):

ventilation (expired air in liters per minute) = frequency $\times$ tidal volume

Consider values for trained and untrained subjects jogging on a treadmill:

untrained: 60 liters per minute = 30 breaths $\times$ 2 liters per breath

trained: 60 liters per minute = 20 breaths $\times$ 3 liters per breath

The trained person moves more air with fewer breaths and is able to move more air at maximal ventilation (150 liters per minute or more, versus 120 or less for the untrained). Slower, deeper breaths are more efficient because they allow more of each breath to reach the portion of the lungs where oxygen and carbon dioxide are exchanged (alveolar sacs). Training also improves diffusion of oxygen from the lungs into the blood. Diffusion depends on good ventilation and adequate blood flow in the capillaries.

Blood Volume

Red blood cells and hemoglobin transport oxygen. We have long known that aerobic fitness is closely associated with total hemoglobin, and that blood volume and hemoglobin improve with training. We have also learned that the loss of blood volume that occurs with detraining is closely correlated with the reversal of important cardiovascular adjustments, leading to a higher resting heart rate and decreased stroke volume (Coyle, Hemmert, and Coggan 1986). Thus the increase in blood volume that occurs with training is likely responsible, at least in part, for so-called cardiovascular changes, and these changes may be secondary to training-induced increases in blood volume. Blood volume may increase 10 to 15 percent with training, raising the volume from 5 liters to 5.5 or even 5.75 liters.

> Training-induced changes in blood volume are likely responsible, at least in part, for so-called cardiovascular changes.

A large portion of the enhanced cardiovascular function of endurance athletes is due to their high blood volume and its effect on cardiac function, increased hemoglobin and stroke volume, and decreased heart rate and blood viscosity (Gledhill, Warburton, and Jamnik 1999). In a recent study, training-induced changes in blood volume accounted for approximately 47 percent of the improvements in $\dot{V}O_2$max, and the results were similar for continuous or interval training (Warburton et al. 2004).

Heart and Circulation

For years we knew that endurance training led to a reduction in the heart rate at rest and at submaximal workloads and to an increase in the stroke volume, the amount of blood pumped with each beat of the heart. That is why we used the term *cardiovascular* to describe training effects. Training leads to an increase in the size of the left ventricle, but only during the filling stage, or diastole (increased left ventricular end diastolic volume [LVEDV]) (see figure 5.3). This change takes place with some thickening of the heart muscle and subtle alterations in its oxidative enzyme capacity. The efficient, trained heart pumps more blood each time it beats, at rest or during exercise, and

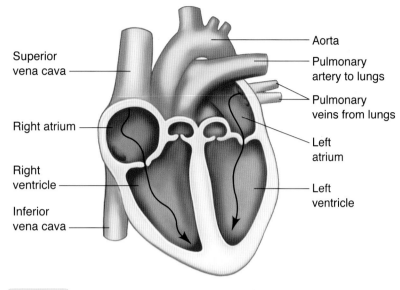

Figure 5.3 The heart.

therefore it can beat at a slower rate. The heart is a pump that ejects much of the blood that enters its chambers; put more blood into the chamber, and more comes out.

The volume of blood that the heart pumps with each beat depends on the blood volume and size of the left ventricle. A fibrous sac (pericardium) encloses the heart, limiting its size. When the sac was removed from dog hearts, the animals were able to train and increase their stroke volume and cardiac output (cardiac output equals heart rate multiplied by stroke volume) a whopping 20 percent (Stray-Gunderson 1986). You can't risk removal of your pericardium (an infection could lead to heart failure), but you can increase blood volume with training, and that seems to lead to increases in stroke volume and cardiac output, and decreases in resting and exercise heart rates. Does the heart rate go down because the stroke volume goes up, or vice versa? You'll soon see.

Heart Muscle Fibers

Adult rats engaged in up to 13 weeks of high-intensity treadmill training and then were detrained. Training led to increases in heart muscle contractile capacity and $\dot{V}O_2$max, and the improvements were correlated to fiber length. When training stopped, training-induced improvements in $\dot{V}O_2$max decreased 50 percent in 2 weeks, and leveled off at 5 percent above sedentary controls after 4 weeks of detraining. Heart muscle fiber length declined along with $\dot{V}O_2$max, and remained 9 percent above sedentary levels after 4 weeks. Other measures of contractile capacity regressed completely within 2 to 4 weeks of detraining (Kemi et al. 2004). A close association exists between heart muscle dimensions, contractile capacity, arterial relaxation, and aerobic fitness. Some portion of this association may be due to training-induced alterations in blood volume.

Aerobic training appears to have subtle effects on the dimensions of heart muscle and on aerobic enzymes and mitochondria. The trained heart is better able to use fat as a source of energy, perhaps because training enlarges the diameter of coronary arteries and improves the oxygen supply to heart muscle. Another important contributor to stroke volume and cardiac output is the redistribution of blood from digestive and other organs to working muscles. Blood vessels in active muscles dilate, whereas those in nonworking muscles and organs constrict, directing blood where it is needed during exercise and helping to maintain high stroke volume. Training improves this ability to redistribute blood. Training also seems to enhance delivery of blood to skeletal muscle fibers by the capillaries. Trained muscles have a higher capillary to fiber ratio (Blomqvist and Saltin 1983). Because trained muscle fibers increase in diameter, the rise in capillaries may be necessary to maintain short diffusion distance from the capillary to the interior of the muscle fiber.

Nervous System

Training has several subtle but important effects on the nervous system. These include improved economy and efficiency of movement and improved efficiency of the cardiovascular system. The economical athlete uses less energy to perform at a given speed. Hours of practice lead to relaxed and efficient use of force to achieve results. This economy is especially evident in skilled tasks such as swimming and cross-country skiing, but it also occurs in running and cycling. Trained distance runners use 10 percent less energy than untrained runners when running at a given speed.

The nervous system, which controls heart rate and the constriction and relaxation of blood vessels, participates in another adjustment that may help solve the question of why heart rate and stroke volume change with training. In 1977 Saltin published a simple but elegant experiment in which subjects trained one leg on a bicycle ergometer, while the other leg served as an untrained

Figure 5.4 Subject trains one leg while the other leg serves as an untrained control.

control (see figure 5.4). Pre- and posttest measures of oxygen intake and oxidative enzyme activity demonstrated that changes occurred only in the trained leg. In other words, the training was specific. Furthermore, the heart rate response to exercise was significantly lower for the trained leg compared with the control, or untrained, leg.

Saltin reasoned that the improvements in the trained muscles were responsible for the lower heart rate response. Mitchell and associates (1977) demonstrated that small nerve endings located in muscle fibers are able to sense conditions in the muscle and modify the heart rate response to exercise through connections to the cardiac control center in the brain. Thus it appears that the influence of training on the muscle may alter cardiovascular responses—that the reduced heart rate can be traced to improved metabolic condition in trained muscles. When the heart beats slower, it has more time to fill, allowing improved stroke volume.

This interpretation suggests that some of the well-documented effects of training are actually by-products of changes in the skeletal muscles. When we consider these changes with the increase in blood volume and redistribution of blood, which combine to put more blood into the heart, we understand why training leads to a decrease in exercise heart rate and an increase in stroke volume. Therefore it appears that some so-called cardiovascular effects of training are due to changes in the muscles being trained, that these changes are specific, and that training doesn't easily transfer from one leg (or one activity) to another. These conclusions also explain why we never use the term *cardio* to describe aerobic exercise.

Endocrine System

The endocrine system includes the many glands whose secretions, hormones, are distributed by the circulation. The effects of training include

- adjustments in hormonal response,
- increased sensitivity to certain hormones, and
- important metabolic adjustments.

Many hormones are involved in the regulation of energy. Epinephrine, cortisol, thyroxine, glucagon, and growth hormone raise blood sugar, whereas insulin is the only hormone capable of lowering blood sugar. The pancreas secretes insulin when blood sugar levels rise, such as after a meal, helping tissues take up the sugar. The others are secreted when blood levels are low, as in vigorous exercise. Epinephrine and growth hormone also are involved in the mobilization of fat from adipose tissue, whereas insulin leads to fat deposition. Endurance training lowers the need for insulin because the muscle can take up sugar during exercise, even in the absence of insulin (as in diabetes). Training seems to increase receptor sensitivity to insulin, leading to more efficient use of hormones and energy.

Fat Metabolism

Years ago animal and then human studies demonstrated improved fat utilization following training. Trained muscle is better suited to use fat as a source of energy, thereby conserving limited supplies of carbohydrate (glycogen) in muscle and the liver. A key finding was the enhancement of beta oxidation, an enzymatic process that systematically chops two carbon fragments from fat (free fatty acids), initiating the release of energy stored in fat to produce ATP. Along with this improvement in fat metabolism is a near doubling of stored fat (triglyceride) in trained muscle fibers. On top of all this, training leads to improvement in fat mobilization.

Fat Mobilization

Epinephrine is available from two sites, the adrenal gland and the nerve endings of the sympathetic nervous system. Like most other hormones, epinephrine acts on receptors located in the surface membrane of its target organ, in this case adipose tissue. The hormone initiates a series of steps leading to the breakdown of triglyceride fat and the release of free fatty acids (FFA) into the circulation (see figure 5.5).

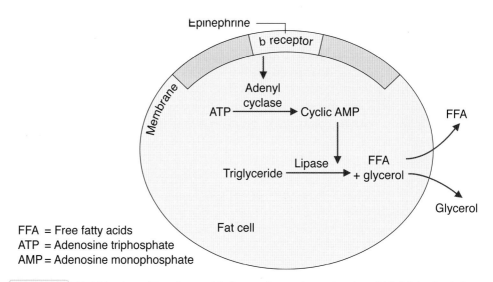

Figure 5.5 Mobilization of free fatty acids from adipose tissue. Lactic acid inhibits the influence of epinephrine on the fat cell and blocks the mobilization of fat.
Adapted from Sharkey, 1975.

The FFA then travel to working muscles or the heart, where they can be used to fuel contractions. During vigorous exercise, lactic acid produced in the muscles seems to inhibit the action of epinephrine, thereby reducing the FFA available for energy. Under these conditions the muscle must use limited supplies of muscle glycogen for energy.

Training improves the oxidative ability of muscles, leading to less lactic acid production and greater fat mobilization and fat metabolism (Holloszy et al. 1986). And trained people appear to be able to mobilize fat even when lactic acid is elevated (Vega deJesus and Siconolfi 1988). The result is improved access to a major source of energy, some 50 times more abundant than carbohydrate! The enhanced utilization of fat has significant health benefits beyond those related to fitness and performance. We'll say it again: The ability to utilize fat may be one of the most important outcomes of the active life and fitness.

> We'll say it again: The ability to utilize fat may be one of the most important outcomes of the active life and fitness.

Other Effects of Training

Training has effects on other tissues, including adipose tissue (fat), bone, ligaments, and tendons. Although some are mere adjustments that counteract the stresses of training, making more activity possible, others have health and cosmetic effects.

Body Composition

Body composition refers to the relative amounts of fat and lean weight. Although the lean body weight (body weight minus fat weight) is relatively unchanged with aerobic training, substantial loss of fat tissue is to be expected. One of the best-documented effects of training is the loss of unwanted fat, a transformation that reveals a trim, pleasing figure. Researchers use underwater weighing or skinfold calipers to measure percent body fat.

If you have 25 percent fat and weigh 120 pounds (54.4 kilograms), you have 30 pounds (13.6 kilograms) of fat and 90 pounds (40.8 kilograms) of lean body weight (LBW). If you jog 3 miles (4.8 kilometers) a day, 5 days a week, you will burn about 1,650 calories per week (3 miles times 110 calories per mile times 5 days equals 1,650 calories). In just 2 weeks you'll burn 3,300 extra calories, almost a pound of fat (3,500 calories equals 1 pound, or .45 kilogram, of fat), or almost 2 pounds (.9 kilogram) a month. In the process you will lower your percent body fat and your body weight with only a slight increase in LBW. We'll say much more about body composition and fat loss in chapters 13 and 14.

Bones, Ligaments, and Tendons

Bones, ligaments, and tendons respond to the stress placed on them. Adaptations follow every change in function. For bones, increased weight-bearing activity leads to a denser, stronger structure designed to counteract the new level of stress. Inactivity leads to reabsorption of calcium and loss of bone density. Increasing age and inactivity create a dangerous combination, especially for females. Bone demineralization, or osteoporosis, begins early in adult life (30 to 40 years of age) and becomes more serious after menopause. Lack of activity hastens the weakening of bones. Weight-bearing activity causes bone tissue to become stronger and denser. But excessive training along with weight loss or menstrual irregularities (amenorrhea, or absence of menstruation) can cause early and possibly irreversible osteoporosis. Calcium intake may be helpful, but it won't do much good without the stress of moderate weight-bearing exercise.

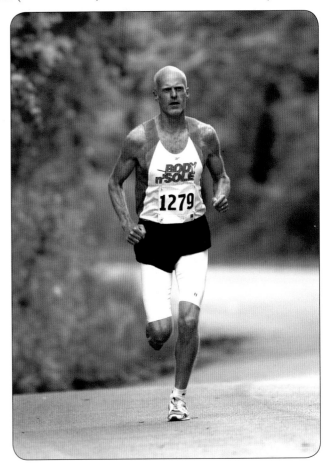

Moderate activity also strengthens ligaments, tendons, and other connective tissue, such as the covering of muscle. By gradually increasing the workload, you can make tissues tough enough to withstand the normal demands of activity and resist damage during slips, trips, and falls.

Specificity of Training

An activity such as jogging recruits muscle fibers uniquely suited to the task. Slow jogging recruits slow fibers. The metabolic pathways and energy sources are also suited to the task. Daily jogging recruits the same fibers and pathways repeatedly, leading to the adaptive response known as the training effect.

Training leads to changes in aerobic enzyme systems in muscle fibers, so it is easy to see why those changes are

Regular, moderate activity can strengthen connective tissues, which can prevent injuries.

specific. In the early stages of training, the inability of the muscles to use oxygen limits performance. Later on, as the fibers adapt and can use more oxygen, the burden shifts to the cardiovascular system, including the heart, blood, and blood vessels. Then the cardiovascular system becomes the factor that limits performance (Boileau, McKeown, and Riner 1984).

Training gains don't automatically transfer from one activity to another. Training effects can be classified as peripheral (in the muscle) and central (heart, blood, lungs, hormones). Central effects may transfer to other activities, but

> The outcomes of training are directly related to the activity employed as a training stimulus.

peripheral changes are unlikely to transfer. Central changes in blood volume and redistribution, however, may aid performance in another endurance activity. But keep in mind that one-leg training studies show that some part of the heart rate (and stroke volume) change is due to conditions within the muscle fibers, conditions that are relayed to the cardiac control center (Saltin 1977). These changes are specific and do not transfer from one activity to another.

Concentrating your training on the movements, muscle fibers, metabolic pathways, and supply and support systems that you intend to use in an activity or sport makes sense. This approach does not imply that athletes should ignore other exercises and muscle groups. Additional training is necessary to avoid injury, to avoid boredom, to achieve muscle balance, and to provide backup for prime movers when they become fatigued. In spite of the widespread affection for the term *cardiovascular fitness* (or *cardio*), the evidence suggests that the concept is overrated. Muscle is the target of training.

Finally, if exercise and training are specific, then testing must be specific if it is to reflect the adaptations that occur with training. This proposition means that you should not use a bicycle to test a runner and vice versa. Training is so specific that the best test for hill runners is an uphill treadmill test. How do we test the effects of training on dancers? We don't. When studies compare runners and dancers on a treadmill test, runners exhibit higher $\dot{V}O_2$max scores. If that is true, why do runners poop out in aerobic dance, cycling, or swimming? The answer is that the effects of training are specific. At present there is no widely accepted way to make an accurate assessment of the effects of aerobic, ballet, modern, or other dance forms.

Summary

In this section we've looked at the effects of aerobic training. We've shown that muscles undergo specific adaptations when an exercise recruits them over a period long enough to overload their oxidative pathways. As aerobic pathways improve, muscles use oxygen more efficiently and burn more fat. Maximal aerobic fitness ($\dot{V}O_2$max) and lactate thresholds rise. The metabolic efficiency is relayed to the cardiac control center in the brain, which results in a slower heart rate, more filling time, and greater stroke volume. Increased blood volume and improved distribution provide ample blood for the heart to pump. Because so many adaptations take place in the muscle, training should be specific to its intended use.

Because training is so specific, you should select an appropriate activity for aerobic training. Fat metabolism and cardiovascular benefits are enhanced in regular, moderate activity that employs major muscle groups for extended periods, but not when different muscles are engaged in a series of short lifting bouts (i.e., circuit weight training). Fat metabolism and cardiovascular benefits are also enhanced in some intermittent "aerobic" activities, in which an ever-changing series of movements maintains aerobic metabolism. Subjecting bones to regular, moderate stress, as in weight-bearing and resistance exercises, maintains bone mineral content.

Choose an activity that you enjoy, or one that you want to improve. Long, slow training improves the ability of slow oxidative fibers to use fat as an energy source. Faster and necessarily shorter training recruits fast-twitch (fast oxidative glycolytic) fibers. High-intensity training may also have more effect on the cardiovascular system. Your approach to training depends on your goals. Train more slowly for distance, faster for speed. You can combine both by going easy and then increasing pace near the end of the workout. German distance coach Ernst Van Aaken advocated a 20:1 slow to fast ratio for his elite athletes (1976). For example, on a 5-mile (8-kilometer) run, you can pick up the pace for the last quarter mile (the last 0.4 kilometer). This short distance provides some speed training at a time when you are well warmed. We like this approach because it limits the discomfort associated with elevated lactic acid. Training doesn't have to hurt to be good, as you'll see in the next chapter.

6

Improving Aerobic Fitness

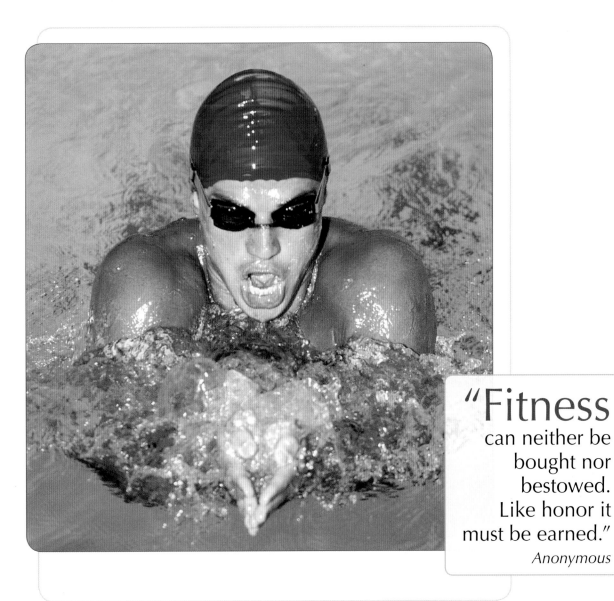

"Fitness can neither be bought nor bestowed. Like honor it must be earned."

Anonymous

Many years ago, before we knew how to prescribe exercise, we chose from a number of unproven training systems that were based on the ideas and experience of well-known physicians, coaches, or educators. Then researchers began to identify the factors associated with improvements in fitness. Exercise prescriptions today are based on the results of thousands of studies. The dose of exercise that safely promotes the training effect is usually represented by the intensity, duration, and frequency of exercise. Research and clinical experience are adding to a carefully developed methodology for safe and effective prescription of exercise.

You earn aerobic fitness minute by minute, day by day, as you engage in appropriate training exercises. As with any treatment or drug, the exercises must be prescribed and taken with care if you are to realize the benefits and avoid potentially harmful side effects.

This chapter will help you

- use your heart rate or perceived exertion to determine exercise intensity;
- determine exercise duration using calories, minutes, or miles (kilometers);
- decide on the appropriate frequency of exercise;
- develop a personalized aerobic fitness prescription based on your level of fitness and training goals; and
- understand how to achieve, maintain, and regain aerobic fitness.

Fitness Prescription Fundamentals

Throughout history people have sought the health benefits believed to be associated with exercise, with prescriptions dating back to centuries-old Chinese and Roman documents. In the late 1800s Dr. Dudley Sargent, physician and director of the Harvard College Gymnasium, tested students and prescribed exercises to rectify weaknesses. Prescriptions improved only slightly until the 1950s, when researchers began to establish the link between lack of activity and heart disease. Since then, we have agreed on a definition of aerobic fitness, identified the factors that contribute to its improvement, and become more aware of the benefits and limitations of exercise as a modality for disease prevention and rehabilitation. We now know how hard (intensity), how long (duration), and how often (frequency) one must exercise to achieve an aerobic training effect. We'll discuss the prescription and then show you how to proceed.

Intensity

Intensity, the most important factor in the development of maximal oxygen intake ($\dot{V}O_2max$), reflects the energy requirements of the exercise, the rate of oxygen consumption, and the calories of energy expended per minute. Although the training heart rate typically defines intensity, other measures can be used (see table 6.1).

Table 6.1   Measures of Exercise Intensity

Intensity	Heart rate[*] (bpm)	RPE[**]	Cal/min[***]	METs[****]
Light	90–120	8–10	5	4.0
Moderate	120–150	11–14	10	8.1
Heavy	150–200	15–18	15	12.2

The number of calories burned per minute depends on body weight; therefore, a heavier person burns more during a given exercise. Each MET equals 3.5 ml · kg^{-1} · min^{-1}, so the MET is adjusted for body weight.

[*]Approximate range for a 20-year-old person. Subtract 1% for every 2 years after age 20.
[**]RPE = Rating of perceived exertion (6–20 scale).
[***]1 L of oxygen is equivalent to 5 cal/min.
[****]The MET, or metabolic equivalent, is a multiple of the resting metabolic rate. The resting rate is 1.2 cal/min (1 MET), so 12 cal/min = 10 METs.

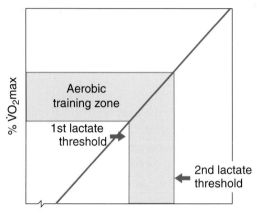

Figure 6.1 Aerobic fitness improves when you exercise within the aerobic training zone. This zone applies to aerobic fitness training. Endurance athletes generally do interval training just above the second lactate threshold and easy training near the first lactate threshold.

Minimum Aerobic Training Intensity

Early studies agreed that training had to exceed a certain minimum metabolic level or threshold if significant changes in aerobic fitness were to occur (see figure 6.1). In an early study we trained young men at heart rates of 120, 150, and 180 beats per minute. The higher-intensity groups improved $\dot{V}O_2$max similarly, but the low-intensity subjects did not (Sharkey and Holleman 1967). Then we learned that training intensity depended on the person's level of fitness, with low-fit subjects making progress at lower intensity whereas high-fit subjects had a higher training threshold (Sharkey 1970). The minimal training threshold, first called the aerobic threshold, is now known as the first lactate threshold (LT1).

Maximum Aerobic Training Intensity

Studies also defined an upper limit to training intensity. They showed that training above that level didn't yield additional improvements in $\dot{V}O_2$max. In recent years we recognized that this upper limit of the training zone coincides with the second lactate threshold (LT2), once called the anaerobic threshold. When the activity exceeds the ability of the muscle to produce energy aerobically and blood lactate accumulates rapidly, the ability to sustain the exercise decreases, and limited aerobic training benefits occur. Stated another way, anaerobic exercise does not contribute substantially to the development of aerobic fitness.

Thus the optimal aerobic training zone ranges from the first lactate threshold on the low end to the second lactate threshold, the point of diminishing returns. Training at the low end of the zone leads to changes in slow oxidative muscle fibers, improvements in fat metabolism, and changes in LT1. Training at the high end of the zone recruits and benefits fast oxidative glycolytic muscle fibers and leads to central circulatory (cardiovascular) benefits. In addition, the high-intensity interval training that athletes use has been shown to raise LT2. This improvement in LT2 can take place without an increase in $\dot{V}O_2$max, especially among those who have already undergone extensive training.

Stated another way, anaerobic exercise does not contribute substantially to the development of aerobic fitness.

Training Heart Rate

Early training studies focused on the metabolic demands of training (liters of oxygen consumed or kilocalories of energy expenditure). Because heart rate is correlated to metabolism, it was used as a simple, inexpensive way to translate training information to the lay public. Unfortunately, over the years the public and some fitness professionals have lost sight of this point. Today many mistakenly consider the training heart rate, not the sustained metabolism of a large muscle mass (e.g., legs), to be the goal of training. They believe that raising the heart rate, no matter how it is done, will improve fitness. For example, the elevation of the heart rate during weight training has led some to believe that circuit weight training can improve aerobic fitness. They ignore the fact that weight training engages each muscle group for only 20 to 30 seconds, far too short a time to prompt changes in the oxidative pathways of muscles. The training heart rate is a convenient external indicator of exercise intensity and oxygen consumption, but it isn't an end in itself. We'll show an alternative to using heart rate later in this chapter.

Training Zone

The aerobic training zone is defined as the training intensity between the first and second lactate thresholds. Both thresholds are related to your level of activity and fitness. Inactive people have a low LT1. If normal daily activity seldom exceeds a slow walk, a brisk walk will exceed the threshold and elicit a training effect. Regular participation in high-intensity activity raises LT2, so highly active people have an elevated threshold and a higher training zone.

In the past, the training zone was based on a percentage of estimated maximal heart rate. Because maximal heart rate declines with age, we used both fitness level and age-adjusted maximal heart rate to determine the training zone.

Fitness (milliliters per kilogram per minute)	Training zone (percent maximal heart rate)
Low (under 35)	60 to 75 percent
Medium (35 to 45)	70 to 85 percent
High (over 45)	75 to 90 percent

If your maximal heart rate (max HR) hasn't been measured, we estimate it with the following formula:

$$\text{max HR} = 220 - \text{age}$$

But because maximal heart rate varies considerably (see chapter 3, page 55), we use estimated heart rate with caution. If the training zone feels too high, we urge people to back off to a more comfortable level. Your maximal heart rate estimate could be lower than expected, so if the zone feels too easy, we move it up a bit. Because of this variability and uncertainty, and because of new research findings, we decided not to emphasize use of heart rate to identify training intensity. Instead, we use the rating of perceived exertion (RPE) to define training intensity. Perceived exertion is determined with a simple rating scale designed to provide an estimate of exercise intensity (see table 6.2).

Table 6.2   Rating of Perceived Exertion (RPE) Scales

Borg scale (6–20)	Intensity	Breathing scale	Distance scale
6	No exertion at all		
7		Can sing full songs	Could continue all day
8	Extremely light		Could continue 4–6 hours
9	Very light	Can sing partial verses	Could continue 3–4 hours
10			Could continue 2–3 hours
11	Light	Can talk in full sentences	Could continue 1–2 hours
12			Could continue 45–60 minutes
13	Somewhat hard	Can talk in short sentences	Could continue 30–45 minutes
14			Could continue 20–30 minutes
15	Hard (heavy)	Breathing hard, thinking clearly	Could continue 15–20 minutes
16			Could continue 10–15 minutes
17	Very hard	Breakaway ventilation	Could continue 5–10 minutes
18			Could continue 2–5 minutes
19	Extremely hard		Could continue 1–2 minutes
20	Maximal exertion		Could continue <1 minute

© Gunnar Borg, 1970, 1985, 1994, 1998.
Breathing and distance scales by the authors.

First developed by Swedish psychologist Gunner Borg (1973), perceived exertion has been validated and used in numerous studies (Robertson 2004). You can use the perceived exertion scale to establish exercise intensity at the start of exercise and maintain it throughout the workout (Kang et al. 2003) We provide the original Borg scale and two additional versions for practical use, along with related information that you can use to define levels of exertion (see table 6.2).

The numbers in the Borg scale, 6 through 20, also relate to exercise heart rate. You just add a zero to the rating to approximate your heart rate, so a 15 on the scale approximates a heart rate of 150. The talk test is another way to determine whether you are within your zone. You should be able to carry on a conversation while you train, at least until you approach your second lactate threshold. Exercise doesn't have to hurt to be good.

Both thresholds are related to your level of activity and fitness. The first lactate threshold is related to activities that you regularly carry out. Sedentary people have LT1s similar to the oxygen cost of activities of daily living (walking, climbing stairs). People who are more active have higher thresholds. The greater the intensity of your long-duration activities, the higher the oxygen cost of your first lactate threshold. In other words, the first lactate threshold for an active person will be higher than that for a sedentary person. The second lactate threshold is related to the highest intensity aerobic activity that you perform regularly for at least several minutes. Regular participation in high-intensity activity raises LT2, so highly active people have elevated thresholds and higher training zones.

You can use perceived exertion to define your training zone. The data from a large multicenter research project indicate that the RPE can be used to estimate the lactate thresholds (Gaskill et al. 2001). The thresholds form the limits of the aerobic training zone.

First lactate threshold	RPE = 11–13	Somewhat easy
Second lactate threshold	RPE = 14–16	Hard

Use table 6.2 to determine your thresholds and aerobic training zone. To determine your first lactate threshold (LT1), complete a warm-up and then find a comfortable intensity (in any aerobic activity) that you can easily maintain for 1 to 2 hours. Hold that pace for 10 minutes and then see whether it fits the somewhat easy category. You should be able to talk in full sentences and keep going for at least an hour. If you want to know your heart rate at LT1, stop, immediately count the rate for 15 seconds, and then multiply by four for the rate per minute. This intensity defines your LT1, the bottom of your aerobic training zone. Generally, your aerobic training zone ranges from the LT1 heart rate to about 25 beats per minute higher.

To determine your second lactate threshold (LT2), increase your intensity until your heart rate is 25 beats above LT1. After about 5 minutes check the RPE chart. If the exertion feels hard, if you can maintain it for another 10 minutes, if you are on the verge of breakaway ventilation, and if you can't talk but can still think clearly, then you are near your second lactate threshold. If necessary, adjust the pace until the effort seems hard. Take your heart rate, note your pace (e.g., miles or kilometers per hour), and how you feel (breathing and so forth). You can carry on a conversation at the lower end of the zone, but you will be able to say only short phrases at LT2. We'll say more about the training zone later in this chapter.

Heart Rates

We have elected to minimize use of heart rates in this edition of the book. For many they are a needless distraction from the pleasures of exercise. If you enjoy the discipline of heart rate measurements, however, continue to use them. You can use a percentage of your maximal heart rate (e.g., max HR = 220 – age) or the heart rate range formula (range = max HR – resting HR) to identify your training heart rate. The heart rate range formula calculates a heart rate equal to the percentage of $\dot{V}O_2$max. For a heart rate equivalent to 70 percent of $\dot{V}O_2$max for a 50-year-old (220 – 50 = 170):

$$HR = [70\% \times (\text{max HR} - \text{resting HR})] + \text{resting HR}$$

$$= [70\% \times (170 - 70)] + 70$$

$$= 140 \text{ bpm}$$

By contrast, 70 percent of the maximal heart rate (170) equals 119 beats per minute, which is approximately equal to 55 percent of $\dot{V}O_2$max. The heart rate range is sometimes used to adjust for measured differences in the resting and maximal heart rates, and to avoid errors in the estimation of the training heart rate.

In time you won't need to check your heart rate because you'll know how it feels to be in the training zone (perceived exertion). We begin with a prescription, but as you learn more about exercise and your body, improve your fitness, and decide on your goals, you will outgrow the need for heart rates and training zones. The RPE is

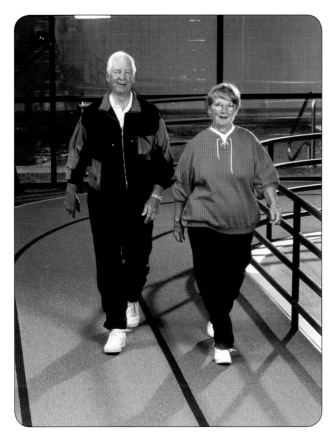

Low-fit people can improve their fitness levels with as little as 10 minutes of exercise per day.

a simple way to judge exercise intensity on a numerical scale that correlates to heart rate, lactate thresholds, and other physiological variables. The RPE is a valid tool for the prescription of exercise (Steed, Gaesser, and Weltman 1994).

Duration

Exercise duration and intensity go hand in hand; an increase in one requires a decrease in the other. Duration can be prescribed in terms of time, distance, or calories. We mention all three to show how they relate, but we prefer to use the calorie because it is so educational. Food labels tell you how many calories you gain when you eat and drink (a double burger equals 550 calories; beer equals 150 calories). You should also know how much exercise it takes to balance your energy intake. Jogging 1 mile (1.6 kilometers) burns 100 calories, so you'd have to jog almost 7 miles (11.2 kilometers) to burn the calories consumed with the burger and beer. Doing the math makes you think!

An early training study showed that low-fit people can improve their fitness with as little as 100 calories of exercise per session (10 minutes at 10 calories per minute) (Bouchard et al. 1966). Low-fit subjects need less intensity and duration than fit subjects do to elicit a training effect. But in time, as fitness improves, they should extend duration to 200 calories or more. Fitness pioneer Dr. Tom Cureton found that people needed higher expenditures to bring about significant improvement in cholesterol levels (Cureton 1969). Additional studies have shown that longer workouts (more than 35 minutes) produce greater fitness benefits (Wenger and Bell 1986), perhaps because the proportion of fat metabolized continues to rise for the first 30 minutes of exercise.

Calorie

The calorie (technically a kilocalorie) is a unit of energy defined as the amount of heat required to raise the temperature of 1 kilogram of water 1 degree Celsius. We store calories when we eat and burn them when we exercise. Body weight influences caloric expenditure during exercise. A 180-pound (81.6-kilograms) person burns more calories running at a certain pace than one who weighs 150 pounds (68 kilograms). The first burns 136 calories per mile (85 calories per kilometer), whereas the second burns 113 calories per mile (70 calories per kilometer). In this book caloric expenditures are based on a weight of 150 pounds (68 kilograms); add or subtract 10 percent for each 15 pounds (6.8 kilograms) over or under 150 pounds. For example, add 20 percent to 113 calories to determine the cost for the 180-pound person (113 times .20 equals 22.6, plus 113 equals 135.6 calories).

A study of 17,000 Harvard graduates provides another way to assess the importance of exercise duration. Paffenbarger, Hyde, and Wing (1986) found significant reduction in the risk of heart disease for graduates who averaged more than 2,000 calories of exercise per week. That translates into about 300 calories daily (400 calories per day in 5 days of exercise per week). Longer duration training leads to improved fat metabolism, which may be the major health benefit of exercise. Increase your training duration to gain significant fitness, weight control, and fat metabolism benefits and to lower blood lipids. But we have no conclusive evidence to recommend workouts that exceed 60 minutes (or 600 calories) for health benefits, other than weight loss. Endurance athletes participate in longer workouts to improve stamina and performance, not for enhanced health benefits. In fact, an epidemiological study suggests that mortality rates, which decline with increasing exercise, begin to rise when energy expenditure exceeds 3,500 calories per week (Lee, Hsieh, and Paffenbarger 1995). Table 6.3 lists some guidelines for exercise duration.

Overload is the key to improvements in training. As fitness improves we need to increase intensity and duration if we hope to continue improvements in $\dot{V}O_2max$ and the lactate thresholds. Now let's see how to adjust training frequency as training progresses.

Table 6.3   Duration per Training Session

Activity level	Walking distance	Calories*
Inactive	1–2 mi (1.6–3.2 km)	100–200
Moderately active	2–4 mi (3.2–6.4 km)	200–400
Very active	>4 mi (6.4 km)	>400

*Add or subtract 10% for every 15 lb above or below 150 lb (or 7 kg above or below 70 kg).

Frequency

For low-fit people, three sessions a week on alternating days are sufficient to improve aerobic fitness (Jackson, Sharkey, and Johnston 1968). But as training progresses in intensity and duration, it must also increase in frequency if improvements are to continue (Pollock 1973). An extensive review of training studies found that changes in fitness are directly related to frequency of training when it is considered independent of the effects of intensity, duration, program length, and initial level of fitness (Wenger and Bell 1986). Six days per week is more than twice as effective as 3 days per week. So for fitness or weight control, consider more frequent exercise. Athletes engage in long sessions, or they train two or more times a day, two or three times a week. But they also observe the hard–easy principle, following hard or long sessions with easy or short ones. Failure to allow adequate time for recovery from training nullifies its effects; overtraining can lead to poor performance, overuse injuries, or illness through suppression of the immune system.

> Overtraining can lead to poor performance, overuse injuries, or illness through suppression of the immune system.

The body needs time to respond to the training stimulus, and some people find that they need more than 24 hours. As one of us reached his 60th year he found that he needed more time to recover from extremely long or strenuous activity. Experiment with schedules to find one that suits you. Work out daily if you prefer, or try an alternate-day plan and increase duration. Whatever you do, be sure to schedule at least one day of relative rest or diversion each week. A colleague and former training partner once wrote, "We should approach running not as if we are trying to smash our way through some enormous wall, but as a gentle pastime by which we can coax a slow continuous stream of adaptations out of the body" (Frederick 1973, 20).

Activity level	Frequency (days per week)
Inactive	3–4 days
Moderately active	5–6
Very active	≥ 6*

*Athletes sometimes do two sessions per day, but always follow a hard day with an easy day.

Your Fitness Prescription

A comprehensive review of training studies showed that maximal gains in aerobic fitness ($\dot{V}O_2$max) were achieved with high intensity (90 percent of $\dot{V}O_2$max or 95 percent of maximal heart rate), a duration of 35 to 45 minutes, and a frequency of four times per week (Wenger and Bell 1986). Less intensity produced respectable increases in $\dot{V}O_2$max with less risk of injury. But keep in mind that all these conclusions were based on changes in $\dot{V}O_2$max, acknowledged as a measure of intensity (Sharkey 1991). Although $\dot{V}O_2$max is important, better measures of endurance are available, such as the first and second lactate thresholds. Sustained training just above LT1 is effective at improving long-term endurance. Shorter (3- to 4-minute) intervals just above LT2 contribute to improvements in the second lactate threshold, the one related to performance in races lasting from 15 minutes to 2 hours or more. But fitness and performance aren't the only goals. People can achieve health benefits, weight control, and improved appearance with moderate levels of intensity, duration, and frequency. Use the prescription in table 6.4 as a starting point but don't be a slave to training. Adapt the program to meet your personal style and goals.

Table 6.4   Aerobic Fitness Prescription

Activity category	RPE	Duration (calories)*	Frequency (days/wk)	Walking or running distance (to meet caloric needs)
Inactive	11–13	100–200	3–4	1–2 mi (1.6–3.2 km)
Moderately active	12–14	200–400	5–6	2–4 mi (3.2–6.4 km)
Very active	13–16	>400	≥6	>4 mi (6.4 km)

*Add or subtract 10% for each 15 lb over or under 150 lb (or 7 kg above or below 70 kg).

Athletes occasionally train at higher intensity or longer duration, and sometimes do two or even three workouts a day. Chapter 15 provides advice on advanced endurance training and insights into cross-training and other ways to make fitness enjoyable. Table 6.5 shows how some popular training activities fit the prescription.

Figure 6.2 illustrates how to carry out the prescription on a given day. Begin every session with a warm-up to minimize soreness and risk of injury. Start with a gradual increase in exercise activity and then stretch. Pay attention to stretching the lower back, hamstrings, calf muscles, and any sore muscles. Muscle soreness shows up 24 hours after the start of a program but diminishes soon thereafter. It won't return unless you lay off for months, increase intensity, or do a new activity. Follow the prescription

Table 6.5   Sample Aerobic Activities

Fitness category (ml · kg⁻¹ · min⁻¹)	RUNNING		JOGGING		CYCLING		WALKING	
	Distance (mi [km])	Time (min)	Distance (mi [km])	Time (min)	Distance (mi [km])	Time (min)	Distance (mi [km])	Time (min)
Inactive	0.8–1.7 (1.3–2.7)	7–14	0.8–1.7 (1.3–2.7)	10–20	1.9–3.9 (3.1–6.3)	12–24	1.0–2.1 (1.6–3.4)	18–36
Moderately active	1.7–3.4 (2.7–5.5)	14–27	1.7–3.4 (2.7–5.5)	20–40	3.9–7.8 (6.3–12.6)	24–47	2.1–4.2 (3.4–6.8)	36–72
Very active	≥3.4 (≥5.5)	≥27	≥3.4 (≥5.5)	≥40	≥7.8 (≥12.6)	≥47	≥4.2 (≥6.8)	≥72

Adapted from Sharkey, 1997.

Figure 6.2   Aerobic training session.

during the aerobic portion of the session and then be sure to cool down before you hit the shower. Easy jogging, walking, and stretching help lower body temperature, reduce metabolic by-products such as lactic acid, and dissipate the hormone norepinephrine, which could cause irregular heart rhythms.

To vary the program, take different routes, work at the upper edge of the training zone for short periods (i.e., hard and short) and the lower edge for longer periods (easy and long), or use another activity for variety (cross-training). As training progresses, the same pace will feel easier and more enjoyable. And as fitness improves, the prescription needs to change, calling for more intensity, duration, or frequency. You'll find yourself going faster at the same level of perceived exertion. By then you will have an idea of what you want to achieve from fitness, and you can decide what works and feels best to you.

Progression

"Make haste slowly" is a philosophy that works well for coaxing the gentle stream of improvements from your body. Training progression refers to how we gradually increase the overall training load. Although studies show the need to overload the body as fitness improves, few provide guidance on how to proceed. Gradual progress allows time for rest, recovery, and adjustments to training. Consider these guidelines. Meet the health goal by doing 30 minutes of moderate activity most days of the week. A brisk walk helps you meet this goal. If you have been sedentary you may have to become active before you begin to train. Begin at the bottom of your training zone (somewhat easy) and find a comfortable duration. Remember, training does not need to be hard. Then, train 3 or 4 days per week, adjusting intensity and duration as you go. When you are ready, increase duration above what you have been doing, while staying at the same intensity. Work up to two longer sessions and one shorter session each week. Then you can increase frequency by adding an extra day with a short workout at a comfortable pace.

When you are feeling good, raise the intensity a bit but try to avoid increasing the load too quickly. To increase intensity, replace a longer workout with one that is slightly harder (RPE of 11 to 13). Reduce the duration by increasing pace for 5 to 10 minutes and then slowing down to recover; repeat a few moderate intervals. Add intensity sessions gradually and pay attention to how your body responds. Then, repeat the cycle. Build on your progress and slowly increase duration, frequency, and intensity until you feel that you are where you would like to be.

After increasing duration, frequency, and intensity over several weeks, you should schedule an easier week for recovery, a process called periodization. You should also be willing to adjust your daily training plan. If you are tired, reduce the load by going shorter, easier, or maybe not at all. By progressing gradually and scheduling rest, you will achieve your goals. We all progress at different rates, so be patient and enjoy the journey.

Periodization of Training

As your training proceeds you'll want to use the progression technique that athletes use. Periodization describes the process of planning systematic variations and rest in the training program. Variation occurs at daily and weekly levels. This process ensures progression along with periods of relative rest and recovery. For example, you can increase training volume for several weeks and then back off for a week to recover. Repeat the pattern as training volume (intensity, duration, frequency) gradually increases. Periodization is used in aerobic and muscular fitness training. We'll show you how to use the technique in chapter 15.

Mode of Exercise

Health benefits occur regardless of the exercise you select. Dr. Michael Pollock and associates compared the fitness and weight-control benefits of walking, running, and cycling. Sedentary middle-aged men trained for 20 weeks, all using the same intensity, duration, and frequency of exercise. Tests administered at the conclusion of the study indicated that all three groups improved similarly in fitness, body weight, and body fat (Pollock et al. 1975). No one mode of exercise is superior to others when the prescription is the same. The best exercise is the one that you enjoy and will continue to do regularly. As discussed earlier, however, improvements in fitness are specific to the manner of training. So if you want to improve your running, that is the way you should train. Swimming and cycling do surprisingly little to improve running, and vice versa, because many of the important changes take place only in the muscles used in training.

Cross-Training

The popular triathlon gave rise to the theory of cross-training and the suggestion that running or cycling could enhance swim performance and so forth. Unfortunately, cross-training doesn't work that way; training must be specific to improve performance (Sharkey and Greatzer 1993). But there are several good reasons to use variety in training. One is to train for a multisport event like the triathlon. Another is to add variety and interest to your training. But the most important reason is to reduce impact and overuse in activities like running.

Over the years, we've found that cross-training relieves the likelihood of nagging overuse injuries. And the variety eliminates the boredom of unrelenting training. We run and mountain bike in summer, with hiking, paddling, swimming, and even golf for diversion. Winter includes cross-country and downhill skiing as well as snowshoeing. Winter diversions include backcountry ski trips. We do one or two weightlifting sessions most weeks to maintain muscular fitness and try to improve or maintain performance. Fall and spring serve as transition periods, enhanced by new activities, new weather, and new locales. Try more than one mode of exercise to train some muscles while resting others. You'll like it!

Achievement

The key to the achievement of fitness goals is to make haste slowly. If you rush the process, the result may be painful, injurious, or worse. You need time to coax that slow, continuous stream of adaptations from the body. You'll experience improved energy and vigor within weeks, improved self-concept and body image will follow, and performance will show change within a month. But don't view these exciting changes as a license for imprudent behavior. Athletes train for years to achieve dramatic results. Don't expect to undo years of inactivity or remove fat that accumulated over a decade in a few short weeks!

What progress can you expect when you follow your prescription? Although the ultimate achievement will depend on your genetic endowment (Bouchard et al. 1988), with time and effort you can achieve your potential. Two factors, age and initial level of fitness, influence the rate of improvement (Sharkey 1970). Training during or just after puberty, a period of intense growth and development, leads to the greatest adaptations in the ability to take in, transport, and use oxygen ($\dot{V}O_2$max). Adolescent training may prompt a 30 to 35 percent improvement in aerobic fitness. Young adults are able to improve 20 to 25 percent. Trainability may decline slowly thereafter, but even a 70-year-old can expect a 10 percent improvement in fitness ($\dot{V}O_2$max). Greater improvements are possible at any age when significant weight loss is involved (Sharkey 1984).

> You need time to coax that slow, continuous stream of adaptations from the body.

Because active people are closer to their genetic potential, they will not improve as much as their less-active and less-fit contemporaries. Complete inactivity, such as prolonged bed rest, provides a clean canvas for the demonstration of dramatic changes, perhaps as much as 100 percent improvement above bed-rest levels. Sedentary folks may improve over 30 percent, whereas already trained athletes may have to accept 5 percent improvement or less, depending on age, proximity to genetic potential, and level of training.

The rate of improvement is dramatic at first, 3 percent per week for the first month, 2 percent per week for the second, and slowing to 1 percent or less thereafter. But although the improvement in aerobic fitness begins to level off after several months, the capacity to perform submaximal work continues to grow (see figure 6.3). Both the capacity for prolonged work (first lactate threshold) and the upper limit of aerobic endurance (second lactate threshold) continue to increase after $\dot{V}O_2$max has reached a plateau. These submaximal capacities, not $\dot{V}O_2$max, define our capacity for work or sport.

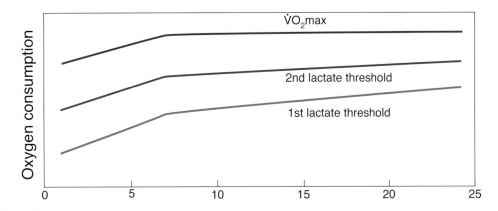

Figure 6.3 | Training, aerobic fitness, and submaximal work capacity. With prolonged training, $\dot{V}O_2$max (aerobic fitness) begins to level off, but the capacity to perform submaximal work at the first and second lactate thresholds continues to improve.

A normally active middle-aged adult male with a fitness score of 40 milliliters per kilogram per minute may improve to 50. If he had started as an adolescent, with a fitness score of 55, and achieved a 30 percent improvement, he may have scored over 70 and been an outstanding athlete. If you started late, don't despair. You can still achieve dramatic improvements in endurance and energy. Most important are the improvements in submaximal capacities, changes that allow a once-sedentary person to climb a mountain or run a marathon. Besides improving your fitness, you are able to sustain a higher percentage of your maximal capacity and continue once-fatiguing activities indefinitely, without fatigue or discomfort. And the benefits extend beyond your regular mode of exercise to all your daily tasks. Fitness expands your horizons.

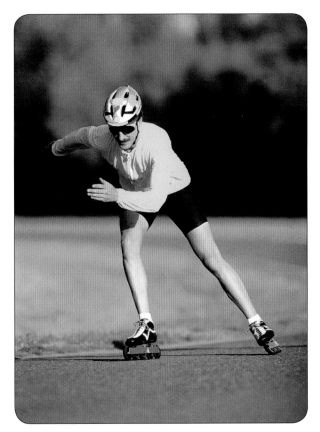

Even if you started late, you can dramatically increase your endurance and energy through training.

Maintenance

If you attain a level of fitness and performance that meets your needs, you may want to switch to a maintenance program. You'll be able to maintain your fitness with three sessions per week, allowing time to apply your newfound fitness in new pursuits. Maintenance has been studied several ways. One is to train to a level of fitness and then use various frequencies of training to see how much is required to remain at that level. Another is to cease training to see how quickly fitness is lost. With some activity, fitness doesn't decline too rapidly, but with complete bed rest it may drop as much as 10 percent a week (Greenleaf et al. 1976). You can maintain fitness with two or three sessions weekly, but the effort must be of the same intensity and duration as that used to achieve the improvements (Brynteson and Sinning 1973). Exercise of lower intensity but longer duration also seems to work, but it won't keep you tuned for a race. One workout of very long duration each week may help maintain fitness for a while; a combination of activities plus two or three training sessions is certain to do the job.

Researchers have used a more complex approach to study maintenance. By observing the effect of a single dose of training on specific aerobic enzymes, the researcher can plot the influence of training and determine its half-life, that is, the time it takes to lose one-half of the benefit. These studies suggest that the half-life of training ranges from 4.5 to 9.4 days (Watson, Srivastava, and Booth 1983). The half-life is used because it is difficult to tell when a biological effect, such as an increase in enzyme activity, returns to pretraining levels. So researchers measure the increase and the time that it takes to return to half that value. If half of the training effect is lost in 4.5 days, you'll want to train more frequently to maintain or improve fitness.

Regaining Fitness

Does a previously fit person regain fitness more quickly than one who has not been fit? Although the limited work in this area says probably not, our experience argues for a tentative maybe. The answer may depend on such factors as genetic potential, level of fitness, and extent of previous training. An extensive period of previous training may lead to changes that are retained longer than are alterations in aerobic enzymes and blood volume. Repetition of training will certainly lead to skill and economy of motion that makes subsequent activity seem easier.

But instead of worrying about how little it takes to achieve, maintain, or regain fitness, find activities that you enjoy and make them part of your life. Then you'll view activity as an essential and enjoyable part of every day. You'll be hooked on activity and fitness, and the rest will take care of itself.

Summary

This chapter summarizes the findings of hundreds of studies that have contributed to our knowledge of the factors associated with the development of aerobic fitness. Manipulation of intensity, duration, and frequency of exercise brings about improvements in fitness. Until recently, virtually all studies relied on the same measure of improvement, $\dot{V}O_2$max, which has been acknowledged as a measure of exercise intensity. So it is not surprising that most studies favor intensity as the most important factor in the training prescription. If your goal is to raise $\dot{V}O_2$max, emphasize intensity, at least some of the time.

But if your goal is health, or the capacity to endure for extended periods, you should give equal attention to another important dimension of fitness—duration, as measured by time or distance. Long-duration exercise raises LT1 and ensures the utilization of fat as a source of energy, a development that has distinct health benefits. If your goal is performance, you should include some training at or near your second lactate threshold. Remember, training must be specific to its intended purpose if you are to achieve optimal results.

Intensity is important, but excessive emphasis on intensity can take the joy out of regular activity. Athletes don't train hard every day, and you shouldn't either. That is why we encourage you to move beyond the objective approach of heart rates and training zones to the subjective, in which you use perceived exertion and listen to your body. Adopt the active life gradually and enjoy the experience, the adaptations, and the amazing results.

7

Implementing an Aerobic Fitness Program

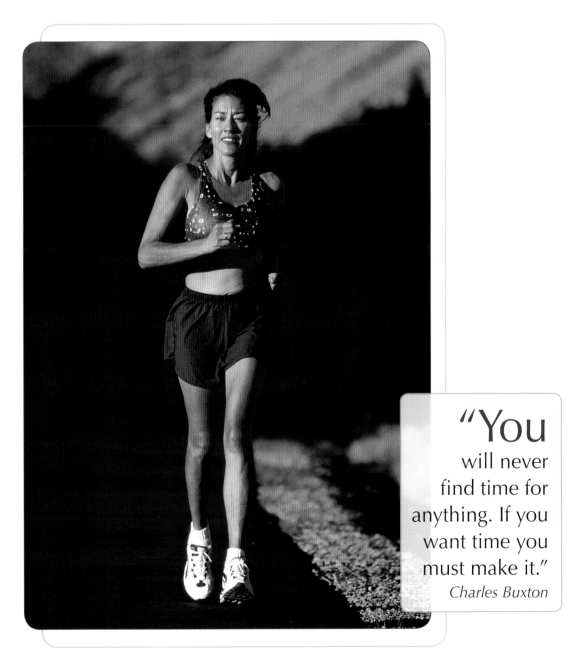

"You will never find time for anything. If you want time you must make it."
Charles Buxton

People tell us that they would like to become more fit but that they just don't have the time. We tell them how others make time for regular exercise, including the last six U.S. presidents and many other busy people. The time has come for you to make time for regular fitness training. This chapter provides training tips, training programs, and other information that you'll need to make training safe, enjoyable, and effective. The programs in this chapter have been proved cost effective, providing maximum benefit for the time invested.

This chapter will help you

- understand how to make training safe and enjoyable;
- apply your aerobic fitness prescription with
   - walk–jog–run programs,
   - cycling or swimming programs, or
   - advanced aerobic training;
- select alternative ways to remain active and fit; and
- deal with common exercise problems.

Training Tips

We'll begin with walking and running as modes of exercise because, for the time and cost, they provide excellent training stimulus. Intensity and duration are easy to control, and you can do the activities at any time, in almost any weather, with little investment in equipment. The equipment is light and easily transported on vacation or business trips. You can participate alone or in a group and can continue throughout life. A recent study of 72,488 female nurses found that brisk walking was inversely associated with the risk of heart disease; the relative risk declined as the amount of walking increased (Manson et al. 1999). The benefits were similar to those achieved with other forms of vigorous exercise, such as running. For these reasons and more, walking and running are fine ways to achieve and maintain aerobic fitness and its benefits.

What to Wear

Nothing is more important to your enjoyment than comfortable shoes, so don't economize when you buy footwear. Go to a reputable sporting goods dealer and seek advice from a knowledgeable salesperson. Avoid sale shoes at discount outlets unless you know something about the product. Buy a training shoe, not one built for competition. A firm, thick sole, good arch support, and a well-padded heel are essential. The sole should be firm but not terribly difficult to flex. A firm heel counter is also important. If blisters are a problem, try tube socks, a thin sock under a heavier one, or a balm on potential hot spots (try bag balm from a livestock outlet).

Walking and jogging don't require fancy clothing. Nylon or cotton shorts and a T-shirt are adequate in summer. For winter, a jogging suit serves until temperatures fall below 20 degrees Fahrenheit (minus 7 degrees Celsius). Some runners prefer tights. Just remember that layers of lighter clothing are preferable to a single heavy garment. Add gloves and a knit cap in cold weather. A cap is important in cold conditions because you lose a large amount of heat from your head. When the wind blows, a thin windbreaker helps reduce heat loss. In extremely cold weather, you can wear tights and wind pants.

> A cap is important in cold conditions because you lose a large amount of heat from your head.

Many runners continue in subzero (Fahrenheit) temperatures (minus 18 degrees Celsius), which is safe if you are properly clothed, warmed up, and sensitive to the signs of windchill and frostbite (see chapter 16). For longer winter outings, we prefer polypropylene underwear to wick perspiration away from the skin, thereby avoiding rapid cooling. Add a pile vest and a windbreaker, and you are ready to go.

Technique

An upright posture conserves energy. Run or walk with your back comfortably straight, your head up, and your shoulders relaxed. When jogging, bend your arms, hold your hands in a comfortable position, and keep arm swing to a minimum. Pumping action will increase with more speed. Swing your legs freely from the hip with no attempt to overstride. Studies show that the stride that feels best is usually the most efficient as well.

We recommend the heel-to-toe foot strike for most new runners. This technique is the least tiring, and most distance runners use it. Land lightly on the heel and roll forward to push off the ball of the foot. For faster running employ a slight forward lean, more knee lift, a quick and forceful pushoff, and more arm action. Check your shoes after several weeks of running. The outer border of the heel will show some wear if you are using the correct foot strike.

Time of Day

Exercise whenever it suits your fancy. Some people prefer to work out before breakfast, and others work out during the lunch hour or after work. A few night owls brave the dark in their quest for fitness; the run and shower help them sleep. Avoid vigorous exercise (except walking, cycling, or cross-country skiing) for 1 to 2 hours after a meal, when the digestive system requires an adequate blood supply. Some like to run during the lunch hour. If you have problems at work you'll often come back with a solution. Unless you need time alone, consider training with a partner. If you find one with similar abilities, interests, and goals, you aren't likely to miss your workout.

Exercise during the time of day that works best for you.

Where to Walk or Run

Avoid hard surfaces for the early weeks of training. Walk or run in the park, on playing fields, on a golf course, or on a running track. Then you'll be ready to try the back roads or trails in your area. Varying your routes will help you maintain interest. When the weather prohibits outdoor exercise, try a mall, YMCA, or school gym, or choose an exercise supplement that you can do at home, such as running in place or skipping rope. We'll suggest other aerobic alternatives later in this chapter.

Sample Aerobic Fitness Programs

Your fitness prescription gives you freedom to tailor a program to meet your specific needs. You have a wide choice of exercise, many options in the length of time that you choose to exercise, and several alternatives for the intensity of the activity. Some people prefer a detailed, step-by-step approach. For this reason, we've included some walk–jog–run programs.

We'll describe programs for three levels of ability: a starter program for those making the transition to activity, an intermediate program, and one for those in higher fitness categories. The President's Council on Physical Fitness and Sport (1975) prepared the starter program, which appeared in the booklet "An Introduction to Physical Fitness."

Starter Programs

This program is suitable for beginner and intermediate exercisers. Use the walk or walk–jog test to determine your current level of fitness and where you should begin. Follow the instructions and you will soon be moving to the next level.

Walk Test

The object of this test is to determine how many minutes (up to 10) you can walk at a brisk pace, on a level surface, without undue difficulty or discomfort. If you can't walk for 5 minutes, begin with the red walking program. If you can walk more than 5 minutes, but less than 10, begin with the third week of the red walking program. If you can walk for the full 10 minutes but are somewhat tired as a result, start with the white walk–jog program. If you can breeze through the full 10 minutes, you're ready for bigger things. Wait until the next day and take the 10-minute walk–jog test.

Walk–Jog Test

In this test you alternately walk 50 steps (left foot strikes the ground 25 times) and jog 50 steps for a total of 10 minutes. Walk at the rate of 120 steps per minute (left foot strikes the ground at 1-second intervals). Jog at the rate of 144 steps per minute (left foot strikes the ground 18 times every 15 seconds). If you can't complete the 10-minute test, begin with the third week of the white program. If you can complete the 10-minute test but are tired and winded as a result, start with the last week of the white program before moving to the blue program. If you can perform the 10-minute walk–jog test without difficulty, start with the blue program.

Red Walking Program

Start with this program, doing each activity every other day at first (see figure 7.1). The first week you'll walk at a brisk pace (RPE = 10–11) for 5 minutes, or for a shorter time if you become uncomfortably tired. Walk slowly for 3 minutes. Then walk briskly again for 5 minutes or until you become uncomfortably tired. The second week of the program is the same, but you increase your pace as soon as you can walk 5 minutes without soreness or fatigue. During the third week of the program you'll increase your brisk walking to 8 minutes. Increase your pace in the fourth week. When you've completed the fourth week of the red program, begin at the first week of the white program.

Figure 7.1   Red Walking Program

Week	Sunday	Monday	Tuesday	Wednesday	Thursday	Friday	Saturday
1	Brisk walk 5 min	Off	Brisk walk 5 min	Off	Brisk walk 5 min	Off	Brisk walk 5 min
	Slow walk/ rest 3 min		Slow walk/ rest 3 min		Slow walk/ rest 3 min		Slow walk/ rest 3 min
	Brisk walk 5 min		Brisk walk 5 min		Brisk walk 5 min		Brisk walk 5 min
2	Off	Brisk walk 5 min	Off	Brisk walk 5 min	Off	Brisk walk 5 min	Off
		Slow walk/ rest 3 min		Slow walk/ rest 3 min		Slow walk/ rest 3 min	
		Brisk walk 5 min		Brisk walk 5 min		Brisk walk 5 min	
3	Brisk walk 8 min	Off	Brisk walk 8 min	Off	Brisk walk 8 min	Off	Brisk walk 8 min
	Slow walk/ rest 3 min		Slow walk/ rest 3 min		Slow walk/ rest 3 min		Slow walk/ rest 3 min
	Brisk walk 8 min		Brisk walk 8 min		Brisk walk 8 min		Brisk walk 8 min
4	Off	Brisk walk 8 min	Off	Brisk walk 8 min	Off	Brisk walk 8 min	Off
		Slow walk/ rest 3 min		Slow walk/ rest 3 min		Slow walk/ rest 3 min	
		Brisk walk 8 min		Brisk walk 8 min		Brisk walk 8 min	

Pedometers

An inexpensive pedometer is an effective way to assess physical activity (Tudor-Locke et al. 2004). Use step goals (e.g., 10,000 steps per day) to motivate increased physical activity. Measure your stride length and set the pedometer. Then begin with a typical day and see how many steps you record. Add additional steps by parking farther from work, taking the stairs instead of the elevator, and taking a walk during your break. You will soon find ways to get 10,000 steps.

White Walk–Jog Program

In this program you'll begin by walking at a brisk pace for 10 minutes, or for a shorter time if you become uncomfortably tired (see figure 7.2). After a slow walk or rest you'll resume the brisk pace. The second week will increase the amount of time spent walking at a brisk pace. The third week takes you to 30 minutes of walking, most days of the week, the minimum level of activity suggested for health by the Centers for Disease Control and American College of Sports Medicine. The fourth week will incorporate jogging short distances, and the fifth week increases the jogging. Do each activity at least four times a week. When you've completed the fifth week of the white program, begin the first week of the blue program.

Blue Jogging Program

In this program you'll increase the amount of time spent jogging each week (see figure 7.3). Do each activity five times a week, as indicated. Although 30 minutes is the minimum time needed for health benefits, the Institute of Medicine has recommended 1 hour of daily activity to achieve greater health benefits and to maintain body weight, so you'll want to work toward the intermediate program.

Figure 7.2   White Walk–Jog Program

Week	Sunday	Monday	Tuesday	Wednesday	Thursday	Friday	Saturday
1	Brisk walk 10 min Slow walk/rest 3 min Brisk walk 10 min	Brisk walk 10 min Slow walk/rest 3 min Brisk walk 10 min	Off	Brisk walk 10 min Slow walk/rest 3 min Brisk walk 10 min	Off	Brisk walk 10 min Slow walk/rest 3 min Brisk walk 10 min	Off
2	Brisk walk 15 min Slow walk/rest 3 min Brisk walk 10 min	Off	Brisk walk 15 min Slow walk/rest 3 min Brisk walk 10 min	Off	Brisk walk 15 min Slow walk/rest 3 min Brisk walk 15 min	Off	Brisk walk 15 min Slow walk/rest 3 min Brisk walk 15 min
3	Brisk walk 10 min Rest 3 min Brisk walk 15 min	Moderate walk 30 min	Brisk walk 10 min Rest 3 min Brisk walk 15 min	Moderate walk 30 min	Brisk walk 10 min Rest 3 min Brisk walk 15 min	Moderate walk 30 min	Off
4	Jog 10 s (25 yd) Walk 1 min (100 yd) 12×	Off	Jog 10 s (25 yd) Walk 1 min (100 yd) 12×	Off	Jog 10 s (25 yd) Walk 1 min (100 yd) 12×	Off	Jog 10 s (25 yd) Walk 1 min (100 yd) 12×
5	Off	Jog 20 s (50 yd) Walk 1 min (100 yd) 12×	Off	Jog 20 s (50 yd) Walk 1 min (100 yd) 12×	Off	Jog 20 s (50 yd) Walk 1 min (100 yd) 12×	Jog 20 s (50 yd) Walk 1 min (100 yd) 12×

Walk briskly at an RPE of 10 to 11. Jog at an RPE of 13 to 15. Meters = yards × .91.

Figure 7.3 Blue Jogging Program

Week	Sunday	Monday	Tuesday	Wednesday	Thursday	Friday	Saturday
1	Jog 40 s (100 yd) Walk 1 min (100 yd) 9×	Jog 40 s (100 yd) Walk 1 min (100 yd) 9×	Off	Jog 40 s (100 yd) Walk 1 min (100 yd) 9×	Jog 40 s (100 yd) Walk 1 min (100 yd) 9×	Off	Jog 40 s (100 yd) Walk 1 min (100 yd) 9×
2	Jog 1 min (150 yd) Walk 1 min (100 yd) 8×	Jog 1 min (150 yd) Walk 1 min (100 yd) 8×	Jog 1 min (150 yd) Walk 1 min (100 yd) 8×	Off	Jog 1 min (150 yd) Walk 1 min (100 yd) 8×	Jog 1 min (150 yd) Walk 1 min (100 yd) 8×	Off
3	Jog 2 min (300 yd) Walk 1 min (100 yd) 6×	Jog 2 min (300 yd) Walk 1 min (100 yd) 6×	Off	Jog 2 min (300 yd) Walk 1 min (100 yd) 6×	Jog 2 min (300 yd) Walk 1 min (100 yd) 6×	Off	Jog 2 min (300 yd) Walk 1 min (100 yd) 6×
4	Jog 4 min (600 yd) Walk 1 min (100 yd) 4×	Off	Jog 4 min (600 yd) Walk 1 min (100 yd) 4×	Jog 4 min (600 yd) Walk 1 min (100 yd) 4×	Off	Jog 4 min (600 yd) Walk 1 min (100 yd) 4×	Jog 4 min (600 yd) Walk 1 min (100 yd) 4×
5	Jog 6 min (900 yd) Walk 1 min (100 yd) 3×	Jog 6 min (900 yd) Walk 1 min (100 yd) 3×	Off	Jog 6 min (900 yd) Walk 1 min (100 yd) 3×	Jog 6 min (900 yd) Walk 1 min (100 yd) 3×	Off	Jog 6 min (900 yd) Walk 1 min (100 yd) 3×
6	Jog 8 min (1,200 yd) Walk 2 min (200 yd) 2×	Off	Jog 8 min (1,200 yd) Walk 2 min (200 yd) 2×	Jog 8 min (1,200 yd) Walk 2 min (200 yd) 2×	Off	Jog 8 min (1,200 yd) Walk 2 min (200 yd) 2×	Jog 8 min (1,200 yd) Walk 2 min (200 yd) 2×
7	Jog 10 min (1,500 yd) Walk 2 min (200 yd) 2×	Jog 10 min (1,500 yd) Walk 2 min (200 yd) 2×	Off	Jog 10 min (1,500 yd) Walk 2 min (200 yd) 2×	Jog 10 min (1,500 yd) Walk 2 min (200 yd) 2×	Off	Jog 10 min (1,500 yd) Walk 2 min (200 yd) 2×
8	Jog 12 min (1,760 yd) Walk 2 min (200 yd) 2×	Off	Jog 12 min (1,760 yd) Walk 2 min (200 yd) 2×	Jog 12 min (1,760 yd) Walk 2 min (200 yd) 2×	Off	Jog 12 min (1,760 yd) Walk 2 min (200 yd) 2×	Jog 12 min (1,760 yd) Walk 2 min (200 yd) 2×

Walk briskly at an RPE of 11 to 12. Jog at an RPE of 13 to 15. Meters = yards × .91.

Intermediate Jog–Run Program

If you've followed the red, white, and blue programs or are already reasonably active, you're ready for the intermediate program (see figure 7.4). You're able to jog 1 mile (1.6 kilometers) slowly without undue fatigue, rest 2 minutes, and do it again. Your sessions consume about 250 calories.

You're ready to increase both the intensity and the duration of your runs. You'll be using the rating of perceived exertion to determine intensity. You'll begin by jogging 1 mile (1.6 kilometers) in 12 minutes, and when you finish this program you may be able to complete 3 miles (4.8 kilometers) or more at a pace approaching 8 to 10 minutes per mile (5 to 6 minutes per kilometer). Each week's program includes three phases—the basic workout, longer runs (overdistance), and shorter runs (underdistance). If the program for a particular week seems too easy, move ahead; if it seems too hard, move back 1 or 2 weeks. On most of the days, you'll jog in intervals and walk to recover. For example, on Tuesday of the first week, begin by jogging .25 to .5 mile (.4 to .8 kilometer) slowly. Then try to jog .5 mile (.8 kilometer) in 5 minutes, 30 seconds, walk to recover, and repeat. Next, jog .25 mile (.4 kilometer) in 2 minutes, 45 seconds, walk to recover, and repeat three times. Finally, jog .25 to .5 mile (.4 to .8 kilometer) as you did in the beginning of the workout. On Thursday, jog 1 mile (1.6 kilometers) in 12 minutes, walk to recover, and repeat. Remember to warm up and cool down as part of every exercise session.

Advanced Aerobic Training

This section is for the well-trained person. We'll provide some suggestions for advanced training, but keep in mind that there is no single way to train. If you enjoy underdistance training, use it. If you find that you prefer overdistance, use that approach. By simply picking up the pace as you approach the end of a long run, you'll receive the optimal training stimulus. Moreover, because the speed work is limited to a short span near the end of the run, discomfort is brief.

Consider the following suggestions to help make your training session safe and productive.

- Always warm up before your run.
- Stretch after warm-up.
- Periodically train at RPE of 15 to 16.
- Vary the location, intensity, and distance of your runs (long or short, fast or slow, hilly or flat).
- Set distance goals:

Phase 1	20 miles (32.2 kilometers) per week
Phase 2	25 miles (40.2 kilometers) per week (ready for 3- to 5-mile, or 4.8- to 8-kilometer, road races)
Phase 3	30 miles (48.3 kilometers) per week
Phase 4	35 miles (56.3 kilometers) per week (ready for 5- to 7-mile, or 8- to 11.3-kilometer, road races)
Phase 5	40 miles (64.4 kilometers) per week
Phase 6	45 miles (72.4 kilometers) per week (ready for 7- to 10-mile, or 11.3- to 16.1-kilometer, road races)
Phase 7	More than 50 miles (80 kilometers) per week (ready for longer races such as the half marathon—13.1 miles, or 21.1 kilometers)

Figure 7.4 Intermediate Jog–Run Program

Week	Monday	Tuesday	Wednesday	Thursday	Friday	Saturday and Sunday
1	1 mi jog (13–14) Walk 3–4 min 2×	1/2 mi slow jog (13) 2× 1/2 mi (14) 4× 1/4 mi (15) 1/2 mi slow jog (13)	2 mi slow jog (13)	1 mi jog (13–14) Walk 3–4 min 2×	1/2 mi slow jog (13) 2× 1/2 mi (14) 4× 1/4 mi (15) 1/2 mi slow jog (13)	2 mi slow jog (13)
2	1 mi jog (13–14) Walk 3–4 min 2× Your mile time should be about 10–15 s faster than week 1.	1/2 mi slow jog (13) 1/2 mi (14) 2× 1/4 mi (16) 2× 1/4 mi (15) 4× 220 yd (15-16) 1/2 mi slow jog (13)	Brisk walk 30–60 min (12)	1 mi jog (13–14) Walk 3–4 min 2× Your mile time should be about 10–15 s faster than week 1.	1/2 mi slow jog (13) 1/2 mi (14) 2× 1/4 mi (16) 2× 1/4 mi (15) 4× 220 yd (15–16) 1/2 mi slow jog (13)	2 1/4 mi slow jog (13) or Brisk walk 30–60 min (12)
3	1 mi jog (13–14) Walk 3–4 min 2× Your mile time should be about 5–10 s faster than week 2.	1/2 mi slow jog (13) 1/2 mi (15) 4× 1/4 mi (14) 4× 220 yd (16) 4× 100 yd (16) 1/2 mi slow jog (13)	2 1/2 mi slow jog (13) or Brisk walk 30–60 min (12)	1 mi jog (13–14) Walk 3–4 min 2× Your mile time should be about 5–10 s faster than week 2.	1/2 mi slow jog (13) 1/2 mi (15) 4× 1/4 mi (14) 4× 220 yd (16) 4× 100 yd (16) 1/2 mi slow jog (13)	2 1/2 mi slow jog (13) or Brisk walk 30–60 min (12)
4	1 mi jog (13–15) Walk 3–4 min 2× Your mile time should be about 5–10 s faster than week 3.	1/2 mi slow jog (13) 2× 1/2 mi (14) 4× 1/4 mi (16) 4× 220 yd (15) 1/2 mi slow jog (13)	2 3/4 mi slow jog (13) or Brisk walk 45–70 min (12)	1 mi jog (13–15) Walk 3–4 min 2× Your mile time should be about 5–10 s faster than week 3.	1/2 mi slow jog (13) 2× 1/2 mi (14) 4× 1/4 mi (16) 4× 220 yd (15) 1/2 mi slow jog (13)	2 3/4 mi slow jog (13) or Brisk walk 45–70 min (12)
5 Easier week	1 mi jog (13–14) Walk 3–5 min 2× Your mile time should be about the same as the previous week.	Off	3 mi slow jog (13)	1 mi jog (13–14) Walk 3–5 min 2× Your mile time should be about the same as the previous week.	1/2 mi slow jog (13) 1/2 mi (15) 4× 1/4 mi (16) 4× 220 yd (15) 4× 100 yd (14) 1/2 mi slow jog (13)	Brisk walk 45–70 min (11–12)
6 Harder week	1 1/2 mi jog (13–15) Maintain same pace as weeks 4 and 5	1/2 mi slow jog (13) 2× 1/2 mi (15) 4× 1/4 mi (16) 4× 220 yd (15) 4× 100 yd (16) 1/2 mi slow jog (13)	3 mi slow jog (13) increasing the pace the last 5–8 min (15)	1 1/2 mi jog (13–15) Walk 5–6 min 2× Maintain same pace as weeks 4 and 5.	1/2 mi slow jog (13) 2× 1/2 mi (15) 4× 1/4 mi (16) 4× 220 yd (15) 4× 100 yd (16) 1/2 mi slow jog (13)	4 mi slow jog (13)

Values in parentheses are RPE units (see table 6.2). Meters = yards × .91. Kilometers = miles × 1.61.

(continued)

Figure 7.4 *(continued)*

Week	Monday	Tuesday	Wednesday	Thursday	Friday	Saturday and Sunday
7 Medium week	1 mi jog (14–15) Walk 3–5 min 2× Your mile time should be about 5–10 s faster than the previous 3 weeks.	1/2 mi slow jog (13) 2× 1/2 mi (15) 3× 1/4 mi (16) 3× 220 yd (15) 1/2 mi slow jog (13)	3 mi slow jog (13)	1 mi jog (14–15) Walk 3–5 min 2× Your mile time should be about 5-10 s faster than the previous 3 weeks.	1/2 mi slow jog (13) 2× 1/2 mi (15) 3× 1/4 mi (16) 3× 220 yd (15) 1/2 mi slow jog (13)	3 1/2 mi slow jog (13)
8 Hard week	1 mi jog (15) Walk 3–5 min 1 mi jog (14) 2× The first mile of each set should be slightly faster than week 7.	1/2 mi slow jog (13) 2× 1/2 mi (15) 4× 1/4 mi (16) 4× 220 yd (16) 4× 100 yd (15) 1/2 mi slow jog (13)	3 1/2 mi slow jog (13)	1 mi jog (15) Walk 3–5 min 1 mi jog (14) 2× The first mile of each set should be slightly faster than week 7.	Off	5 mi slow jog (13)
9 Easy week	1 mi jog (14) Walk 3–5 min 2× Your mile time should be about the same as week 7.	1/2 mi slow jog (13) 2× 1/2 mi (15) 3× 1/4 mi (15) 4× 220 yd (16) 4× 50 yd (16) 1/2 mi slow jog (13)	3 mi slow jog (13)	1 mi jog (14) Walk 3–5 min 2× Your mile time should be about the same as week 7.	1/2 mi slow jog (13) 2× 1/2 mi (15) 3× 1/4 mi (15) 4× 220 yd (16) 4× 50 yd (16) 1/2 mi slow jog (13)	4 mi slow jog (13)
10 Harder week	1 1/2 mi jog (13–15) Walk 4–6 min 2× Maintain same pace as week 9.	1/2 mi slow jog (13) 2× 1/2 mi (16) 3× 1/4 mi (14) 4× 220 yd (17) 1/2 mi slow jog (13)	4 mi slow jog (13), increasing the pace the last 8–10 min (15)	1 1/2 mi jog (13–15) Walk 4–6 min 2× Maintain same pace as week 9.	1/2 mi slow jog (13) 2× 1/2 mi (16) 3× 1/4 mi (14) 4× 220 yd (17) 1/2 mi slow jog (13)	6 mi slow jog (13)
11 Medium week	1 mi jog (14–15) Walk 3–5 min 3× Your mile time should be about 10 s faster than week 10.	1/2 mi slow jog (13) 4× 1/2 mi (15) 4× 1/4 mi (16) 2× 220 yd (17) 1/2 mi slow jog (13)	4 mi slow jog (13)	Off	1/2 mi slow jog (13) 4× 1/2 mi (15) 4× 1/4 mi (16) 2× 220 yd (17) 1/2 mi slow jog (13)	5 mi slow jog (13)
12 Hard week	1 1/2 mi jog (13–15) Walk 4–6 min 2× Maintain same pace as week 11.	1/2 mi slow jog (13) 5× 1/2 mi (16) 4× 1/4 mi (15) 4× 220 yd (16) 2× 100 yd (17) 1/2 mi slow jog (13)	4 mi easy jog (13), increasing the pace the last 8–10 min (15)	1 1/2 mi jog (13–15) Walk 4–6 min 2× Maintain same pace as week 11.	1/2 mi slow jog (13) 5× 1/2 mi (16) 4× 1/4 mi (15) 4× 220 yd (16) 2× 100 yd (17) 1/2 mi slow jog (13)	6 mi slow jog (13–14)

Values in parentheses are RPE units (see table 6.2). Meters = yards × .91. Kilometers = miles × 1.61.

- Don't be a slave to your goals, and don't increase weekly distance unless you enjoy it.
- Run 6 days per week if you like. Otherwise, try an alternate-day schedule with longer runs.
- Try one long run (not more than one-third of weekly distance) on Saturday or Sunday.
- Try two shorter runs if the long ones seem difficult. Try 5 plus 5 instead of 10.
- Every third or fourth week do an easier week as a way to recover physically and mentally.
- Keep records if you like. You'll be surprised! Record date, distance, and comments. Note morning pulse and body weight. At least once per year, check your performance over a measured distance to observe progress. Use a local road race or the 1.5-mile (2.4-kilometer) run test (see chapter 4, pages 83-84). Check your fitness several times per year.
- Don't train with a stopwatch. Wear a wristwatch so that you'll know how long you've run.
- Increase speed as you approach the finish of a run.
- Always cool down after a run.

Cycling and Swimming Programs

This section provides training programs for cyclists and swimmers. The programs combine the training concepts outlined earlier and the principles of training described in chapter 15 to provide safe, effective, and interesting approaches to fitness. Use the programs to improve fitness, but when you are satisfied with your level of fitness, switch to a maintenance program. You need not improve fitness to a high level; health benefits are available to those who remain active.

Cycling Program

This program uses a training menu to guide your progress (see figure 7.5). The weekly training menu includes the following:

Monday	Easy distance—ride at a comfortable pace (RPE = 13).
Tuesday	Pace—cycle at a brisk pace (RPE = 15).
Wednesday	Hills—include hills to build stamina (RPE = 14).
Thursday	Intervals—push harder for brief intervals (RPE = 15). Increase to RPE = 16 after 4 weeks.
Friday	Overdistance—go easy to develop endurance (RPE = 11).
Saturday	Variety—try a different activity (e.g., tennis or hiking) or ride a trail.
Sunday	Rest—or try a light activity (e.g., gardening or walking).

After 8 weeks design your own program using elements from this plan or others that you enjoy. Plan a long trip with friends and do your training rides together.

Figure 7.5   Weekly Cycling Program

	WEEK							
	1	**2**	**3**	**4**	**5**	**6**	**7**	**8**
Monday	30 min	40	50	40	50	60	70	60
Tuesday	2 × 10 min	2 × 15	2 × 20	3 × 10	3 × 15	3 × 20	4 × 10	4 × 15
Wednesday	15 min	20	25	20	2 × 15	2 × 20	2 × 25	3 × 20
Thursday	3 × 3 min	3 × 4	3 × 5	3 × 6	4 × 3	4 × 4	4 × 5	5 × 5
Friday	60 min	70	80	75	90	100	110	120

Always wear a helmet; ride easy to warm up.
Pace: Ride 10 min, relax and recover, ride another set. Hills: Include some standing but try to keep RPE = 14. Intervals: Ride one, cycle easy to recover, and ride the next. Overdistance: Ride easy; stop for rest and fluids every 30 min.

Note: When using a stationary bicycle, use a fan for ventilation or place the bicycle in a cool room to enhance the experience and allow a full workout (VanSchuylenbergh, VandenEynde, and Hespel 2004).

Swimming Program

This program assumes a certain amount of skill in swimming (see figure 7.6). If the program seems too difficult for your level of ability, scale it down and take lessons to improve your skill and efficiency.

The weekly training menu includes the following:

Monday	Easy distance—go easy at a comfortable pace (RPE = 12).
Tuesday	Pace—swim at a firm pace (RPE = 15).
Wednesday	Arms or legs—swim with arms or legs only (RPE = 13).
Thursday	Intervals—swim harder for brief intervals (RPE = 15). Increase to RPE = 16 after 4 weeks.
Friday	Overdistance—relax on a longer swim (RPE = 11).
Saturday	Variety—try a different activity or water games (e.g., water polo).
Sunday	Rest—try a light activity (e.g., gardening or walking).

Figure 7.6   Weekly Swimming Program

	WEEK							
	1	**2**	**3**	**4**	**5**	**6**	**7**	**8**
Monday	15 min	20	25	20	25	30	35	30
Tuesday	2 × 5 min	2 × 6	2 × 7	2 × 8	3 × 6	3 × 7	3 × 8	4 × 5
Wednesday	5 min/each	6/e	7/e	8/e	9/e	10/e	11/e	12/e
Thursday	3 × 3 min	3 × 4	3 × 5	3 × 4	4 × 3	4 × 4	4 × 5	5 × 4
Friday	25 min	30	35	40	35	40	45	50

Use good goggles; warm up well on Tuesday, Wednesday, and Thursday; and swim easy laps after these workouts.
Pace: Swim slowly or walk in the water to recover between sets. Arms and legs: Use a kickboard or flotation device for support. Intervals: Swim slowly or walk to recover between sets.

When you have completed 8 weeks, design your own program using the types of training that you most enjoy. You could even decide to engage in cross-training or train for the triathlon (see chapter 15).

Aerobic Alternatives

When you are unable to engage in your regular activity because of weather or injury, consider an alternative. These examples can also serve as a form of cross-training to reduce the impact of running. Many types of exercise devices are on the market; most end up gathering dust in the basement. Before you buy, use the device for several days and don't buy features that you don't need, such as fancy electronics (for good advice, go to www.acsm.org, the Web page for the American College of Sports Medicine). Finally, use a fan to make the indoor experience more enjoyable.

- **Bicycle.** A good stationary bicycle should be comfortable and offer good adjustment and controls and sufficient resistance to provide a training stimulus, now and in the future. Of course, the bike should also fit your significant other if he or she plans to use it. Some stationary bikes combine cycling with arm exercise, a good idea for someone with a condition like multiple sclerosis. The best allow leg, arm, or combined arm and leg exercise and include a flywheel for resistance and a fan for cooling. A low-cost alternative is a stand for your outdoor bike.

- **Treadmill.** Treadmills range from less expensive nonmotorized devices to sturdy motor-driven machines and devices that combine some arm exercise. Be sure that you like the feel of the machine, that it is well built and guaranteed, and that it is capable of sufficient elevation and speed to provide a training stimulus, now and in the future. Also, be aware that some machines may require a new electrical circuit in your home.

- **Cross-country ski device.** Ski simulators are widely advertised. Be sure that you try before you buy. Then buy a reputable brand known for durability. Consult the want ads in your local paper for a secondhand device.

- **Rowing machine.** Better-quality models use a flywheel instead of adjustable shock absorbers to control resistance. Rowing machines combine upper- and lower-body work (as do other devices such as ski simulators). The combined exercises allow you to burn more calories per minute than you do with leg-only exercise, without raising the perception of exertion.

- **Stair climber.** Popular in health clubs, these are now available for home purchase. Look for a sturdy, brand-name model with a good warranty.

- **Elliptical device.** An effective device for reducing impact forces during aerobic exercise, elliptical trainers are becoming popular at health clubs. Again, look for a brand-name device with a good warranty.

- **Rope skipping.** A skipping rope is inexpensive, easy to transport, can be done anywhere, and accommodates a wide range of intensity and skill. The ends of the rope should reach your armpits when you stand on the center of the rope. Use a length of number 10 sash cord or buy a jumping rope and go for it. Just be careful to avoid overexertion while you are learning the skills.

- **Racewalking.** This Olympic event is an interesting alternative to running. The distinctive heel-to-toe gait is a complex skill that takes time to learn properly. For instructions and training programs consult a good book, such as *USA Track & Field Coaching Manual* (2000) from Human Kinetics (www.hkusa.com).

> You have no excuse for stopping exercise because of weather or injury.

■ **Other alternatives.** Other aerobic alternatives include slide boards; aerobic dance; step aerobics; some martial arts; swing or Western dance; and the best low-impact activity, swimming. Runners can swim, or they can run in the deep end of the pool while they wait for injuries to heal. In other words, you have no excuse for stopping exercise because of weather or injury.

Exercise Problems

Previously inactive adults often encounter problems when they begin exercise. You can avoid such problems if you make haste slowly. It took you years to get out of shape, and you won't be able to reverse the trend overnight. Plan for gradual progress; at the start, too little may be better than too much. After several weeks, when your body has begun to adjust to the demands of vigorous effort, you'll be ready to increase your exercise intensity or duration. Another way to avoid exercise problems is to warm up before each session. Careful attention to warming up and stretching eliminates many of the nagging complications that plague less patient people. Don't forget to cool down after each workout.

Prevention is the best way to deal with exercise problems. When a problem arises, treat the cause, not just the symptom. If your knee hurts, put ice on it, but don't stop there. Find out why it hurts (e.g., old shoes) and correct the problem.

Common Injuries

You can deal with many of the injuries that threaten to diminish your enjoyment of training. People who engage in regular exercise may experience the following problems, but by taking a few precautions, you can prevent minor injuries before they arise.

■ **Blisters.** Blisters are minor burns caused by friction. You can prevent them by using properly fitted shoes, appropriate socks (double-layer or tube socks), and a lubricant (e.g., bag balm) on potential hot spots. At the first hint of a potential blister, cover the area with duct tape, that's right, duct tape. We've found that a tape job can last for several days of backcountry hiking or skiing. Treat advanced cases with a sterilized hollow needle. Release the fluid, treat with an antiseptic, circle the area with a foam rubber donut, and go back to work. Keep a blister prevention kit in your locker or gym bag and always carry the kit on hiking trips.

■ **Muscle soreness.** Delayed-onset muscle soreness (DOMS) develops about 24 hours after you perform a new or more vigorous exercise. DOMS occurs in the muscles involved and may be due to microscopic tears in the muscle or connective tissue, to swelling, or to localized contractions of muscle fibers (Armstrong 1984). You can minimize the soreness by phasing into a sport gradually. Mild stretching and warming up make subsequent activity less painful. Massage seems to reduce the discomfort. The good news is that DOMS is a temporary inconvenience that inoculates you from further discomfort for several months—at least until you start a new sport.

- **Muscle cramps.** A cramp is a powerful involuntary contraction that results when the muscle refuses to relax. Normally, the nervous system tells muscles when to contract and when to relax, but when the normal control fails, the result can be painful. Immediate relief comes when you stretch and massage the cramped muscle. But that process does not remove the underlying cause of the involuntary contraction. Salt and calcium are involved in the chemistry of contraction and relaxation. Hot temperatures and dehydration seem to predispose muscles to cramps. Attend to fluid and electrolyte replacement during activity in hot weather.

- **Bone bruises.** Hikers and joggers sometimes get painful bruises on the soles of their feet. You can avoid such bruises with careful foot placement and quality footwear. Cushioned inner soles and gel- or air-sole shoes can aid in reducing the repetitive shocks that lead to bruises. A bad bruise can last for weeks. Ice may lessen discomfort, and padding may allow some activity. When bruises occur, examine your shoes. It may be time to replace them or try a cushioned heel cup or inner sole.

- **Ankle problems.** Treatment for a sprained ankle involves RICES (see the subsequent list). Ice the ankle immediately, preferably in a bucket of ice water. Ice several times a day, and in between, rest and elevate the ankle. Use a wrap to stabilize and maintain compression. When possible, use high-top shoes to prevent ankle problems. Tape or lace-on supports may allow some activity after the swelling subsides.

Rest

Ice

Compression

Elevation

Stabilization

- **Calf or Achilles tendon injuries.** Do not ignore a pulling sensation in the calf or Achilles tendon. Treat minor pulls with rest, ice, and gel heel cups. Return to activity cautiously; a serious pull can take weeks to heal. Prevent calf or Achilles problems with adequate stretching, good footwear, and a gradual warm-up.

- **Shin splints.** Pain on the front portion of the shinbones is known as shin splints. It can be caused by inflammation of the tibialis anterior muscle, its membrane, or the bone it attaches to, or a spasm of the inflamed muscle. Rest, compression wraps, deep massage (toward the heart), ultrasound, and anti-inflammatory drugs (e.g., ibuprofen) provide some relief. Prevention involves gradual adjustment to training, avoidance of hard running surfaces, occasional reversal of direction when running on a curved track, use of the heel-to-toe foot strike, resistance exercises, and stretching.

- **Knee problems.** Research suggests that running doesn't harm healthy knees. Unfortunately, many of us run on less than healthy knees, knees already afflicted with osteoarthritis. Heavy physical loading (occupation or sport) increases the risk of knee osteoarthritis and cumulative physical stress has a deleterious effect on the joint (Manninen et al. 2002). A high school football injury left one of us with an arthritic knee. The knee is ACL deficient, and the cartilage was removed 40 years ago. Surprisingly, Brian continues to run with the help of several aids: weight training to stabilize thigh and hamstring muscles, cycling to add strength and endurance without trauma, orthotics (foot supports), and a nonsteroidal anti-inflammatory drug (NSAID) such as

Prevent pain from interrupting your training by correcting the causes and treating the symptoms of knee problems.

aspirin or ibuprofen to quiet inflammation and discomfort in the degenerative joint. Overuse (e.g., a long hike or run) calls for a bit more of the NSAID until things cool down. Recently, glucosamine has decreased the need for NSAIDs.

If you experience runner's knee or some other problem, correct the cause while you treat the symptom. Try new shoes or arch supports. Alternate between two pairs of shoes if you run a lot, one with padding for sore feet and the other with a flexible sole for sore legs. If these ideas don't help, consult an athletic trainer or a podiatrist who specializes in sports medicine. Specialists may recommend orthotics to alleviate your problem. These plastic inserts can correct pronation and reduce some knee pain.

■ **Stitch.** The side pain called a stitch, usually blamed on food or fluid in the digestive system, may be due to tugging of ligaments that attach the gut to the diaphragm. A treadmill study induced the stitch by giving the subjects a drink and then used several techniques to reduce their discomfort. Bending forward while tightening the abdominal muscles, exhaling through pursed lips, or tightening a belt around the waist were dramatically effective treatments. The authors suggested that the results were consistent with a ligamentous origin for the stitch (Plunkett and Hopkins 1995).

Overuse Syndromes

If you go too far or too fast too soon, if you forget to stretch or warm up, if you have muscle imbalances, if one leg is shorter than the other, or if you have weak feet, you are bound to have overuse problems now and then. Use ice for all acute strains and sprains. Keep an ice "Popsicle" in the freezer and use it several times a day to reduce inflammation and hasten recovery (tape a tongue depressor upright in a Styrofoam cup of water and put it in the freezer). Rub the problem area with ice until it becomes numb. You'll be amazed by your rapid return to activity.

Exercise Hazards

Regular, moderate physical activity is an established aid to health, fitness, weight control, and longevity. All of us understand the term *regular*, but the concept of *moderate* requires definition. Moderate exercise for an athlete may be hazardous for the sedentary adult. We can define moderate exercise as a level likely to bring about improved fitness without exposing the person to the hazards of strenuous effort.

Nonsteroidal Anti-Inflammatory Drugs

The careful use of the nonsteroidal anti-inflammatory drugs (NSAIDs) aspirin and ibuprofen helps minimize many nagging problems and some big ones. With a doctor's advice, one of us started taking aspirin more than 30 years ago to quiet that painful knee. Then we learned that one pill a day reduces blood clotting and the risk of heart attack. Aspirin also reduces the little strokes (transient ischemic attacks) that become more prevalent with age. Ibuprofen, which is good for muscle and joint pain, has been associated with lower risk of Alzheimer's disease. Both drugs cause stomach irritation, and some people are allergic to aspirin. When taken in small doses with food to minimize stomach irritation, however, aspirin or ibuprofen offers amazing relief for the price.

Aspirin reduces pain and inflammation by inhibiting the production of cell hormones called prostaglandins. Exercise can cause prostaglandin production, which may lead to soreness. A single NSAID before exercise can reduce the need for larger doses afterward. Judicious use of NSAIDs keeps many aging athletes active long after others have given up. Because ibuprofen interferes with some beneficial aspects of aspirin, you should not take them at the same time.

Sudden Vigorous Exercise

Failure to warm up before vigorous exercise can result in electrocardiogram abnormalities, regardless of the fitness or age of the subject. Dr. Barnard found such abnormalities in 31 of 44 apparently healthy firefighters tested on a vigorous treadmill test. The findings indicated inadequate blood flow in the coronary arteries and lack of oxygen to the heart. A warm-up consisting of a 5-minute jog prevented the problems (Barnard et al. 1972). Athletes aren't the only ones who need to warm up. Anyone performing vigorous work or exercise can benefit. Callisthenic warm-ups are common among factory workers in Europe and Japan but less common in the United States. Although most workers can and should warm up, it is hard to see, for example, how law enforcement officers can do so before chasing a suspect. For this reason police officers should do all they can to keep fit and healthy.

Stressful Exercise

Stress is something that a person perceives as a threat. The body reacts to the threat by secreting a group of hormones that assist the mobilization of energy and prepare the body for combat or retreat (fight or flight). The body does not differentiate between physical and mental threats; it reacts similarly to each. An important exam may be stressful to a medical student, and a canoe trip could be stressful to a nonswimmer. Stress accelerates clotting time of the blood, which is good for a soldier in battle or a boxer in the ring, but bad for an adult with atherosclerosis, for whom a clot could block the flow of blood to the heart. Although exercise is not inherently stressful, studies indicate that unfamiliar, exhausting, and competitive exercise can be stressful for some people.

UNFAMILIAR EXERCISE   A person's first skiing or mountain-climbing experience may be stressful, but the stress diminishes as skill and confidence grow. We found faster clotting time on a subject's first treadmill test but normal clotting after weeks of experience, when the test was no longer perceived as a threat (Whiddon, Sharkey,

Learn new types of exercise gradually to avoid potential hazards.

and Steadman 1969). Early experiences in unfamiliar or threatening exercise situations, such as whitewater kayaking, should be preceded with less-threatening introductions, such as a session in a pool.

EXHAUSTING EXERCISE   In experiments on dogs, a Japanese researcher found that exhaustion could be stressful (Suzuki 1967). A bike-riding attendant took the animals for runs of various intensities and durations. Only exhausting runs increased the secretion of stress hormones. The researcher concluded that nonexhausting exercise need not be stressful. Of course, the dogs' fears of being left behind may have caused at least some of the stress associated with exhaustion.

COMPETITIVE EXERCISE   Years ago, researchers at Harvard University studied stress responses to various types of competition in rowers. Crew members did not perceive the strenuous effort of practice as a threat, but they did demonstrate increased hormone levels after either a time trial or a competitive race. The nonexercising coxswain also exhibited a stress response after the competitive event. The researchers concluded that exercise, by itself, was not stressful, but the excitement of competition did elicit the response, with or without exertion (Hill, Goetz, and Fox 1956).

The hormones of the stress response are required for the full mobilization of resources and the maximal performance of the athlete. We would never suggest that healthy men or women avoid the excitement of unfamiliar, exhausting, or competitive activity. Previously inactive people, however, should prepare for participation with gradual adaptation to the stress involved. In time, the unfamiliar becomes familiar, training reduces exhaustion, and the athlete within learns to cope with the physical and psychological requirements of competition.

> For many, the excitement of sport keeps them active.

Indeed, adults regularly engage in stressful activities. For many, the excitement of sport keeps them active. Those who thrive on challenge, excitement, or exhaustion do so after long periods of preparation. Aging athletes continue to practice and train so that they can remain competitive. If you want to become involved in competitive tennis, distance running, or mountain biking, give yourself time to adjust to the demands. Improve your fitness and skill as you prepare for your first exposure. Set reasonable goals and never take the results too seriously.

Summary

This chapter has presented training tips; walking, running, and other training programs; aerobic alternatives; and advice on how to handle some common problems. You are welcome to adopt one of the programs or to use your aerobic prescription and fashion your own approach. We're often amazed by the ingenious and personal approaches that some folks devise—such as the retired zoology professor who regularly climbed the mountain behind our campus, both for exercise and to observe the flora and fauna. Years ago, before it was in vogue, he used ski poles to exercise his arms while lowering the load on his legs. The poles become even more important on the return trip, relieving stress on his knees during the steep descent. His creative adaptation extended his range and saved his knees for many years of enjoyable outdoor exercise.

Another way to avoid common problems is to include attention to muscular fitness training. We'll see how it can help you in the next chapter.

Part III

Muscular Fitness

Not too many years ago, muscular fitness occupied an awkward position on the fringe of the fitness movement. We recognized its contributions to performance in sport and some forms of work, but we lacked conclusive evidence linking muscular fitness with health and the quality of life. That situation has now changed, and we can say with confidence that both aerobic fitness and muscular fitness contribute substantially to health. Muscular fitness training increases muscle mass, the furnace that burns fat. Exercises that improve muscular fitness help you avoid the crippling bone demineralization known as osteoporosis. Attention to muscular fitness is essential if you are to avoid the low-back problems and repetitive motion injuries that plague millions of Americans. Continued participation ensures the capacity for independence and mobility in your postretirement years.

The essential components of muscular fitness are strength, muscular endurance, and flexibility. Other important components include power, speed, agility, and balance. With most physiologic capabilities, you either use them or lose them, and that is certainly true for muscular fitness. Strength, endurance, flexibility, power, agility, and balance all decline with age. But the rate of decline is much slower for those who remain active. And numerous studies show that we have the capability to build strength even into our 90s (Fiatarone et al. 1994)!

But don't wait until you are 90 to experience the pleasures and rewards of muscular fitness. Begin now. You will soon notice that tasks are easier, your muscles are firmer, your tummy is flatter, and you feel better about yourself and life in general.

Understanding Muscular Fitness

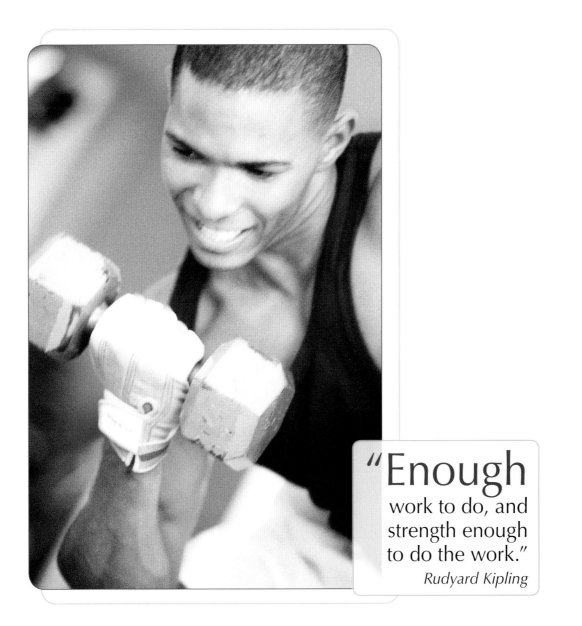

Enough work to do, and strength enough to do the work."

Rudyard Kipling

For many years muscular fitness didn't get the respect it deserves, partly because of images of overdeveloped, muscle-bound physiques. Now we can honestly say that aerobic and muscular fitness both contribute to health, but they do so in different ways and at different times. Young folks use muscular fitness to improve performance in a favorite sport or activity, or to look good in a bathing suit. Middle-aged individuals rely on abdominal tone and flexibility exercises to prevent or minimize low-back problems. Older folks employ strength and endurance activities to retain bone density and to remain active and independent, capable of performing important activities of daily living. Muscular fitness is essential if you are to avoid the low-back problems that plague millions of Americans. In recent years we have learned that muscular fitness training (e.g., resistance or weight training) is a good way to avoid the crippling bone demineralization known as osteoporosis. And we've learned that muscular fitness helps maintain the muscle that you need to burn fat and to sustain mobility well into retirement years. So if you intend to remain active after retirement, you'd better add muscular fitness training to your fitness program.

We begin with a consideration of the primary components of muscular fitness—strength, muscular endurance, and flexibility. These are called primary components because they are the ones most related to health. We'll cover other components, such as speed, power, agility, balance, and coordination, later in the chapter. First, let's briefly consider the structure of the muscle.

This chapter will help you

- identify the components of muscular fitness;
- understand the factors that influence strength;
- differentiate between strength and muscular endurance;
- understand the importance of flexibility; and
- determine how muscular fitness contributes to health, total fitness, and performance.

Muscle Structure

Each muscle contains many thousands of spaghetti-like muscle fibers, ranging from 1 to over 30 centimeters (.4 to 12 inches) in length. The fibers contain the contractile proteins actin and myosin. Muscles shorten and produce movement when the actin and myosin filaments creep or slide along each other. Cross-bridges extending from the thicker myosin to the thinner actin filaments perform this creeping. The cross-bridges reach out, make contact, and pull like oars. The barely perceptible movement produced in one location adds to movement produced along the length of the fiber, and visible motion takes place. Because the muscles attach to bony lever systems, the modest muscle shortening is multiplied to produce familiar movement patterns (see figure 8.1).

Muscle fibers contract at the command of the motor nerve. Because each motor nerve branches many times, the typical nerve activates 150 individual muscle fibers simultaneously. The motor nerve and the muscle fibers it commands make up a motor unit.

Human muscle is composed of two fiber types. All the fibers in a motor unit are of the same type—either fast twitch or slow twitch. Fast-twitch fibers are fast contracting and fast to fatigue. They are larger and have fewer capillaries than slow-twitch fibers do and seem best suited to short, intense effort. Slow-twitch muscle fibers contract somewhat more slowly but also are slow to fatigue. They have a rich capillary supply and a generous stock of the internal chemistry required for long-duration endurance activities. When the nervous system commands a motor unit to contract, all the fibers respond together. The way that the nervous system uses muscle fibers (for short, intense effort or for long-duration effort) seems to dictate their characteristics (see table 8.1).

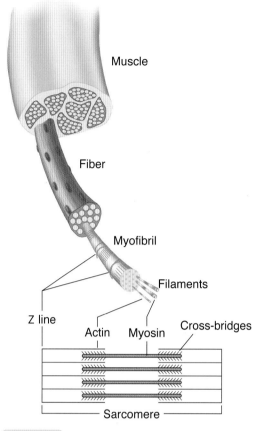

Figure 8.1 Architecture of the muscle.
Reprinted from Sharkey, 1975.

Table 8.1   Characteristics of Muscle Fibers

Characteristics	Slow oxidative (SO)	Fast oxidative glycolytic (FOG)	Fast glycolytic (FG)
Average fiber percentage	50%	35%	15%
Speed of contraction	Slow	Fast	Fast
Force of contraction	Low	High	High
Size	Smaller	Large	Large
Fatigability	Fatigue resistant	Less resistant	Easily fatigued
Aerobic capacity	High	Medium	Low
Capillary density	High	High	Low
Anaerobic capacity	Low	Medium	High

Reprinted from Sharkey, 2002.

Muscular Strength

Strength is important when your occupation demands it, in certain sports, and—surprisingly—for those over 60 years of age. During the early part of our lives, as we age, strength declines at a slow pace, especially if we use it. But sometime after 55 to 60 years of age, the rate of decline accelerates. Throughout our years we need some strength to avoid acute or chronic injury, to meet emergencies, and to engage fully and independently in life. We need strength to change a flat tire; to shovel the walk; and to lift and carry infants, laundry, or groceries. Lack of muscular fitness leads to less activity, which hastens the loss of strength, and so on in a vicious cycle that ends in a nursing home. But you can reverse this cycle and remain strong and independent well into your eighth decade.

Strength is defined as the maximal force that can be exerted in a single voluntary contraction. Most of us possess more strength than we are able to demonstrate. In a fascinating experiment, Ikai and Steinhaus (1961) showed that significant increases in strength could be elicited with a gunshot, shouting, drugs, or hypnosis during a contraction. Untrained individuals inhibit the full expression of strength. Inhibitions reside in the brain and in inhibitory muscle receptors. One effect of strength training is to reduce inhibitions and allow a fuller expression of available strength.

> Most of us possess more strength than we are able to demonstrate.

Strength, then, is not an absolute value. It is subject to change, and this makes the subject of strength training extremely interesting. When strength improves, how much of the improvement is because of reduced inhibitions and how much is from changes in muscle tissue? Can we find a way to increase strength without spending a lot of time with weights?

Factors Influencing Strength

The force that you exert in a maximal voluntary contraction depends on a number of factors, such as inhibitions, muscle mass or cross-sectional area, the number of contracting fibers and their contractile state (length, fatigue), and the mechanical advantage of the bony lever system. Most of these are easy to explain. More fibers equal more girth and more force, the stretched muscle exerts more force (probably because of elastic recoil and favorable alignment of contractile proteins), the rested muscle exerts more force than a fatigued one, and mechanical factors conspire to magnify force or speed. Several other factors, including gender, age, fiber type, and training deserve more attention.

Gender

Until 12 to 14 years of age, boys are not much stronger than girls. Thereafter, the average male gains an advantage that persists throughout life. Is the difference due to the increase in the male hormone testosterone at puberty? Perhaps; the average male has 10 times the testosterone of the average female. Testosterone is an anabolic (growth-inducing) steroid that helps muscles get larger. College women have 50 to 60 percent of the arm and shoulder strength and 70 percent of the leg strength of their male counterparts. But a relationship doesn't imply cause and effect. The relationship of strength and testosterone might also be related to a third factor. For example, the hormone may make men more aggressive and willing to train harder.

Consider another confounding possibility—body fat. Young women average twice the percentage of fat as men (25 percent versus 12.5 percent). When you look at strength

Strength training can greatly improve women's upper body strength.

per unit of lean body weight (body weight minus fat weight), women have slightly stronger legs, whereas their arm strength remains 30 percent below the values for men. Wilmore (1983) suggests that because women use their legs as men do (walking, climbing stairs, bicycling), their leg muscles are similar in strength. Because fewer women use their arms in heavy work or sport, their strength lags behind in this area. Thus, judging women the weaker sex may be a mistake. As more women engage in upper-body strength training for sport or occupational purposes (law enforcement, firefighting, construction), their strength will certainly come closer to that of men. In fact, recent research with cross-country skiers showed that elite female athletes had 97 percent of the strength of male athletes per unit of lean body mass. When women train their upper bodies, they are comparable with men (Gaskill, personal data from U.S. Ski Team and elite junior skiers).

Muscle size and strength do go together for both genders, however, and the average male is larger than the average female. Most studies indicate a force of 4 to 6 kilograms per square centimeter of muscle girth. To estimate muscle girth in the upper arm, we should measure subcutaneous fat and bone size as well, because they will be part of the total circumference. All other things being equal, the larger muscle is the stronger one, but not necessarily the most successful in work or sport.

Age

Strength reaches a peak in the early 20s and declines slowly until about age 60. Thereafter the rate of decline usually accelerates, but it doesn't have to. When people use their strength, it hardly declines at all, even into the 60s. Champion weight lifters have achieved personal records in their 40s. Auto mechanics retain grip strength into their 60s. Training before puberty leads to improvements that are mostly due to changes in the nervous system (neurogenic factors include reduced inhibitions and learning how to exert force). Training after puberty combines nervous system changes with changes in muscle tissue (myogenic changes). Because testosterone levels decline in old age, many physiologists thought that older people would be able to achieve only neurogenic changes when they engaged in strength training. A study of very elderly people (72 to 98 years), however, has shown that resistance training leads to increased strength, muscle mass, and mobility (Fiatarone et al. 1994). Elderly people who perform strength training achieve increases in protein synthesis, strength, muscle size, and improvements in activities of daily living (Frontera and Bigard 2002). Training at any age maintains or improves strength, especially when diet is adequate. We'll say more about both later on.

> Training at any age maintains or improves strength, especially when diet is adequate.

Muscle Fiber Types

Earlier we noted the presence of two fiber types, slow twitch and fast twitch. The larger, faster contracting fast-twitch fibers have greater potential for rapid development of tension. People with a higher percentage of fast-twitch fibers have greater potential for power development. Studies of human muscle tissue reveal that power lifters have twice the area of fast-twitch fibers that nonlifters do. The size can be attributed to heredity and to training. The effect of strength training on muscle fiber types has yet to be completely resolved. Current evidence indicates that both types grow larger with training, but growth of the fast fibers is more pronounced. Strength training improves the capabilities of both types but doesn't seem to change one type into another.

Although resistance training may not change slow fibers into fast fibers, we are learning that, besides heredity and training, several other factors may influence muscle mass and strength. A recent study shows a positive correlation between birth weight and adult grip strength for 2,775 men and women, even when adjusted for adult body size and social class. The study suggests that birth weight has an important influence on the number of muscle fibers established at birth, and that even in middle age (53 years of age), compensating hypertrophy may be inadequate. As the inevitable loss of muscle fibers proceeds with aging, the deficit in fibers could threaten the quality of life (Kuh et al. 2002).

Measures of Strength

Maintaining adequate strength throughout life is important to our ability to live independently and enjoy life to the fullest. We can measure and develop strength in several ways, each of which is highly specific to how we will use strength and should dictate the mode of training and testing.

Using muscular power during movement is called dynamic strength. Dynamic strength, also called isotonic, is defined as the maximal weight that a person can lift one time. This amount is actually a measure of strength at the hardest part of the lift, usually the beginning. Because the mechanical advantage of your muscle-lever system changes, a lift such as a forearm curl becomes easier after you overcome the initial resistance and angle of pull. Dynamic strength measurements are related to performance in sport and work. Weightlifting with machines or free weights is the common form of isotonic training. (Iso means "same," and tonic means "tone," so isotonic means "same tone.")

Another measure of strength is static strength. A person demonstrates static strength by exerting maximal force against an immovable object. Also called isometric

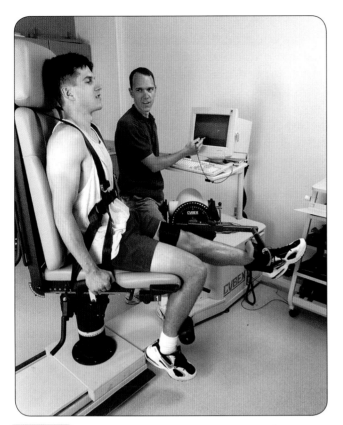

Figure 8.2 Isokinetic strength testing is important for sports medicine and rehabilitation.

strength, it is specific to the angle at which it was trained. Static strength doesn't necessarily reflect dynamic strength or strength throughout the range of motion. You train by exerting near maximum force against an immovable object. (*Metric* means "length," and *isometric* means "same length"—the muscle doesn't change length appreciably during the contraction.)

A popular measure of strength in clinical and rehabilitation settings is isokinetic strength, which is measured with expensive electronic or hydraulic apparatus. The equipment allows the exertion of maximal force throughout the range of motion, as well as the control of the speed of contraction. Although such devices have become popular testing aids, it is not yet clear to what extent strength throughout the range of motion is related to performance. (*Kinetic* means "motion" or "speed," and *isokinetic* means "same speed.") A number of sophisticated devices are available for isokinetic measurement of muscle force and power. Sports medicine specialists test knee extension and flexion strength, power, and endurance and use isokinetic devices to rehabilitate athletes following knee surgery. Variable and accommodating resistance devices are used to strengthen muscles and to prevent injuries (see figure 8.2).

Athletes may use free weights, isokinetic machines, and even isometric contractions to improve performance. Keep in mind that strength is specific to the method of training, to the speed of contractions, and to the angle used in training. Therefore, to obtain an accurate assessment of the effects of training, the method of testing should be specific to the mode of training. In other words, a static strength test will not accurately measure changes from dynamic strength training or vice versa.

Muscular Endurance

An additional component of muscular fitness is muscular endurance. Muscular endurance means the ability to persist. We define and measure it as the repetition of submaximal contractions or submaximal holding time (static or isometric endurance). Muscular endurance is essential for success in many work and sport activities. When you have the strength to perform a repetitive task, additional improvement in performance will depend on muscular endurance, the ability to persist. As mentioned earlier, stronger fast-twitch fibers fatigue more readily. Thus endurance and strength are not highly related, except when a very heavy load is used in an endurance test.

> Muscular endurance is essential for success in many work and sport activities.

We use the term *muscular endurance* to differentiate it from other uses of the term, such as aerobic endurance. A person may develop considerable endurance in small muscles, such as a barber who develops the finger flexors, without achieving any noticeable effect on the heart or respiratory systems. Although a barber is likely to have great endurance in the muscles of the fingers, his or her aerobic fitness may be poor. Muscular endurance resides in metabolic adaptations and neuromuscular efficiency of the fibers used in the activity.

Let's spend a moment contrasting muscular endurance and strength, which are quite different in physiological terms. We achieve muscular endurance by repetitive contractions of muscle fibers. Repetitive contractions require a continuous supply of energy, and muscle fibers with aerobic (oxidative) capabilities (slow oxidative and fast oxidative glycolytic fibers) are suited to the job. Repetitive contractions enhance aerobic enzymes, mitochondria, and fuels needed for repetitive contractions.

Strength comes from lifting heavy loads a few times. As we have said, the effects of strength training are most noticeable in fast-twitch fibers. Training effects include increases in contractile proteins (actin and myosin) and tougher connective tissue. Increased strength comes from greater cross-sectional area, which means that more contractile protein is available to exert force. The type of training and the physiological effects of endurance and strength training are quite different. Keep that in mind as you plan your program. Endurance is important for practice, training, and performance. Repetition leads to skill, and repetition requires endurance, so endurance is one of the keys to success in sport or work.

Flexibility

Flexibility is the range of motion through which the limbs are able to move. Skin, connective tissue, and conditions within joints restrict range of motion, as does excessive body fat. Injury can occur when a limb is forced beyond its normal range. Improved flexibility reduces this potential. Range of motion increases when joints and muscles are warm. Stretching exercises are most successful after some warm-up but

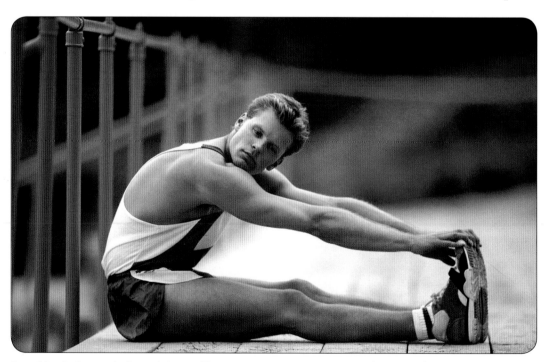

Stretching before and after training and between training sessions can reduce muscle soreness.

before vigorous effort. Stretching after exercise, during the cool-down period, may reduce delayed-onset muscle soreness and improve flexibility for the next workout. Stretching before subsequent activity certainly reduces feelings of tightness and discomfort. Flexibility exercises are important when you are training for strength or endurance. They help you maintain the range of motion that might otherwise decrease. Most runners turn to stretching to make the pastime more enjoyable. Calf, hamstring, groin, and back muscles can become tight and sore, especially after an increase in intensity or duration of training. Daily stretching may mean the difference between enjoyment and discomfort. We have found that the need for stretching increases with age.

Yoga has gained popularity as a way to achieve relaxation and meditative states. When stripped of its mystical elements, yoga emerges as a safe, enjoyable, and relaxing flexibility program. The benefits are typically limited to flexibility. Little evidence supports claims of improved aerobic fitness or significant gains in strength or muscular endurance.

Many fitness instructors believe that flexibility contributes to success in work and sport. It certainly is important in activities like gymnastics, figure skating, and diving, in which range of motion is essential. Lack of flexibility is implicated in the development of acute and chronic injuries, repetitive trauma, and low-back problems. Studies of military recruits show that static stretching did not influence total injury rates. But the incidence of muscle and tendon injuries and low-back pain were significantly lower in the stretching group (Amako et al. 2003). The value of stretching in injury prevention may be more problematic. When the sport demands high range of motion in a joint, stretching seems to be valuable. But when the activity consists of low intensity or contraction cycles (jogging, cycling, swimming), the need for a very compliant muscle–tendon unit is less. In these cases stretching has no beneficial effect on injury prevention (Witvrouw et al. 2004). In addition, when 34 elite runners were examined for flexibility (sit-and-reach test) and running economy, the least flexible runners were the most economical (Jones 2002). Evidence is insufficient either to endorse or to disapprove of routine stretching before or after exercise to prevent injuries in competitive or recreational athletes (Thacker et al. 2004). Some of us may profit from regular stretching exercises. Older folks have a special need, because connective tissue becomes less elastic with age.

> Lack of flexibility is implicated in the development of acute and chronic injuries, repetitive trauma, and low-back problems.

Other Components of Muscular Fitness

Besides strength, muscle endurance, and flexibility, muscular fitness also includes speed, power, agility, balance, and neuromuscular coordination. These components, especially agility and balance, are often important to success in sport or work and may help you avoid serious injury. See whether you need to add them to your program.

Speed

Speed may be the most exciting ingredient in sport. It requires rapid acceleration, which involves the contraction of fast-twitch muscle fibers. Speed of movement includes reaction time and movement time. Reaction time (the time from the stimulus, such as a starting gun, until the beginning of the movement) is a function of the nervous system. We can't change the speed of nerve impulse transmission along a neuron.

Thus the only way to achieve significant improvement in reaction time is by increasing awareness of important stimuli and by repeating appropriate responses, which reduces central nervous system processing time. In sports, coaches use special drills to improve reaction time.

speed of movement = reaction time + movement time

Movement time, the interval from the beginning to the end of the movement, may improve (decrease) with appropriate strength and power training. The key to success lies in the principle of specificity: The movement must be specific to the sport. If you want to throw a baseball with greater velocity, train with light weights at a fast speed (e.g., throw a weighted ball). If you are a shot-putter, throw heavier weights as fast as possible. Specificity applies to the rate of movement and the resistance employed, which means that training should simulate the action as closely as possible.

How much can you improve? Remember what we've said about fast-twitch fibers: You'll need a high percentage to be fast. If you don't have over 50 percent fast fibers, don't despair. You may never be as fast as those with a high percentage, but you can improve your movement time by following the principles presented in the next chapter. But don't conclude that continued improvements in strength will always lead to improvements in movement time. Strength is related to speed when movement is resisted (as in football and shot put), but less so when resistance is light (as in the tennis serve). And remember, speed—like strength—is task specific. The speed of arm movement is not necessarily related to leg speed. Some people may be quick with their hands but, because of lack of training or skill or because of excess weight, may be slow of foot. Improved skill and strength training reduce the time it takes to complete a movement.

Power

Football coaches often talk about power. Power is a combination of strength (force) and velocity or speed. A lineman needs explosive power to move his opponent. But power is important in every sport that requires speed and acceleration. Even cycling and cross-country skiing require power. Lance Armstrong wins because he generates more power in sprints and uphill climbs. Power is defined as work divided by time, or the rate of doing work.

power = force $\times$ distance $\div$ time, or $F \times D \div T$ = force $\times$ velocity (velocity = $D \div T$)

Power combines strength (force) and velocity or speed (distance divided by time). A person who is able to do more work than someone else in the same unit of time has more power. A person who moves 100 kilograms 1 meter in 1 second has done 100 kilogram-meters of work per second. If you move the same load 2 meters in 1 second or 1 meter in .5 second, you've exhibited twice as much power. Thus power is related to strength and velocity (distance divided by time). Improve them and you'll increase power.

Power is important in a number of sports, but nonathletic adults seldom need it. If you want to increase your power for cycling, skiing, basketball, or some other sport, remember the principle of specificity. Even runners can increase power by lifting weights, running uphill, and running against resistance. They can increase speed by using high-speed repetitions in power training or by running downhill. We'll provide a prescription for power training in chapter 10.

Agility

Agility is the ability to change position and direction rapidly, with precision and without loss of balance. It depends on strength, speed, balance, and coordination. Agility is undeniably important in the world of sport, but it is also useful in helping people avoid embarrassment or injury in recreational activities and in potentially dangerous work situations. Because agility is associated with specific skills, no one test predicts agility for all situations. You can improve agility with practice and experience. Excess weight hinders agility, for obvious reasons. Extreme strength isn't a prerequisite, nor is aerobic fitness. But because agility deteriorates with fatigue, aerobic and muscular endurance can help maintain agility for extended periods, such as a long tennis match.

Balance

Balance can be static or dynamic. Static balance, as measured by a test such as the stork stand (standing on one foot with hands on hips and eyes closed), measures the ability to maintain balance while stationary. Balance is important in activities like diving, gymnastics, and mountain climbing. You can improve balance with specific training, and balance may decline with age or inactivity, or as the result of illness or even head trauma. Dynamic balance is the ability to maintain equilibrium while in motion. Balance depends on the ability to integrate visual input with information from the semicircular canals in the inner ear and from muscle–joint receptors. Although measuring and predicting its role is difficult, dynamic balance certainly contributes to sport performance.

Evidence indicates that people can improve their balance through participation in sports and a variety of movement experiences, especially during childhood. Leg strength is a factor in dynamic balance, especially in the elderly (Spirduso 1995). Elderly practitioners of tai chi exhibited better joint proprioception and balance control than sedentary subjects did, but when they were compared with elderly golfers, the active groups were similar in dynamic standing balance control (Tsang and HuiChan 2004). Active older males subjected to a 6-week balance intervention program showed little improvement in static or dynamic balance. An active life appears sufficient to maintain balance, even in older adults (Lail et al. 2004).

Because balance is probably task specific, practice of the specific activity is likely the best way to improve balance and performance. Having football or basketball players engage in aerobic dance or ballet classes is likely to result in a profound cultural experience for both the players and the teacher, and the classes are sure to make the athletes

Childhood participation in sports and other movement experiences can improve balance.

better dancers. Whether the classes will improve the players' performance on the field or court has yet to be demonstrated. We can safely say that few, if any, top basketball professionals developed their moves around an arabesque, entrechat, or glissade. And none whom we've seen shoot fouls in the fifth position!

Coordination or Skill

Coordination implies a harmonious relationship, a smooth union or flow of movement in execution of a task. In striking the tennis serve, one develops force sequentially. As momentum from the body turn approaches its peak, the arm extends at the elbow, and maximum racket speed finally occurs with the snap of the wrist. If the forces are added in the wrong sequence, the movement appears uncoordinated.

Although a certain amount of coordination may be inherited (as with the natural athlete), skill is achieved with practice, practice, and more practice. Repetition of a skill leads to decreases in synaptic resistance in the nervous system, increasing the likelihood and accuracy of the practiced movement and eventually making the movement automatic. Correct practice is crucial. Repetition of the wrong movement will form a bad habit that is hard to break. Seek professional instruction as you endeavor to improve your skill.

"Practice makes permanent: Perfect practice makes perfect."

Because every skill is specific, we must learn each individually. Ability in tennis doesn't ensure success in badminton, squash, or racquetball. Skill doesn't transfer between sports as readily as we once thought it did. Another feature of coordination or skill will become apparent as you train for fitness. Skilled performers work efficiently; they don't waste movement or energy. A skilled runner uses less energy at a given speed. A skilled worker often can outproduce a stronger, more fit coworker. We can learn skill, coordination, and technique. With proper skill we make best use of leverage and large-muscle groups, thereby avoiding injury and fatigue of smaller muscles.

> Because every skill is specific, we must learn each individually.

Summary

We've introduced the components of muscular fitness and discussed their contributions to health and performance. We hope that you have decided to integrate muscular fitness into your activity program. You won't be sorry that you did. With improved muscular fitness you are better able to do yard work, to hike with a pack, to cycle or run uphill, to paddle a canoe, to cross-country and downhill ski, and more. The effects become more pronounced with every passing year. See what muscular fitness can do for you!

You may wonder how you stack up in terms of muscular fitness (see table 8.2). If you want to assess your muscular fitness, be sure to warm up and do some stretching before you attempt a vigorous test. Or you may prefer to engage in some training before you do these or other tests. In the chapters that follow we'll describe the effects of training and provide training prescriptions to help you improve your scores.

Table 8.2 Muscular Fitness Tests

			MEN			WOMEN		
			Low	Medium	High	Low	Medium	High
Upper body	Strength	Chin-up[*]	<6	6–10	>10	<20	20–30	>30
	Endurance	Push-up	<20	20–40	>40	<10	10–20	>20
Trunk	Endurance	Sit-up	<30	30–50	>50	<25	25–40	>40
Leg	Strength	Leg press[**]	<220%	220–320%	>320%	<220%	220–300%	>300%
Flexibility (sit and reach)	Reach toes		No	Yes	Beyond	No	Yes	Beyond
Power	Vertical jump[***]		<17 in.	17–23 in.	>23 in.	<10 in.	10–15 in.	>15 in.
Speed (40 m)	Seconds		>7.5	7.5–6.0	<6.0	>9.0	9.0–7.5	<7.5

[*]Women do modified chin-up.

[**]Percent of body weight.

[***]Low vertical jump is associated with a low percentage of fast-twitch fibers.

Benefits of Muscular Fitness

"Power waits upon him who earns it."
John Burroughs

How does training lead to changes in muscle fibers? How does a muscle fiber know the difference between strength and endurance training? Part of the answer to these questions is related to the training stimulus, the characteristic of training that leads to specific adaptations. Strength improves when you apply sufficient tension to the muscle fiber and its contractile proteins. The tension required seems to be above two-thirds of the maximal force of the muscle. If you do contractions that require little tension, you won't gain much strength. Contraction time, the total number of repetitions, also seems to influence the development of strength (Smith and Rutherford 1995). By doing more contractions you obtain better results, up to a point. The number of contractions probably depends on your level of training, nutrition, and genetic endowment. You will receive benefits from any form of strength training, as long as you exert enough tension for a sufficient number of repetitions (or time).

$$\text{strength} = \text{tension} \times \text{time (number of sets and repetitions)}$$

This chapter will help you

- understand how a bout of training leads to changes in muscles,
- identify the specific changes that result from strength or endurance training,
- recognize the importance of flexibility exercises,
- understand how to minimize muscle soreness,
- see how speed and power training improve performance, and
- see how core training contributes to health and performance.

Muscular Fitness Training

In training we often speak of the overload principle, which states the following:

- For improvements to take place, workloads have to impose a demand (overload) on the body system (above two-thirds of maximal force for strength).
- As adaptation to loading takes place, more load must be added.
- Improvements are related to the intensity (tension for strength), duration (repetitions), and frequency of training.

Overload training leads to adaptations in the muscles according to the type of training. Here again, the principle of specificity applies, as it did with aerobic training. The adaptation to strength training includes increased size because of increases in contractile proteins (actin and myosin) and tougher connective tissue. These and other adaptations allow the muscle to exert more force.

The specific adaptations to muscular endurance training include improved aerobic enzyme systems, larger and more numerous mitochondria (increased mitochondrial density), and more capillaries. All these changes promote oxygen delivery and utilization within the muscle fiber, thereby improving endurance (Jackson and Dickinson 1988). Fatiguing repetitions somehow stimulate the muscle fiber to become better adapted to use oxygen and aerobic enzymes for the production of energy (adenosine triphosphate, or ATP) to sustain contractions. If you perform many repetitions, you become better able to use fat as a source of energy.

We do not entirely understand how the strength or endurance training stimuli bring about the appropriate changes. But from what we know about how cells work, the training stimulus probably signals the nucleus to make messenger RNA (mRNA). This messenger is shaped by the DNA and sent into the muscle fiber to order the production of specific proteins (contractile protein for strength training, aerobic enzyme protein for endurance training). Structures in the muscle fiber called ribosomes receive the message and begin to produce the protein needed to adapt to the training stimulus. Another RNA (transfer RNA, or tRNA) gathers up the amino acids needed to construct the desired protein, transports them to the ribosome, and places them in the growing chain of amino acids that become a specific protein. Because DNA forms RNA, the training stimulus must somehow influence the nuclei (one muscle fiber has many). We don't know whether tension, metabolic activity, hormones, or a combination of factors signal the nuclei; therefore, we are unable to trick the muscle into getting stronger or building endurance without training. So you'll have to pursue the prescriptions in chapter 10 to improve your muscular strength or endurance.

Table 9.1 reviews the effects of each type of training. The table shows that high-resistance training leads to the development of strength and that low-resistance repetitions lead to muscular endurance, and it suggests that questions remain regarding the effects of training that falls between strength (high resistance and low repetitions) and endurance (low resistance and high repetitions). Use the table to help identify your training goals. Later in the chapter we will explain how to add power to your muscular fitness training program.

Muscular Strength Training

Strength contributes to performance in work and sport, and strength training puts stress on bones, which leads to stronger bones and lower risk of osteoporosis. You can also use strength training to tone muscles, to improve your appearance, and, within hereditary limits, to enhance your shape. In addition, strength training will certainly

Table 9.1   Strength–Endurance Continuum

	Strength	Short-term (anaerobic) endurance	Intermediate endurance	Long-term endurance
For	Maximum force	Brief (2–3 min) persistence with heavy load	Persistence with intermediate load	Persistence with lighter load
Prescription	4–8RM (slow) 3 sets rest >3 min	15–25RM 3 sets rest 1–3 min	30–50RM 2 sets rest <1 min	Over 100RM 1 set
Improves	Contractile protein ATP and CP Connective tissue	Some strength and anaerobic metabolism (glycolysis)	Some endurance and anaerobic metabolism Slight improvement in strength (for untrained)	Aerobic enzymes Mitochondria Oxygen and fat utilization
Doesn't improve	Oxygen intake Endurance	Oxygen intake		Strength

RM = repetitions maximum
ATP = adenosine triphosphate
CP = creatine phosphate

help you lead an active and vigorous life, well beyond retirement years. How does this simple mode of exercise produce such remarkable results?

Strength training, also called resistance training or weight training, involves high resistance and low repetitions and leads to the following adaptations:

- Increased contractile protein (actin and myosin)
- Tougher connective tissue
- Reduced inhibitions
- Contractile efficiency
- Possible increase in number of muscle fibers
- Increase in muscle mass and cross-sectional area (hypertrophy)

CONTRACTILE PROTEIN   Years ago, Gordon (1967) compared the effects of strength and endurance training on muscle proteins. Researchers throughout the world have since corroborated the results. Strength training adds to the portion of the muscle that generates tension, the contractile proteins. Endurance training, on the other hand, enhances the energy supply system, the aerobic enzymes (all enzymes are constructed of proteins). But the most surprising outcome of Gordon's study was the observation that strength training brought about a decline in endurance enzymes, and that endurance training led to a decline in contractile protein. Thus if you train only for strength or endurance, you could lose a bit of the other. This aspect of specificity shouldn't surprise us too much—the size and strength of your thigh muscles increase during weight training but decline somewhat when you return to distance running.

> Strength training adds to the portion of the muscle that generates tension, the contractile proteins.

CONNECTIVE TISSUE   Connective tissue and tendons grow in size and toughness when you place them under tension. This increased toughness in tendons may help quiet the inhibitory influence of the muscle receptor known as the tendon organ, a receptor sensitive to stretching. The increase in thickness of connective tissue contributes some to the growth, or hypertrophy, of the muscle.

NERVOUS SYSTEM   Some of the effects of strength training occur in the nervous system. With experience we seem to have fewer inhibitions, both in the central nervous system and from muscle receptors. Practice (repetition) allows us to be more efficient, more skilled in the application of force. Thus practice alone accounts for some of the improvement in the early stages of training. This notion may explain why involuntary contractions brought on by an electrical stimulator do not equal the results obtained with voluntary contractions. Involuntary contractions may elicit changes in the muscle, but they don't teach the nervous system how to contract (Massey et al. 1965).

MUSCLE FIBERS   The ability to look at samples of human muscle before and after training has led to some fascinating questions. Can strength training lead to the formation of additional muscle fibers?

Studies on human muscle suggest that we may be able to increase the number of muscle fibers when overloaded fibers split to form new fibers. This finding, however, is still the subject of scientific debate. And we would never suggest that you will form new fibers as the result of ordinary strength training. But those athletes who spend hours each day lifting weights or use hormones (anabolic steroids, growth hormone) to promote extra growth may be able to increase the number of muscle fibers (note, however, that anabolic steroids have been found to lower HDL cholesterol and increase the risk of heart disease).

New Fibers?

We once believed that the number of muscle fibers was set at birth and was not subject to change. Van Linge (1962) transplanted the tendon of a small rat muscle into a position where it would have to assume a tremendous workload. He studied the rat muscle after he had subjected it to a period of heavy training and found that the transplanted muscle had doubled its weight and tripled its strength. Furthermore, the heavy workload stimulated the development of new muscle fibers. Recent research indicates a role for satellite cells in muscle hypertrophy. They seem to aid regeneration of injured cells and may contribute to the formation of new fibers (Barton-Davis, Shoturma, and Sweeney 1999).

Muscular Endurance Training

Endurance training, which involves low resistance and high repetitions, leads to the following adaptations:

- Increased aerobic enzymes
- Increased mitochondrial density
- Increased capillaries
- More efficient contractions
- Possible changes in fiber type (e.g., fast twitch to slow twitch)

We've already mentioned the effects of endurance training on aerobic enzymes, particularly those involved in fat metabolism; on mitochondria; and on capillaries. Aerobic pathways that are more efficient are able to provide more energy from fat, thereby conserving muscle glycogen as well as blood glucose, which is the preferred fuel of the brain and nervous system. As a result, muscles that once fatigued in minutes become able to endure for hours. Some of the effects of endurance training take place in the nervous system. Skilled, more efficient movement conserves energy, thereby contributing to endurance. But most documented effects of muscular endurance training seem to focus on muscle fibers.

Fiber Type Transformation

Evidence suggests that the aerobic enzyme improvements noted in endurance training may be an early stage in the eventual transformation of fast-twitch to slow-twitch muscle fibers. Pette (1984) has reported metabolic (enzyme) and then structural changes in muscle following prolonged endurance training (electrical stimulation). Studies of rat and rabbit muscle show that fast fibers first take on improved oxidative capabilities and eventually assume the contractile properties of slow-twitch fibers. We do not yet know if these fiber type changes occur in humans.

We do know that successful distance runners have as high as 80 percent slow-twitch fibers. Is that high percentage due to fiber type transformation or to heredity? At present it appears that endurance training can improve the aerobic or oxidative capabilities of all fibers, and that fast-twitch fibers become more able to use oxygen. These studies demonstrate that muscle is extremely adaptable and can adjust to the demands imposed on it.

Methods of Training

What is the best method to train for strength or endurance: static, dynamic, or isokinetic? The answer depends on what you are training to accomplish, the goal of your training. If you just want to get stronger, almost any method will work. If you want to gain strength to improve performance in work or sport, your training should be specific to your goal. We conducted a study in which college women trained with weights (isotonic), isokinetic devices, or calisthenics. The isotonic group did best on lifting tests, and the calisthenics group scored best on calisthenics tests. The isokinetic training group, which gained strength on the isokinetic devices, came in third on the other two tests. This study showed the importance of training in the manner in which you will eventually use the strength (Sharkey et al. 1978).

STATIC (ISOMETRIC) TRAINING   Based on an early study conducted in Germany (Hettinger and Müller 1953), static training was popular until studies finally compared isometrics with traditional weightlifting and found that static contractions came in a distant second. Isometric contractions don't provide a sense of accomplishment through lifting something, they elevate blood pressure, and they are seldom specific to the training goal. Isometrics do have some uses: in rehabilitation, when that is all that the patient can do; for work at the sticking point of a lift; and for activities that require static strength or endurance (e.g., archery or rock climbing). More recently, isometric contractions have been used in conjunction with weightlifting to produce better results.

DYNAMIC (ISOTONIC) TRAINING   Isotonic contractions (weightlifting) gained popularity when DeLorme and Watkins (1951) outlined a formula for success. Simply stated, the formula called for high-resistance, low-repetition exercise. People still use variations of that formula to develop dynamic strength. Free weights and weight machines are readily available in most health clubs. And weightlifting with free weights remains the method of choice for most serious athletes and bodybuilders.

ISOKINETIC TRAINING   Isokinetic exercises combine the best features of isometric (near maximal force) and isotonic (full range of motion) training. With the appropriate device the exerciser can overload the muscles with a near maximal contraction throughout the range of motion and control the speed of contraction. The problem, if one exists, seems to be the lack of specific devices for many sports skills (see figure 9.1) and the cost of sport-specific equipment. But as more devices are developed for specific sports, isokinetic training may become even more popular.

WHICH METHOD IS BEST?   No single method is best for strength or endurance training. Free weights are inexpensive and versatile but require more supervision for safety and to prevent theft. Weight machines are convenient and require less supervision. Isokinetic devices are effective but costly and limited in application. But unlike weightlifting, isokinetic training doesn't cause muscle soreness. Thus people can do it in conjunction with other activities without adversely affecting performance.

A note of caution before we go on: Be sure that the training program you adopt is appropriate to your level of fitness and ability. What is best for beginners doesn't

Figure 9.1 *(a)* The swim bench provides a sport-specific way to train swimming strokes.
Photo *a* courtesy of www.vasatrainer.com

work for athletes, and vice versa. In psychology, many theories are based on research conducted on college freshmen and rats. In exercise physiology, numerous studies have been conducted on "gym rats," college students enrolled in activity classes. Studies that compare various forms of strength training on gym rats all seem to yield similar results: With beginners who follow the prescription, anything works. But that finding doesn't predict how the method will work on athletes or others with high levels of strength, and it doesn't prove that the increased strength will improve performance. We know how to improve strength. Now we need to find out how much strength a person needs to improve performance and how best to train to get results (chapter 10).

Flexibility

To consider the effect of training on range of motion, first we must consider the limits of flexibility. The tough connective tissue that covers muscles is a major restriction to range of motion, as are the joint capsule and tendons. Thus training must concentrate on altering these limits. Flexibility decreases with age and inactivity. Some injuries may be more likely as flexibility decreases, and low-back problems are associated with poor flexibility (back, hamstrings) and weak abdominal muscles. On the other hand, enhanced flexibility may improve performance in some sports, especially those with obvious flexibility components (gymnastics, diving, wrestling).

Increased muscle and joint temperatures increase flexibility, as do specific stretching exercises. Stretching gradually leads to minor distensions in connective tissue, and the summation of these small changes can dramatically improve range of motion.

Years ago, flexibility exercises conjured up images of vigorous bobbing and jerking movements, but times have changed. Today we engage in static stretching or, at most, light bobbing movements. The reason for the change is the stretch reflex. A rapid stretch invokes a stretch reflex, and the reflex calls forth a vigorous contraction of the muscle. Because a vigorous contraction is the opposite of what we are seeking, we must avoid this explosive stretching and learn the gentle art of static stretching.

Stretching Exercises

To complete your stretching exercises effectively, warm up a bit with light exercise or calisthenics and then do your stretching. Finish the warm-up with more vigorous effort or, if you prefer, begin your run or other exercise at a slow pace. Never substitute skill rehearsal, such as tennis strokes, for stretching. Do your warm-up and stretching before you begin to compete. You can use several different types of stretching exercises to achieve your goals.

- **Static stretching.** Static stretching involves using slow movements to reach a point of stretch, holding the position (for 5 to 10 seconds), and relaxing. You may repeat the stretch and perform very light bobbing.

- **Contract and relax stretching.** A variation of the static stretch is the contract and relax technique. Do a static stretch, relax, and then contract the muscle for a few seconds. Then repeat the static stretch. When performed on muscles like those in the calf, the technique seems to help the muscle relax so that you can better stretch the tendon.

- **Dynamic stretching.** This method requires moving through the range of motion and working at either end of the range to increase the reach. This stretching technique mimics sport movements and uses controlled motion. Use care to remain gentle in your motions.

Static stretching and the contract and relax variation are at least as effective as dynamic stretching and provide other advantages such as low risk of injury and reduction of tightness and lingering muscle soreness. When you do flexibility training correctly, the results are quite persistent. You should retain improved range of motion for at least 8 weeks. But after you have learned to enjoy stretching, you may get hooked on its subtle sensations and move on to advanced forms such as yoga. If not, just remember to do the stretches that you need to minimize soreness, reduce the risk of injury, and avoid low-back problems.

The following common stretching exercises are best done to the point of mild discomfort and then held for 10 to 20 seconds. Choose exercises that help you increase the range of motion for joints and movements that are limited.

Shoulder and Arm Stretch

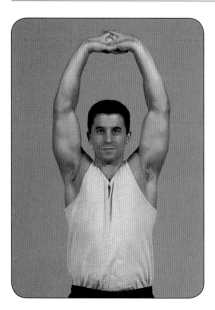

Intertwine your fingers above your head with your palms facing upward. Push your arms upward and slightly to the rear. Feel a stretch in your arms, shoulders, and upper back.

Hand Stretches

With the wrist and fingers of one hand extended, use your other hand to gently increase the extension of the fingers. Repeat with opposite hands. Other options for stretching the hands include extending the wrist and flexing your fingers at the same time or extending your wrists and at the same time abducting (spreading out) the fingers as far as possible.

Neck Stretch

Lean your head sideways toward the right shoulder while reaching down with your left arm. To increase the stretch, use your right hand to pull your left arm downward behind your back. Repeat on the opposite side.

Shoulder Stretch

Intertwine your fingers together behind your back with palms facing inward. Start the stretch by turning your elbow while maintaining straight arms. For a second stretch, maintain an erect posture and raise your arms up behind you until you feel a mild stretch.

Upper Chest Stretch

Stand in front of a door jam or a similar structure. Place your hands about shoulder height on the door jam and gently lean forward, feeling a stretch across the front of your shoulders and chest. If you need a little more stretch, step back further from the door jam and relax your shoulders to let gravity increase the stretch.

Trunk Stretch

Standing upright, look over your right shoulder and turn your upper torso as far as possible. Try to keep your hips facing forward. Repeat to the left. As an alternative, stand about 18 inches from a wall and face away from it. Keeping your hips facing forward, rotate both hands and shoulders and touch the wall. Go only as far as is comfortable.

Back Stretch

Place both hands shoulder width apart on a bar or other solid support that is about chest height. With slightly bent knees let your torso droop forward. Keep your hips directly above your feet. Try bending your knees a little more to increase the stretch and experiment with different height objects to hold onto.

Side Bend Stretch

Stretch your left arm up and behind your head. Grasp the left elbow with your right hand as you bend to the right and pull your left arm simultaneously. Feel the stretch from the elbow down though the upper arm and upper torso. Repeat on the right side.

Lower Back and Shoulder Stretch

While standing or sitting, place your hands on your lower back. Bring your shoulders back and your elbows toward one another while pushing your back forward.

Standing Groin Stretch

With feet spread, bend your left knee while keeping your right leg straight. Push your hip down and toward the left foot until you feel a modest stretch along the inner thigh of the right leg. Repeat on the other side.

Groin and Hamstring Stretch

Stand with your left side to a table or bench. While facing forward, place your left foot out to the side with your toe up on the bench. Gently lean towards the bench and hold. You should feel a stretch in the medial hamstrings and groin areas. Repeat on the other side.

Groin, Hamstring, and Hip Stretch

Place your right knee directly above the ankle and extend your rear leg behind you as shown. Weight should be on the toes and ball of the rear foot. Hold an easy stretch by letting your torso relax forward past the front knee. Use your hands for balance. Repeat on the other side.

Groin, Hamstring, and Front of Hip Stretch

Place the ball of your foot on a secure support such as a table. Keep the support leg pointed forward. Push your hips toward the front foot while bending the front knee. Feel the stretch in the groin and hamstring of the elevated leg and in the front of the hip on the side of the support leg. Repeat on the opposite side.

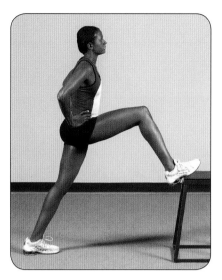

Calf Stretches

Leaning against a wall or solid support, place most of the weight on the rear foot and push your hips down and forward while keeping the rear leg straight and the heel on the ground to cause a stretch in your upper calf. An additional stretch you can do in this position is to relax the hips and focus on pushing the rear knee forward and down while keeping the heel on the ground to stretch the lower calf. Repeat on the other leg.

Knee and Quad Stretch

While balancing against a wall, hold the top of your right foot with your left hand and gently pull your foot upward and toward your buttocks. Repeat on the opposite side.

Squat Stretch

This stretch will be felt in the lower legs, knees, back, ankles, Achilles tendons, and groin. Squat down with your feet flat, knees above the toes, and toes pointing out slightly. Changing the width of your feet and knees will change the areas stretched.

Single Leg Hamstring Stretch

Sitting on the floor with your torso upright, tuck the sole of one foot in by your inner upper thigh and relax the knee to the floor. Slowly bend forward from the hips toward the foot of the extended leg until you feel a modest stretch. Keep your back straight for this stretch. Repeat on the other side.

Upper Hamstring and Hip Stretch

Sitting on the floor (if necessary, sit with your back to a wall), hold onto the outside of your ankle (and/or knee) and foot as shown. Gently pull the entire leg toward your torso until you feel a slight stretch in the back of your upper leg. Repeat on the other side. An additional stretch that you can do in this position is to use your hand to gently rotate the foot through its full range of motion to stretch tight ligaments.

Sitting Groin Stretch

Sitting on the floor, place the soles of your feet together as shown and gently hold onto your toes. Gently pull to bring your torso forward by bending at the hips. You may also use your elbows to gently push the knees toward the floor to increase the stretch. Be gentle.

Outer Hip Stretch

Sitting on the floor as shown with one leg extended and the other bent and placed over the extended leg, gently pull the knee across your torso into the opposite shoulder. Repeat on the other side.

Spine Stretch

This stretch may be felt across the entire back, outside of the hips, and in the ribs. Sit upright on the floor with the right leg out in front. Bend the left leg and place the foot on the floor across the extended right leg. Bend your right elbow and place it on the outside of the left thigh near the knee. Use the left arm for balance as shown and twist, looking over your left shoulder while maintaining pressure with the right arm on the left knee. Repeat on the other side.

Ankle and Quad Stretch

Lie on one side with the lower arm supporting your head. Hold the top of the upper foot with the free hand as shown. First, gently pull your heel toward your buttocks to stretch your ankle and quadriceps. Second, push the top of your foot into your hand and upward by contracting the gluteus (buttocks) muscles. This movement should further stretch the quadriceps. Repeat on the other side.

Quad and Gluteus Stretch

Lie on your back with your head and shoulders contacting the floor with one leg extended and the other knee and hip flexed. Use both hands to hold the lower thigh behind your knee and gently pull your knee toward your chest. Repeat on the other side.

Groin Stretch

Lie on your back with your head and shoulders contacting the floor. Place the soles of your feet together and pull them in toward your buttocks. Gently let your knees droop toward the floor, letting gravity do the work. Relax and breathe.

Muscle Soreness

The muscle soreness that becomes evident 24 hours after you overdo training (delayed-onset muscle soreness, or DOMS) may be due to slight tears in connective tissue, to uncontrolled contractions or spasms of individual muscle fibers, to muscle fiber damage, or to the lingering effects of metabolic by-products. We are reasonably certain that soreness is not due to leftover lactic acid, which is eliminated within an hour of cessation of effort. We do know that certain types of exercise (but not isokinetic) lead to soreness that often persists for days and can make subsequent activity less enjoyable. Komi and Buskirk (1972) compared two types of strength training: concentric (as in ordinary flexion) and eccentric (in which the muscle is under high tension as it lowers an overload). Subjects in the eccentric group, the group that lowered the weight, complained of muscle soreness, whereas the other group did not. So if you begin a weightlifting program and plan to lower the weights, be prepared for some soreness.

You may be surprised to know that the eccentric group in the Komi and Buskirk study gained a bit more strength, a common finding in eccentric training studies, probably because you can let down more weight than you can lift (hence the muscle is under more tension). But before you get excited about eccentric training, remember what we keep saying about specificity: Unless your sport or job calls for letting down heavy loads, the training may not help performance as much as regular weight training will, and you are certain to get muscle soreness with eccentric contractions.

You can diminish soreness by beginning with light weights and progressing gradually. Avoid maximal lifting, all-out running, or ballistic movements such as hard throwing or serving at the start of the season. Be patient. Experience shows that we are seldom patient enough; therefore, we need a way to reduce soreness. Stretching has been shown to reduce muscle discomfort (deVries and Housh 1994), so stretch after a warm-up and after exercise and whenever you feel tight or sore. If your legs are stiff and sore during a long plane flight, go to the rear of the plane and stretch. If other passengers see you trying to push down the wall of the galley, don't be embarrassed. Fitness enthusiasts will understand that you are experiencing the pleasure and relief of a good static stretch.

Muscle soreness is correlated with submicroscopic muscle damage, accumulation of fluid (edema), and diminished strength that may persist for up to 2 weeks. The damage may occur in older or otherwise susceptible muscle fibers. Recovery is faster and soreness diminishes after successive bouts of exercise. Leakage of the muscle enzyme creatine kinase (CK) suggests membrane damage. Because soreness peaks 1 to 2 days after the effort and the enzyme levels peak 2 to 3 days later, the cause of muscle soreness is still unclear (Newham 1988). Fortunately, DOMS occurs only during the start-up phase, and the symptoms disappear within a few weeks, reappearing only after a long layoff or the vigorous start of a new activity. Indeed, exercise-induced muscle soreness seems to inoculate the body from subsequent discomfort for up to 6 months following the initial soreness (Nosaka et al. 2001).

> Muscle soreness is correlated with submicroscopic muscle damage, accumulation of fluid (edema), and diminished strength that may persist for up to 2 weeks.

Speed and Power

Years ago, while attempting to make some sense of the confusing and sometimes contradictory research on strength and speed, we noticed that strength and speed seemed to be related when heavy loads were used in the test of speed. When little resistance was used, strength and speed were not related. In an effort to generalize the findings to other areas of work and sport, we turned to a well-known physiological principle: the force–velocity relationship.

Force–Velocity Relationship

It has long been known that velocity of shortening in a contraction is greatest with no load or resistance. As the resistance increases, the velocity of shortening decreases (see figure 9.2). We thought that the force–velocity relationship could help simplify basic principles about how and why muscles should be trained for force, speed, or power. From reading the available literature we concluded that strength training would improve heavily loaded movements but would have little effect on the velocity of unloaded movements, and vice versa. Imagine our delight when we happened upon studies that confirmed the hypothesis!

Ikai (1970) demonstrated that training for strength alone led to increased strength and velocity with heavy loads. He also found that training for speed alone improved velocity

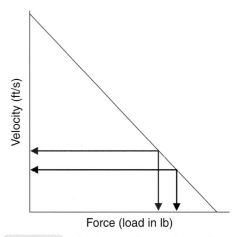

Figure 9.2 The force–velocity relationship. The benefits of strength training are more pronounced in events involving loaded or resisted movements.
Adapted from Sharkey, 1975.

with light loads but did nothing for strength or velocity with heavy loads. Most interesting of all was the finding that training with intermediate loads (30 to 60 percent of maximal strength) at the highest speed possible led to improvements in force, speed, and power. Years later, this finding was corroborated when Kanehisa and Miyashita (1983) confirmed the specificity of velocity in training. They trained three groups at either slow-, medium-, or high-speed contractions. The slow-speed group improved in leg extension strength at slow speeds, and the fast group improved in the force that they could exert at fast speeds. But only the intermediate-speed group was able to improve at all speeds. Power training (15 to 25 repetitions at 30 to 60 percent of maximal strength, as fast as possible) may be the way to train when you desire speed or power (see table 9.2). Does that throw out the concept of specificity?

If you are preparing for the shot put, a sport in which both force and speed are important, you will need considerable strength, so train for strength. If high speed is your primary goal, as in pitching a fastball, train for speed. Power training could help performance in both. The power prescription is ideal for sports like cross-country skiing, a power and endurance sport that requires hundreds of little explosions to power the skier uphill. The principle of specificity does not imply that you should avoid other types of training, only that training must eventually mimic the movements of the sport to obtain the best results.

A final note concerning the use of isotonic and especially isokinetic training for speed, strength, and power development is in order. Both techniques adapt to the

Table 9.2 Training for Power

	Power with heavy load	Power with moderate load
Prescription	8–12RM FAP*	15–25RM FAP
	60% of max	30% of max
Sets	3 sets	2–3 sets
Rest	3 min	1–2 min
Improves	Some strength	Some muscular endurance
	Neural recruitment	Neural recruitment
	ATP and CP	Strength
	Connective tissue	
Doesn't improve	Oxygen intake	Oxygen intake

*FAP = fast as possible. Training is sport or activity specific and may require specialized equipment to allow explosive movement.

advice that we've just provided. By reducing resistance below 30 percent of maximal, you can increase the velocity of contractions. By increasing resistance above 60 percent, you'll focus on force development.

When power (force times velocity) is required, contract as fast as possible with weights in the range of 30 to 60 percent of maximal. Although isokinetic contractions seem ideally suited for strength or power development, it is possible that you can develop both strength and power with weight-training equipment or even with calisthenics and plyometrics that follow prescriptions provided in chapter 10.

Preload and Elastic Recoil

Before we leave the subject of power, we want to acquaint you with one of the secrets of athletic performance. It took us years to realize that a well-known fact of muscle physiology—that a muscle exerts more force when it is stretched just before contraction—describes how muscles are meant to work. The stretch, or preload, does several things: It aligns contractile elements (cross-bridges) in muscle for maximal force, takes slack out of the system, and stores elastic energy in the muscle–tendon complex. Studies of the force and efficiency of contraction indicate that this stretch-shortening cycle is the way that muscle works most efficiently (Komi 1992).

> Studies of the force and efficiency of contraction indicate that this stretch-shortening cycle is the way that muscle works most efficiently.

Here's how it works in a vertical jump. First, you sink at the knees to put the thigh muscles on stretch. Then you immediately contract the stretched muscles and quickly convert the preload into elastic recoil as you jump. To see how effective the combination of preload and elastic recoil is, compare that jump with one in which you eliminate the preload. Sink to the starting position, stop for a full second, and then jump. Without preload and elastic recoil, the results are inferior. The preload and elastic recoil combination works whenever you are able to preload just before contraction. It happens in running, at the ankle and thigh; in cross-country skiing; in tennis during the serve; and, of course, in weightlifting, where it has been called cheating! Often, the preload and elastic recoil combination happens automatically, but if it doesn't, see whether you can use it to provide more power, or the same power with less effort. Done properly, it contributes to power and economy of movement.

Core Training

A recent development in muscular fitness training is a focus on the core. Core exercises recruit one or more large-muscle areas (abdominal, back, chest, shoulders, hip), involve two or more primary joints (multijoint), and are a high priority for health and performance (Baechle, Earle, and Wathen 2000). Core training focuses on the central portion of the body, an area that many consider the foundation for performance in sport. A moderate amount of core training seems to be important for low-back health, but the relationship of core fitness to performance in sport is less well established. Logic tells us that we must develop the core muscles as we train the muscles of the arms and legs. Strong and balanced muscles of the trunk permit better transfer of power from one part of the body to another or to an external object.

You can train the core in a number of ways, ranging from old-fashioned calisthenics and medicine balls to Swiss balls and Pilates. Popular core exercises are shown in figure 9.3. Video programs, books, and magazine articles will help guide your use of core exercises. As we await the results of research studies, remember that past generations of athletes survived with calisthenics and medicine balls. You don't need to spend a lot to achieve the benefits of core training.

a

b

c

Figure 9.3   Other popular methods of developing muscular fitness include: *(a)* Pilates, *(b)* yoga, and *(c)* balance-ball exercises. Interested readers are encouraged to buy one of the many fine guides to these activities that are available. These activities focus on core trunk muscles and provide a stable base for further resistance training.

Summary

Research has shown that tension multiplied by time is the stimulus for strength development. How the tension is produced doesn't seem to matter. Legend tells of Milo from Crete, who began daily lifts of a young calf. As time passed and the animal grew, so did Milo's strength. More recently, study subjects have lifted weights, pulled rubber bands, squeezed bags of water, and suffered electrical stimulation to build strength, and all worked. We are beginning to understand how the stimulus leads to stronger, tougher, more efficient muscles. More important is our growing understanding of the distinction between strength and endurance, in terms of training and cellular outcomes. We may soon be able to say how much strength or endurance is required to perform optimally in a sport or job.

By now you know enough to design and carry out a muscular fitness program that will improve your appearance, health, and everyday performance. If you want to improve performance in work or sport, you'll find more help in chapter 15.

10

Improving Muscular Fitness

> "The two kinds of people on earth . . . are the people who lift and the people who lean."
>
> *Ella Wheeler Wilcox*

By now you have some idea of the benefits and applications of muscular fitness. First are the health benefits. All of us need to do flexibility and abdominal exercises to prevent low-back problems. Try to maintain a regular schedule. If you don't, you are likely to become one of the millions of Americans whose days are diminished by this preventable problem. Those at risk for osteoporosis should plan a prevention program that consists of moderate weightlifting along with weight-bearing aerobic activity. Middle-aged people must understand how muscular fitness contributes to muscle mass, mobility, and the quality of life after retirement, and realize that they should begin long before they retire and continue the rest of their days.

Of course, people seek to improve muscular fitness for many other reasons. Some become involved to correct posture or perceived deficiencies of figure or physique (e.g., to look good at the beach). Body shaping and bodybuilding motivate others. To decide on a program, you may want to evaluate your current level of muscular fitness. If you are dissatisfied, if you have room for improvement, or if you want to enhance performance in work or sport, use the prescriptions, select your mode of exercise, and get going. You'll be happy to learn that muscular fitness doesn't require a lot of time. Unless you are seeking high levels of strength or endurance, you should be able to achieve health and other goals with two to three weekly sessions of 30 minutes each. And you can maintain muscular fitness with one or two sessions per week.

This chapter will help you

- develop training prescriptions for muscular strength, endurance, and power;
- take precautions and follow guidelines to make training safe and effective; and
- adopt a program to improve or maintain low-back fitness.

Warm-Up

Warm-up is as important for you as it is for your car. During winter months you can't just jump into the old pickup and expect instant performance. You start the engine and wait a few seconds while the oil pressure rises. Then you drive slowly to avoid overloading the engine until it heats up. In the case of the body, muscle is the engine, and increased muscle temperature improves enzyme activity and combustion. By slowly increasing heart rate, respiration, and muscle temperature, you avoid wasteful and uncomfortable anaerobic metabolism early in the workout. And by slowly warming and stretching the muscles, you reduce the risk of injury. Begin with a brisk walk, increasing to an easy jog. Use any aerobic exercise, or do light lifting exercises to warm up and then do your stretching (use the exercises in chapter 9).

A 5-minute warm-up before exercise and a cool-down afterward will enhance your enjoyment of the experience and increase the likelihood that you will be able to participate tomorrow, without discomfort. Remember that muscular fitness is only part of total fitness. No program is complete without a well-planned aerobic fitness regimen.

Prescriptions for Muscular Strength

Research has identified safe, proved prescriptions for each component of muscular fitness. You may fulfill the prescription with calisthenics, weights, or weight machines. You'll get results with hydraulic devices, accommodating or variable-resistance equipment, or old-fashioned free weights. The key to improving strength is to place the muscle under tension for a sufficient amount of time (repetitions and sets). Your level of muscular fitness and how you intend to use the strength will dictate how you should train. If you are untrained, use 60 percent of maximal strength (one repetition maximum, or RM). Increase to 80 percent RM as you become trained (Rhea et al. 2003). Training is specific in terms of angle, range of motion, and even velocity of contractions. Train the muscles and movements that you want to improve. In designing your program, consider the factors described in the following sections.

Repetitions

We've known how to prescribe strength training since the early 1950s, when DeLorme and Watkins (1951) published their analysis of progressive resistance exercise. This report and more recent studies have confirmed the need for lifters to use a resistance that they cannot lift more than 10 to 12 times (10RM). When more repetitions are possible, the load must be increased, hence the term *progressive resistance*. A comprehensive review of the literature leads to the conclusion that there is no optimal number of repetitions. Anything between 2 and 12RM yields success, as long as each set is in fact the maximal number of repetitions possible (Fleck and Kraemer 1997). Of course, working at the higher end of that range is safer, so 8 to 12 repetitions are usually prescribed for all but the most serious lifters.

Move the weight at a slow to moderate rate, always maintaining control. Breathe out as you lift and inhale as you lower the weight. Although some have recommended very slow lifts (10 seconds per repetition), studies have not been done to confirm the value of this approach.

Sets

Although a study with adult recreational lifters suggests that a single set provides an adequate training stimulus (Hass et al. 2000), other studies show that three sets of up to 10RM yield as much as 50 percent more stimulus (Kramer et al. 1997). A recent review of 140 training studies showed that four sets per muscle group elicited maximal strength gains in trained and untrained people (Rhea et al. 2003). In chapter 16 we'll show how you can use even more sets in advanced weight training. A prudent approach for the newcomer is to begin with one set of each exercise, progress to two, and then perform three sets as strength develops. Proceed to four sets if you have specific training goals, such as an improvement in leg strength for alpine skiing.

Allowing time to recover after each set of repetitions is important. For strength training, 2 to 3 minutes is recommended. For muscular endurance, 1 minute is recommended. Inadequate rest will diminish strength gains.

Frequency

One of the early studies to compare different training frequencies (Barham 1960) found that 3- or 5-day-per-week formats were superior to 2 days per week but that the 3- and 5-day programs were not significantly different from each other. In their 1997 review, Fleck and Kraemer concluded that the majority of research indicates that three training sessions per muscle group per week is the minimum frequency that causes maximum gains in strength. Apparently, untrained individuals need 48 hours to recover from a training bout and to adapt to the training stimulus. The most recent analysis indicated that untrained people can achieve maximal gains by training each muscle group 3 days a week, whereas trained people do best with 2 days per week (Rhea et al. 2003). Of course, trained athletes participate in a more demanding program (see advanced strength training in chapter 15).

The basic prescription for strength is

- three sets of 8 to 12RM (with slow movement and adequate recovery time) and

- three times per week (every other day).

In practice many lifters prefer to vary the program by changing the number of repetitions per set. Some begin at 10RM, then go to 8, and end at 6. Others prefer to begin low and go up (e.g., 6, 8, and 10RM). For safety, we recommend that you begin with more reps and less weight and avoid high weights (low RM) (see table 10.1). Just remember to increase the resistance when you are able to do more than 10 reps in all three sets. Progressive resistance training suggests that you always try to increase the load, and in general this is true. We recommend that you add resistance as necessary (to stay below 10RM) for 2 to 3 weeks and then do a week with lighter weights and reduce the frequency to two sessions per week. This easier week promotes muscle recovery and long-term gains.

Table 10.1 Prescriptions for Components of Muscular Fitness

Component	% 1RM	Reps	Sets	Recovery	Speed of movement
Strength	70–90%	6–12**	3–4	2–3 min	Slow
Endurance—short term	<60%	15–25	3	1–2	Moderate
Endurance—intermediate	<50%	20–30	2–3	1	Moderate
Endurance—long term	<40%	>30	1–3	<1	Sport specific
Power	30–60%	15–25	3	2–3	Fast as possible
Hypertrophy*	50–75%	10–20	3–6	1	Moderate

*Sought by bodybuilders, hypertrophy is an increase in muscle mass and cross-sectional area.
**Trained athletes may use 1–5RM with longer rest.

Strength-Training Guidelines

If you engage in calisthenics, weight training, or isokinetics, keep the following points in mind:

- Ease into the program with lighter weights and fewer sets. Begin with 15 to 25RM and gradually increase the load to 10RM resistance.

- Avoid holding your breath during a lift. Doing so can cause a marked increase in blood pressure and the work of the heart. Holding your breath also restricts the return of blood to the heart and the flow of blood in the coronary arteries that serve the heart muscle (just when your heart needs more oxygen, it gets less—a dangerous situation, especially for older, untrained people). Severe breath holding and straining can increase intra-abdominal pressure and cause a hernia.
- Exhale during the lift and inhale as you lower the weight.
- Always work with a companion or spotter when using free weights.
- Alternate muscle groups during a session; alternate arm and leg exercises. Allow 2 to 3 minutes of recovery time between sets of the same exercise.

You should keep records of your progress. Test for maximum strength every few weeks (see figure 10.1 for a log to keep track of progress). Also record body weight and fat, and important dimensions (chest, waist, biceps, and so on). Vary the program; each fourth week should be somewhat easier to allow recovery.

Experienced lifters use a process called periodization that usually includes several cycles of training. Athletes may train strength in the off-season, endurance in the preseason, and power in the early competitive season. Because progress begins to level off after 2 months, you may want to change the program every 8 weeks, or when you reach a plateau or get bored. In chapter 15 we will show you how to periodize muscular fitness training for performance in sport.

Strength Improvements

Although strength doesn't increase rapidly, you can expect the following:

- Your rate of increase will range from 1 to 3 percent per week, with previously untrained individuals increasing at a faster rate. With hard training, some people may temporarily achieve a rate of 4 to 5 percent improvement per week.
- The rate of improvement will decrease or level off as you approach your potential maximal strength. Take 1 or 2 easy weeks and then resume strength training (at less than 10RM) to reach a higher plateau.
- The rate of improvement may decrease if you combine strength training with strenuous aerobic training.
- Improvement will take place only in the muscle groups that you train.
- Your gains will be smaller if you fail to maintain adequate protein and energy in your diet. Increase protein intake if you are on a weight-loss diet.

A previously sedentary person on an adequate diet can expect to increase strength 50 percent or more in 6 months. Hard training could lead to similar gains in less time.

Maintenance and Detraining

You can maintain strength with lower volume and frequency of training, as long as intensity (resistance) remains high. One session per week will maintain strength for 6 weeks or more. Two sessions will ensure maintenance for a prolonged period, depending on the level of strength that you achieved before beginning the maintenance program.

Figure 10.1 Muscular Fitness Log

Date | Chin-ups | Sit-ups | Push-ups | | | | | Other | | | | |

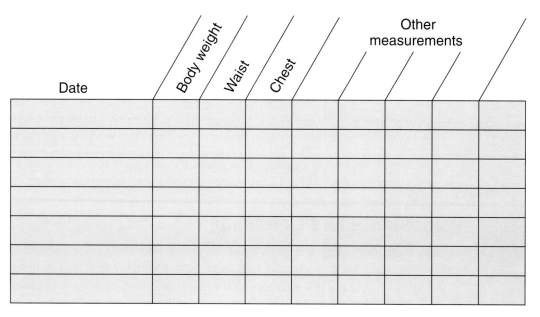

Date | Body weight | Waist | Chest | | | Other measurements | | |

From *Fitness and Health, Sixth Edition* by Brian J. Sharkey and Steven E. Gaskill, 2007, Champaign, IL: Human Kinetics.

Nutrition and Muscular Fitness

Diet can exert positive effects on the development of muscular fitness. Carbohydrate and protein intake significantly alters circulating metabolites and the hormonal environment, including insulin, testosterone, growth hormone, and cortisol, thereby influencing muscle protein response to training (Volek 2003). Postexercise intake of carbohydrate and protein is associated with muscle growth. Furthermore, the need for protein increases in strength training. Although sedentary people need .8 gram of protein per kilogram of body weight per day, serious weightlifters can use 1.4 to 1.8 grams per kilogram, as well as sufficient energy to avoid breakdown of muscle mass (Lemon 1995). You should take energy or protein snacks after a training session. Consume sufficient protein and carbohydrate calories and avoid rapid weight loss during muscular fitness training. We'll say more about diet and nutrition in chapter 11.

With normal activity, you will retain most of your newly gained strength for up to 6 weeks after cessation of training, and you will retain half the strength that you gained for up to 1 year. When you resume training, you'll return to previous levels with less effort, perhaps because of the learning that took place in earlier training. Studies on older people show that strength declines very slowly in muscle groups that they use regularly. Thus an investment in strength could pay dividends later in life. Of course, we recommend that you set aside at least 8 to 12 weeks each year to maintain or improve strength, and to continue a maintenance program (one to two times per week) thereafter. Find a season that suits your schedule and follow a program. As the years pass, you'll be glad that you did.

> Studies on older people show that strength declines very slowly in muscle groups that they use regularly.

Strength and Aerobic Training

A 1980 study concluded that combining strength training with aerobic training diminished strength, but not the aerobic outcomes (Hickson 1980). Strength training is most effective in fast-twitch muscle fibers, whereas endurance training is likely to influence slow and fast fibers. Endurance training interferes with maximal strength development by causing fast glycolytic to FOG fibers and attenuated hypertrophy (Putman et al. 2004). Yet other work indicates that concurrent strength and aerobic endurance training does not impair adaptations in strength or muscle hypertrophy (McCarthy, Pozniak, and Agre 2002). And in studies of older subjects, concurrent strength and aerobic training was as effective as either strength or endurance training. The authors suggested that combining strength and aerobic training for older subjects may be more effective in optimizing functional fitness than are programs that involve only one component of fitness (Wood et al. 2001). Yet a recent study on untrained subjects found that concurrent strength and endurance training did not interfere with strength development but might hinder development of aerobic capacity (Glowacki et al. 2004). We recommend that you do both, at least some of the time, unless you are a competitive weight lifter or runner.

How Much Strength?

Strength may be related to performance in your work or sport. Don't assume, however, as many have, that if some is good, more is better. In most activities, performance improves with strength, but only to a point. Thereafter, you may be wasting your time or diminishing performance with excessive attention to strength. The trick is to know how much is enough. When strength is optimal for the sport, move on to other important phases of training. Just be sure to maintain the necessary strength with one or two sessions each week.

How much strength is sufficient? The answer differs according to the sport. For an endurance sport such as swimming or cross-country skiing, strength is adequate when the force needed in a single contraction (e.g., the arm pull in swimming) is below 40 percent of your maximal for that movement. If you exert 20 pounds of force in the average arm pull, you need approximately 50 pounds of force (2.5 times 20 pounds) in a single maximal pull. More strength will not contribute to performance; if the arm pulls through too quickly, you'll go slower, not faster. So if strength is adequate, move on to endurance training. For daylong work, strength is adequate when the force that you need is at or below 20 percent of your maximal. If a loaded shovel weighs 10 pounds, you'll need 50 pounds of force (5 times 10). We'll say more about strength and performance in chapter 15.

Prescriptions for Muscular Endurance

We've pointed out how strength and endurance are different and why endurance may be more important than a high level of strength, presuming that you have adequate strength. The main difference between training for strength and training for endurance is the level of tension in the muscle and, consequently, the resistance used and number of repetitions possible. Lighter weights (less than 66 percent of maximum strength) don't provide much stimulus for strength development, but if you do enough repetitions, you will develop muscular endurance.

Years ago it was believed that training with fewer than 10RM developed strength, whereas training with more than 10RM developed endurance. We wondered if the body really made such fine distinctions. Recent studies have added to our knowledge of strength and endurance and the territory that lies between. Studies in our lab (Washburn et al. 1982) and others (Anderson and Kearney 1982) show that 15 to 25RM will still develop some strength (1 percent per week versus 2 to 3 percent with 6 to 10RM for strength training), along with short-term or anaerobic endurance. Table 10.1 summarizes muscular fitness prescriptions for strength, endurance, and power. As the number of repetitions increases, less strength and more endurance develops.

The number of repetitions that you need depends on several factors. What are you training for? Are you training for short-term (anaerobic) endurance or long-term endurance? Your training should be specific to the way in which you will use it. Emphasize speed when necessary. Do many repetitions when you need long-term endurance with less resistance. When the activity involves moderate resistance, lift heavier weights and do fewer repetitions. For short (less than 2 minutes) and intense activities, train with 15 to 25RM to get short-term or anaerobic endurance. If your goals are vague and time is short, use fewer repetitions to avoid boredom. Follow the appropriate endurance prescription and observe the precautions mentioned for strength training. Because the loads are lighter, muscle endurance training is safer than strength training, and it is probably more suited to the everyday activities of the average adult.

Endurance Improvements

Muscle endurance is trainable. Although going from two to four chin-ups is difficult (that takes strength), improving from 20 to 40 push-ups is easy (that takes endurance). When you have sufficient strength for the task, gains in endurance come with relative ease. Subjects in the Washburn study improved 10 percent per week in short-term endurance when they trained with 15 to 25RM. On an upper-body endurance test, short-term (anaerobic) endurance training was more effective than strength training was, improving short-term endurance 70 percent versus 50 percent for strength training. When strength is adequate, improvement in endurance enhances most adult activities. Tennis and skiing require hours of practice, and good practice requires endurance. The fatigued tennis student usually practices a sloppy version of the skill, and a fatigued skier carries a higher risk of injury.

> Improvement in endurance enhances most adult activities.

How do you know if your strength is adequate for an activity? If you can perform an activity 10 times, the way you would in the sport, you probably have adequate or functional strength. If you have enough strength to hit 10 tennis shots, or ski a series of turns down the slope, you may want to work on muscular endurance. If you struggle with the activity, you may need to develop additional strength and then concentrate on endurance.

Of course, your genetic endowment and your devotion to training will dictate your ultimate progress. If you have a high percentage of slow-twitch muscle fibers, your potential for muscular endurance is excellent. If you do not, don't despair. Training will improve the endurance capabilities of slow and fast fiber types. Although you may not be a world-class endurance athlete, you will come closer to your potential.

Adequate endurance enables you to maintain good technique during practice.

Diet and Endurance

The best endurance performances occur when muscle fibers are well supplied with glycogen. And glycogen levels are highest when you follow a high-carbohydrate diet. Scandinavian studies have shown that a full day of alpine skiing can deplete muscle glycogen stores. If you dine on steak and salad after skiing, your muscles will not be ready to perform the following day. By doing all that you can to replace muscle glycogen, you will be able to ski all day and still have energy for après-ski. More important, you will be less likely to fatigue, fall, and be injured. Take energy snacks throughout the day and begin energy replacement immediately after activity, with several hundred calories of a carbohydrate–protein mix (ratio of 4 grams of carbohydrate for 1 of protein) (Ivy et al. 2002). Then continue with the high-carbohydrate performance diet indicated in chapter 11.

Circuit Weight Training

Circuit weight training (CWT) involves a series of resistance exercises designed to promote strength and muscular endurance. The CWT circuit, with short rest intervals between sets, is intended to raise energy expenditure and heart rate and, according to some fitness practitioners, to improve aerobic fitness. Although this popular technique will improve strength and muscular endurance, its effect on aerobic fitness is slight (3 to 5 percent). A set of 10 repetitions of an exercise such as a forearm curl is not sufficient to overload the oxidative system of the muscle. So its effect on aerobic fitness is far less than the 20 to 25 percent improvement derived from sustained large-muscle activity such as cycling or running. Aerobic fitness improvements are greater when you jog between sets.

CWT is an effective way to achieve muscular fitness goals, but whether the rest interval between sets is short (20 seconds) or long (60 seconds), the effect on energy expenditure or aerobic fitness is modest at best (Haltom et al. 1999). Do CWT if you like, but if you want the most from muscular and aerobic fitness training, focus on each one individually.

Calisthenics

Calisthenics include a wide range of exercises, such as push-ups, chin-ups, and sit-ups. The strength-training prescription calls for high resistance and low repetitions, so you may have to add additional resistance when you are able to do more than 10 repetitions (more than 10 repetitions will build short-term endurance but not much strength). You can overload the push-up in several ways. For example, have someone place a hand on your back to increase the resistance or put your feet on a chair to place more weight on the arms. You could also do variations, such as fingertip push-ups or power push-ups (push up and clap hands). Just remember that as the number of repetitions exceeds 10, you are shifting toward endurance training. You can use calisthenics to train for both.

Knee Push-Up

A good chest and triceps exercise for beginners is the knee push-up. With hands outside your shoulders and knees bent, push up, keeping your back straight. Do as many as possible.

Push-Up

The push-up is an intermediate exercise. With hands outside your shoulders, push up, keeping your back straight. Return until your chest almost touches the floor. Do as many as possible.

Chair Dip

The chair dip is an advanced exercise. Make sure that the chair you use is stationary. Grasp the sides of the chair and slide your feet forward while supporting your weight on your arms. Lower your body and return. Do as many as possible. You can also use parallel bars if available.

Modified Chin-Up

A good biceps and back exercise for beginners is the modified chin-up. Stand with the bar about chest height. With an underhand grasp, hang from the bar with the body straight and feet on the ground. Pull up and return. Do as many as possible.

Chin-Up

The standard chin-up is the intermediate version of the exercise. With the underhand grasp, pull up until your chin is over the bar and return. Do as many as possible. Variations include using an overhand grip or climbing a rope.

Pike Chin-Up

The pike chin-up is an advanced exercise. Perform the chin-up from the bar with legs in a pike position.

Basket Hang

The basket hang is an advanced abdominal exercise. Hang from the bar with an underhand grasp. Raise your legs into a "basket" and return. Do as many as possible.

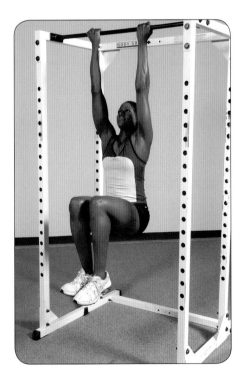

Sit-Up With Arms Crossed

A good exercise for abdominal strength and endurance is the sit-up with arms crossed. On your back with arms crossed on the chest and knees bent, curl up to a semisitting position and return. Do 10 to 15 times. Variations include doing repetitions very fast, doing the exercise on an inclined board, and holding a weight on your chest.

Leg Lift

The leg lift is a good exercise for back strength and endurance. Lying facedown on the floor with a partner holding your trunk down, raise your legs 5 to 10 times. Avoid hyperextension.

Hills

Power walk up a steep hill, stadium steps, or office stairs. For a variation, use ski poles for balance, to aid the downhill trip, or to exercise arms. Wear a weighted pack for added resistance.

Trunk Lift

Lying facedown on the floor with fingers laced behind your head and ankles anchored to the ground, raise your trunk 5 to 10 times. Don't overextend.

Bench Stepping

Step up and down on a bench as fast as possible for 30 seconds. Switch to lead with the other leg and repeat. You can also do bench stepping with a loaded pack.

Half Knee Bend

The half knee bend is good for leg strength and endurance. With feet apart and hands on hips, squat until your thighs are parallel to the ground and return. Do as many as possible. Try a 2-inch (5-centimeter) block under the heels to aid balance. For variety, do this exercise with a weight on your back (e.g., a backpack).

Heel Raise

Stand erect, hands at sides or on hips, feet close together. Rise up on your toes 20 to 40 times. You can do heel raises with your toes on a 2-inch (5-centimeter) platform or with a loaded pack.

Weight Training

Weight training, sometimes called resistance training, has emerged as an essential part of the program to improve performance, fitness, and even health. Use a weight-training apparatus (stack weights) or free weights (bar and weights). Although machines are expensive, they have several advantages over free weights: They are safer and more versatile, they save time, and they eliminate equipment theft. Using a machine also makes it much easier to change resistance as you move from one exercise to another. On the negative side, a machine restricts you to a set series of lifts and movements, and you don't learn to balance the load as well. But for general training, and especially for groups, machines are probably the best bet. Try the weight-training exercises that follow the descriptions of the apparatus in this section. Use the exercise prescriptions found in table 10.1 on page 176.

Weight-Training Machines

A number of companies manufacture weight machines. Some devices use a cam to adjust resistance throughout the lift. Most clubs have stations for triceps, chest exercises, leg press, leg flexion and extension, abdomen and trunk, military press and curls, lat pull-down, leg flexion and extension, biceps curl, bench press, and much more. A variety of variable-resistance devices are specifically designed for sports such as football, basketball, volleyball, and swimming.

Free Weights

Advanced programs often use free weights to isolate and overload specific muscles. Use the appropriate prescription to achieve your goal (e.g., 6 to 10RM for strength, more repetitions for endurance).

Isokinetics

Isokinetic devices, as well as accommodating or variable-resistance machines, are available in health and fitness clubs, in recreation centers, in schools and colleges, and even in private homes. The good ones allow you to exert near maximum force as the device moves through a full range of motion. You can vary the speed and resistance to suit specific training needs. You can use low-cost home devices in a variety of ways. Least expensive of all is isokinetic exercise with a friend (counterforce). Your partner provides resistance throughout the range of motion. For example, as you attempt forearm flexion, your partner provides resistance. You can do fast, medium, or slow isokinetics, depending on the goal of your training. But recent studies indicate that moderately fast training against resistance is more likely to develop strength and power.

Follow the program on an alternating-day schedule. Select the program to suit your needs, not those of the club. If you need medium or fast contractions for your sport, do them. Also, if the club recommends that you do one set, follow that advice for the first few weeks. But when your strength levels off, as it will with one set, progress to two and then three sets. Fitness clubs like lifters to use slow contractions that save wear and tear on the machines, and they advise one set because it eliminates long waits to use the apparatus.

Pull-Down

The pull-down works the lats. Kneel on one or both knees, or sit on a bench if one is available, and grasp the handles. Pull the bar down and return to the starting position.

Leg Press

Leg presses work the quadriceps. Place your feet on the pedals and grasp the handles of the seat. Press your feet forward to elevate the weight and return. Inhale while lowering the weight and exhale while lifting it.

Leg Flexion

The leg flexion exercise works the hamstrings. Lie facedown on the table with your heels positioned behind the padded bar. Flex your legs to elevate the weight. Return to the starting position. Watch for leg cramps.

Leg Extension

The leg extension works the quadriceps. Sit on the bench with your instep under the padded bar. Extend your legs to elevate the weight. Return to the starting position.

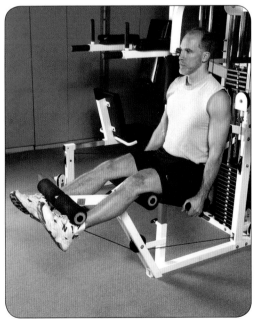

Bench Press

Bench presses exercise the chest and arm extensor muscles. Lie flat on your back with your feet on the floor astride the bench. Grasp the bar wider than shoulder-width, with arms extended. Lower the bar to your chest and then press it back up to the starting position. Inhale while lowering the weight and exhale while pressing it. A partner should assist with weights before and after the exercise.

Triceps Extension

Sit astride a bench with your back straight. Grasp the bar with your hands about 2 inches (5 centimeters) apart, using an overhand grip. Move the bar to full arm extension above your head. Lower the bar behind your head, keeping the elbows stationary.

Bent Rowing

Work the back muscles with bent rowing. Stand in a bent-over position; your back is flat and slightly above parallel with the floor. Spread your feet shoulder-width apart, with your knees comfortably bent. Grasp a barbell with an overhand grip. Your hands should be slightly wider than shoulder-width. Keep your buttocks lower than your shoulders. Pull the bar to your chest and then lower it to the starting position. Keep your upper body stationary.

Military Press

The military press works the arm and shoulder muscles. Stand erect with feet comfortably apart. Grasp a barbell with an overhand grip and raise it to your upper chest. Then press the bar overhead until your elbows are fully extended. Lower the bar to chest position and repeat.

Biceps Curls

For the biceps curl, stand erect with your feet comfortably apart and knees slightly flexed. Hold the bar in front of your thighs with an underhand grip shoulder-width apart and the arms straight. Flex your elbows fully, lifting the bar toward your chest. Keep your elbows close to your sides and avoid raising your shoulders. Don't lean backward or bounce the bar with your leg motion. Repeat.

Arm Flexion

As you try to lift your arms, a partner resists the movement. Your partner should allow movement to progress slowly (through range of motion in 3 seconds). Do three sets of eight repetitions.

Arm Extension

As you try to extend your arms down, a partner resists the movement. Your partner should allow movement to progress slowly (through range of motion in 3 seconds). Do three sets of eight repetitions.

Push-Up

As you do a conventional push-up, a partner provides resistance. Do three sets of eight repetitions. Switch places between sets to allow time to rest.

Leg Flexion

As you try to flex your leg, a partner resists the movement. Your partner should allow movement to progress slowly (through range of motion in 3 seconds). Switch legs and repeat. Do three sets of eight repetitions each. Switch positions between sets. Watch out for leg cramps.

Leg Extension

As you try to extend your leg, a partner resists the movement. Your partner should allow movement to progress slowly (through range of motion in 3 seconds). Switch legs and repeat. Do three sets of eight repetitions each. Switch positions between sets.

Prescriptions for Speed and Power

As with other types of training, the key to speed and power training is specificity. Try to pattern the training after the intended use. To throw a baseball faster, train with a weighted ball or simulate the motion with pulley weights or an isokinetic device. To improve jumping ability, do half squats with weights, jump while wearing a weighted vest, or use an isokinetic jumping device. When in doubt, be specific. Here are some ideas on speed and power training.

- **Speed (velocity).** Do high-speed contractions with low resistance. Sprinters have gained speed by running down slight grades, running against resistance, and performing assisted running (being towed). For more on speed training consult a good book on the subject (e.g., Dintiman and Ward 2003).

- **Power (force times velocity).** Do three sets of 15 to 25 high-speed contractions with 30 to 60 percent of maximal resistance. You can use accommodating resistance devices to do power training, but free weights are not well suited for high-speed training. Athletes use sport-specific devices, higher resistance (e.g., 8RM), and explosive contractions to improve power for brief, intense efforts (e.g., football).

Another approach, a popular technique borrowed from European coaches, is plyometrics. Plyometrics are explosive movements designed to improve power. Sprinters do one- and two-leg hops to gain power. High jumpers, broad jumpers, volleyball and basketball athletes, and even cross-country skiers use plyometrics to improve performance. Proponents have said that plyometrics train the capacity for preload and elastic recoil, and build strength and explosive power (Radcliffe and Farentinos 1985). Unfortunately, the research concerning the value of plyometrics for various sports and for athletes at different levels of development is not extensive. Moreover, excessive use or poor technique can lead to painful knee problems.

We recommend that you try plyometrics, if only because of the effect on skill and economy of movement. Start with a modest number, on a soft surface, and quit at the first sign of discomfort in the knees. Even if you don't gain additional power, you may become more effective in using the power that you possess (In chapter 9 we described the phenomenon called preload and elastic recoil, and explained how it contributes to power and performance.) When training for speed or power, or doing plyometrics, consider the following precautions. Before you do speed or power training, establish a strength and endurance base to avoid injury.

- Warm up and stretch before fast or explosive efforts.
- Start relaxed and gradually increase the intensity and speed of movement.
- Start with light resistance and increase gradually.
- Do not use free weights.
- Use machines and devices designed for high speed.

Start slowly with plyometrics. Use easy jumps and few repetitions. Increase repetitions and intensity gradually. When overdone, plyometrics can cause joint pain and delayed-onset muscle soreness.

Squat Jumps

Stand with one foot a step ahead of the other. Squat (drop quickly) until your front thigh is at a 90-degree angle to the lower leg. Then immediately jump as high as possible, extending the knees. Switch position of your feet on the way down, land, squat, and jump again. Perform 15 to 25 repetitions. Start gently and increase numbers and intensity slowly.

Two-Leg Jumps

Jump as high as possible from both legs. Do 10 to 20 explosive two-leg jumps.

Hops

Do one-leg hops, alternating legs with a balance step between hops. Do 10 with each leg. Work up to two sets of 20.

Low-Back Health

More than 30 million Americans are afflicted with low-back pain, and an estimated 24 million (80 percent) of these problems are due to improper posture, weak muscles, or inadequate flexibility. Weak abdominal muscles cannot counter the forward tilt of the pelvis, which can displace the vertebrae and cause pain. Lack of flexibility in back and hamstring muscles has also been associated with low-back pain, which is a hypokinetic disease, one that results from a lack (hypo) of movement (kinetic).

Back-care specialists continue to explore new approaches, including greater use of back exercises to strengthen extensor muscles and maintain trunk flexibility. Sophisticated back-testing devices allow measurement of flexion and extension strength and range of motion. In one study using specialized equipment, isolated lumbar extension exercise with the pelvis stabilized led to increases in strength and vertebral bone mineral density, reductions in pain and symptoms, and less reutilization of the health care system. Achieved with low-volume training, the results were long lasting and independent of initial diagnosis (Carpenter and Nelson 1999).

Now, many health clubs have back-extension devices. If you have a low-back problem, ask your physician or physical therapist about these and other approaches to the prevention, diagnosis, and treatment of low-back disorders. If you decide to improve back-extension strength, avoid hyperextension. When you do have a problem, consider the results of a study of patients with acute low-back pain. The outcomes of treatment, recovery from pain, and return to function and work were similar whether the care came from primary care physicians, chiropractors, or surgeons. Care by the primary care physician, however, was the least expensive (Carey et al. 1995). Prevention is even cheaper, so begin your back health program today.

Low-Back Fitness Tests

The simple tests that follow, developed at the Sun Valley Health Institute, will help identify areas that need additional attention. Take the tests again after several months to monitor your progress.

Curl-Up

Lie on your back and bend your knees to a 90-degree angle with feet on the floor. Using one of the following arm positions, slowly curl up to a sitting position. Don't swing your arms or allow your feet to come off the floor. If successful, try a more difficult position (higher number). If not, try an easier one (lower number). Your score is the highest number achieved.

1. Arms at side, unable to curl up without aid of partner
2. Arms at side, hands pull back of thighs
3. Arms at side
4. Arms folded across chest
5. Hands behind neck
6. Arms extended overhead, fingers intertwined, with arms pressing against ears

This test indicates abdominal muscle strength and flexibility of back muscles. If you can't do number 5, you need more than a maintenance program. Do repetitions of number 3 and number 4 so that you can achieve number 5.

Leg Lift

The leg lift test evaluates the strength of the lower abdominal muscles. Lie on your back, head on floor, legs straight, and hands under the hollow of your back. Flatten your back and then attempt to raise both feet 10 inches (25 centimeters) and hold the position for 10 seconds.

1. Unable to lift both legs
2. Back rises immediately
3. Back rises after several seconds
4. Able to hold back flat

If you can't do number 4, you need more abdominal tone. Use the basket hang and other exercises to improve abdominal tone.

Sit and Reach

The sit-and-reach test evaluates low-back and hamstring flexibility. Sit with your legs flat on the floor. Place one hand over the other and point the toes to the ceiling. Reach forward and try to touch your toes or beyond. Hold for several counts. Score as follows after several warm-up trials.

1. Well short of toes (more than 3 inches, or 7.6 centimeters, short)
2. Touch toes (or come within 2 inches, or 5 centimeters)
3. Touch well beyond toes (more than 3 inches, or 7.6 centimeters, beyond)

Although extreme flexibility isn't necessary for a healthy back, the lower-back and leg muscles need adequate flexibility. A score of 2 is adequate. With practice you may be able to score a 3.

Hip Flexion

Lie on your back with your legs straight and flat. Keep your head on the floor throughout the test. Bend your right leg and pull your knee to your chest. Test both sides and score as follows.

1. Knee to chest but left leg completely off the floor
2. Knee to chest but left leg lifts somewhat
3. Knee completely to chest with left leg flat on the floor

Tight hip flexors may cause an exaggerated lumbar curve, which predisposes the back to injury. Do this test and other stretching exercises to improve flexibility of the hip flexors. In time you should be able to score a 3 with both legs.

Low-Back Exercises

Low-back pain is a huge problem for industry, responsible for numerous lost workdays and sky-high worker's compensation and medical costs. Yet in many cases, people can prevent low-back problems by assuming good posture and adhering to a regular program of flexibility, back, and abdominal exercises. Maintaining proper weight and a trim waistline also helps. To avoid injury to the lower back, use your legs instead of your back when lifting heavy objects and avoid carrying heavy objects above the level of the elbows. Other suggestions for prevention of low-back problems include the following:

- Sleep with the knees somewhat flexed. Avoid lying flat on your back or belly. Use a firm mattress or sleep with a piece of plywood under the mattress.
- Sit with one or both knees above your hips. Cross your legs or use a footrest.
- Keep your knees bent while driving. If your car seat doesn't provide lumbar support, use a cushion.
- When standing, place one foot on a stool, especially while ironing, washing dishes, or working at a counter or workbench.

Regular practice of the following exercises will help prevent or improve low-back problems and maintain low-back health (Williams 1974). Remember, when low-back pain does arise, the best treatment is not bed rest but a return to normal activity as soon as possible (Malmivaara et al. 1995).

Knee to Chest

With knees bent and arms above your head, move one knee as far as possible toward your chest while straightening the other. Return to the starting position and repeat, switching leg positions. Relax and repeat.

Flat Back

Bend your knees, with your feet flat on the floor and arms above your head. Tighten the muscles of your lower abdomen and buttocks at the same time, keeping your back flat on the floor. Hold 10 seconds, relax, and repeat.

Double Knee Pull

Starting in the same position, with your arms at your sides, draw your knees to your chest and clasp your hands around your knees. Keeping your shoulders flat against the floor, pull your knees tightly against your chest, hold 10 seconds, relax, and repeat. Repeat and touch your forehead to your knees.

Curl-Up

Bend your knees with your feet flat on the floor. Lift one leg and rest the ankle on the knee of the opposite leg. Lock your hands behind your head. Raise your head and shoulders from the floor. With chin to chest and with your back rounded, curl up as far as possible, trying to touch your elbow to the opposite knee. Be sure to pull with the abdominal muscles. Lower slowly. Do 5 to 10 repetitions, switch position, and repeat. Increase until you can do 20.

Angry Cat

Kneel and place your hands on the floor. Lower your head and contract your abdominal and buttocks muscles, arch your lower back, hold 5 seconds, and relax.

Seated Back Stretch

With your knees bent, bend forward at the waist to bring your head between your knees. Pull in your abdomen as you curl forward. Keep your weight back on your hips. Release your abdominal muscles and reach to stretch your lower back. Come up slowly. Relax and repeat. Move forward to involve and stretch the hamstring muscles.

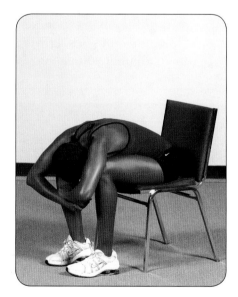

Summary

This chapter has provided prescriptions and guidelines for the development of muscular strength and endurance. We've suggested ways to train, shown what progress you can expect, explained how to maintain muscular fitness, and described what happens when training stops. We also provided prescriptions for speed and power. Be certain to precede vigorous speed or power training with at least 8 weeks of a sport-specific buildup (strength and progressively faster running, throwing, and jumping) to avoid excessive soreness or injury. An important part of the chapter dealt with the important issue of low-back health and the essential contributions of muscular fitness.

Besides the obvious benefits of strength and endurance to appearance and performance, other important reasons for muscular fitness include avoidance of crippling osteoporosis and lifelong maintenance of mobility. Avoidance of osteoporosis, the weakening of bone through loss of bone minerals, requires regular weight-bearing activity, such as walking or jogging, as well as moderate resistance exercises for the upper body. Normal household tasks, such as lifting, vacuuming, mowing grass, shoveling snow, and others, will help avoid the problem. Research shows, however, that people achieve the best results by a combination of weight-bearing and resistance exercise, along with a diet that includes adequate calcium and vitamin D (exposure to sunlight is a natural way to form vitamin D). Postmenopausal women may need strength training to slow the loss of bone density and improve muscle strength and balance (Nelson et al. 1994).

Finally, living the active life, which includes engaging in aerobic and muscular activities, preserves mobility and independence. Anyone, regardless of age, can restore mobility and independence by becoming active. Studies of older adults and frail older people indicate that resistance training improves strength as well as performance of activities of daily living. These activities include getting out of a chair, walking, climbing stairs, and carrying groceries. If you can't perform these activities, you will be relegated to family care or a nursing home. Start now to maintain or improve your muscular fitness.

Activity and Weight Control

Ours is a nation of paradoxes. We boast more dieters, diet books, diet foods, and diet centers than any other country on earth, yet we have become the fattest nation on earth. The reason for this is simple—dieting. What a paradox—the more we diet, the fatter we get! Part IV reviews basics of good nutrition, deals with the importance of activity in weight control, and discusses the contributions of fitness to fat metabolism and weight control. We'll show how diet alone is a recipe for failure and how the active life provides a positive approach to weight control while allowing enjoyment of your favorite foods. These ideas are not new; they appeared in Brian's first book, published in 1974. But in the years that followed, overweight and obesity—and their consequences—have been, so to speak, expanding.

We'll provide a plan to help you gain control of your weight and then show you how the active life will keep you there. But you don't just want to lose weight. You want to lose fat. The active life and fitness help you attain that goal by making muscle cells efficient users of fat. Diet leads to the loss of muscle, the furnace in which fat is burned. Activity conserves muscle while it burns fat, and improved fitness increases muscle tissue while further enhancing its ability to consume fat. You'll find all this and more in part IV.

11

Nutrition and Health

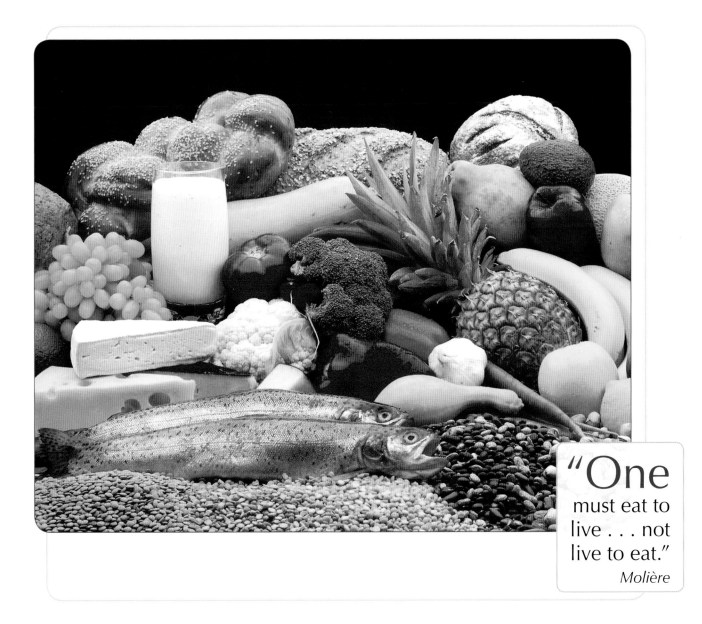

"One must eat to live . . . not live to eat."
Molière

As people work longer hours, less time is available for the selection and preparation of food, leading to increasing reliance on prepared food, fast food, ordering in and eating out, and loss of control over the quantity and quality of food that we eat. We select the item but have little influence over its preparation. Consequently, we eat more calories, more saturated and hydrogenated fat, and more salt, and we run the risk of being shortchanged in other areas of nutrition.

Work once implied physical exertion, but today few of us burn many calories at work or after work. Many of us spend leisure time in front of a TV set, a computer, or a video game. Few people walk or engage in vigorous activity. Kids ride a bus to school and stay inside after school. The convergence of these changes in eating and activity make good nutrition more important than ever before.

This chapter will help you

- understand the basics of good nutrition,
- identify sources of energy and their contribution to performance and health,
- consider your need for vitamin and mineral supplements,
- understand the relationship between diet and health, and
- select foods that are good for your health.

Energy

Energy from the sun grows plants that animals eat. Our sources of energy—carbohydrate, fat, and protein—originate from plant and animal sources. We ingest the food, digest it, and absorb it into the bloodstream for transport to cells. Using enzyme catalysts aligned in metabolic pathways, we convert these energy sources into molecules of ATP (adenosine triphosphate), the high-energy compound that fuels muscular contractions and many other cellular functions. The pathways control the

The Calorie

A calorie is the amount of heat required to raise 1 cubic centimeter of water 1 degree Celsius. The kilocalorie is 1,000 calories, or the heat required to raise 1 kilogram of water 1 degree Celsius. In this book, we use the term *calorie* as nutritionists use it; 1 calorie in nutrition refers to the kilocalorie, the standard of measurement in nutrition and exercise. For example, you take in 100 calories with one light beer, and burn 100 calories when you jog 1 mile (1.6 kilometers).

You always expend some energy, even when you're asleep. If you stay in bed for 24 hours and do nothing at all, you will expend about 1,600 calories (for a 154-pound, or 70-kilogram person). This energy is used by heart and respiratory muscles, for normal cellular metabolism, and for maintenance of body temperature. Heavy thinking does little to raise energy requirements, but as soon as you begin to move, energy expenditure increases dramatically. Caloric expenditure can go from 1.2 calories per minute at rest to more than 20 calories per minute during vigorous effort. Physical activity has the greatest effect on energy needs. Walking burns about 5 calories per minute, jogging about 10, and running more than 15 calories per minute.

SELF-EVALUATION FOR GOOD NUTRITION

To evaluate how well you meet your nutritional needs on a daily basis, consider the following questions:

- How many servings of fruits and vegetables do you eat?
- How many calories do you consume?
- What percentage of your caloric intake comes from fat? From protein? From carbohydrate?
- What percentage of each should you get?
- What percentage of your fat intake comes from saturated fat?
- Do you meet your vitamin and mineral needs?
- How many times per week do you eat out, order in, or eat prepared foods?
- Do you regularly eat rich sauces, fatty meats, or desserts?

You can evaluate your responses later in this chapter, using information from the section on food choices.

---

combustion of the fuels that we burn, and we measure energy needs with a unit for measuring heat, the calorie.

Carbohydrate

Throughout the world carbohydrate provides the major source of energy. Carbohydrate is available in simple and complex forms. Simple sugars such as glucose, fructose, and sucrose (refined sugar, composed of molecules of glucose and fructose) contain energy but few nutrients (i.e., vitamins and minerals). Complex carbohydrates found in beans, rice, whole-grained products (bread, pasta), potatoes, and corn come with important nutrients and fiber. Unfortunately, the average American gets half of his or her dietary carbohydrate from concentrated or refined simple sugars, packed with so-called empty calories (empty because they lack nutrients). Fresh fruits contain simple sugars, but they also provide important nutrients.

Digestion of complex starch molecules begins in the mouth where an enzyme (salivary amylase) reduces complex carbohydrates to simple sugars. Digestion temporarily ends in the stomach when gastric secretions inactivate the enzyme. In the small intestine, another enzyme (pancreatic amylase) helps to digest starches further. Enzymes secreted by the wall of the intestine and absorbed into the bloodstream complete the final breakdown to glucose. The absorption is rather complete; most of the sugar that you eat gets into the blood. Surprisingly, some complex carbohydrates, like potatoes, can enter the blood as quickly as table sugar does (Jenkins, Taylor, and Wolever 1982).

Because carbohydrate is important for muscular contractions and because it is not stored in large quantities, we should consume a sizable percentage of daily calories from complex carbohydrate and fruit. The performance diet recommended for active people and athletes suggests that 55 to 60 percent of calories should come from carbohydrate, which is more than the 40 to 50 percent that the average American consumes (see table 11.2).

Glycemic Index

The glycemic index describes the rate of carbohydrate digestion and its effect on the rise of blood glucose. Foods that digest rapidly and cause a pronounced rise in blood sugar have a high glycemic index, whereas those digested and absorbed more slowly, because of fiber or fat, have a low index. As you might expect, foods with a high glycemic index include sugar and honey, as well as corn, white bread, refined cereals, and baked potatoes. Foods with a moderate glycemic index include pasta, whole-grained breads, rice, oatmeal, bran, and peas. Foods with a low glycemic index include beans, lentils, and fruits (apples, peaches, and grapefruit). High-index foods lead to a rapid rise in blood sugar and a greater rise in insulin, the hormone responsible for lowering blood glucose (Foster-Powell and Miller 1995).

> Foods that digest rapidly and cause a pronounced rise in blood sugar have a high glycemic index.

People with insulin resistance, a condition often associated with overweight, hypertension, low HDL cholesterol, and elevated triglycerides and blood glucose, are wise to select low-index foods. High-index foods prompt an insulin surge from the pancreas, stimulating body cells to store glucose. Over time the cells become less sensitive to insulin, eventually contributing to adult-onset (type 2) diabetes. Insulin resistance is linked to heart disease, obesity, age, and inactivity. Weight loss and regular, moderate activity reduce insulin resistance.

Should you avoid foods with a high glycemic index? No, they are useful when you want to speed glucose into cells to replace muscle glycogen after prolonged exertion. Also, when you consume a high-glycemic carbohydrate such as potatoes in a mixed meal, along with fat and protein, you slow the entry of glucose into the bloodstream (see table 11.1).

After a meal, absorbed sugars are taken up by the blood and by cells in the heart, skeletal muscle, and liver, in that order. After blood sugar levels are restored, heart and skeletal muscles accept glucose. The constantly working heart uses it for energy, and the skeletal muscle can store glucose for use when energy is needed. Granules of stored glucose are called muscle glycogen. The liver accepts glucose and stores it as glycogen. When sufficient glucose has been stored in the liver (about 80 to 100 grams, or 2.8 to 3.5 ounces), the leftover glucose suppresses fat oxidation and is itself used for energy. Thus an excess intake of carbohydrate does not become a supply of quick energy; it is oxidized, thereby conserving fat (Swinburn and Ravussin 1993). The glucose stored in the liver is readily available when needed, but muscle glycogen can be used directly only by the muscle in which it is stored. Nerves, muscles, or other tissues in need of energy also use blood glucose.

Table 11.1   Glycemic Index of Common Foods

High glycemic
Glucose
Sucrose
Cane, maple, and corn syrup
Honey
White breads including bagels
Potatoes
Cornflakes and most cold cereals
Raisins and bananas
White rice

Moderate glycemic
Whole-grain breads
Spaghetti
Corn
Oatmeal
Oranges

Low glycemic
Milk products and yogurt
Nuts including peanuts
Legumes (peas and beans)
Apples and peaches

Table 11.2   Performance Diet

Component	Performance diet (% of total calories)	Typical diet (% of total calories)
Carbohydrate	55–60*	45–50
Fat	25–30**	35–40
Protein	15	10–15

*Increase before long-distance event (see "Carbohydrate Loading," page 310).
**No more than one-third of fat calories from saturated fats (avoid intake of hydrogenated or trans fatty acids).

As we've noted, carbohydrate is stored in muscles and the liver as granules of glycogen, a compound consisting of many linked molecules of glucose. We use this stored carbohydrate at the start of exercise, and its contribution to energy metabolism increases as exercise intensity increases. During prolonged exercise, when muscle glycogen stores become depleted, we are forced to use blood glucose that is supplied from the liver. When that limited supply runs out, we bonk—a term that cyclists coined to describe the utter fatigue, confusion, and lack of coordination that results when blood glucose falls below the level required by the nervous system (see figure 11.1). To avoid bonking, distance athletes consume energy bars and drink beverages containing 6 to 8 percent carbohydrate (60 to 80 grams per liter).

Finally, be aware that chronic ingestion of a high-carbohydrate diet, especially a diet high in simple sugars, without an active lifestyle, may lead muscle to become insulin insensitive, adipose tissue to convert excess carbohydrate to fat, and the liver to increase production of very low density lipoprotein (VLDL) cholesterol (Graham and Adamo 1999). With regular physical activity, insulin sensitivity increases, the carbohydrate is burned, and blood lipids are lowered.

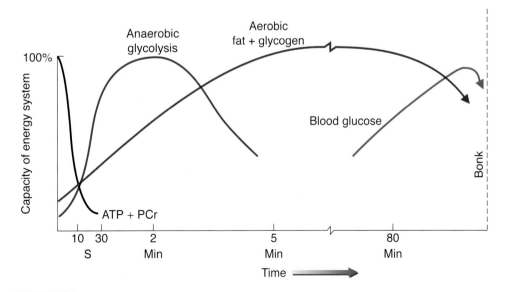

Figure 11.1   Patterns of energy use. We use short-term energy sources (ATP plus PCr) at the start of exercise, and then anaerobic glycolysis or nonoxidative breakdown of glycogen (glycogen is carbohydrate stored in the muscle). After several minutes, more efficient aerobic pathways take over, with more glycogen use at higher intensities. As muscle glycogen is used up, blood glucose temporarily fills the demand for carbohydrate.
Adapted from Sharkey, 1984.

Fat

Fat is the most efficient way to store energy, with 9.3 calories per gram versus the 4.1 and 4.3 calories for carbohydrate and protein, respectively. The small intestine breaks down and absorbs dietary fat, which then travels through the lymphatics, a system of tiny vessels and nodes that transports and filters cellular drainage. The fat clumps (chylomicrons) eventually dump into the circulation for transport to cells for energy or to adipose tissue for storage. But dietary fat intake isn't the only way to acquire this source of energy. Excess carbohydrate or protein can be converted to fat and stored in adipose tissue. We have many ways to acquire fat but only one good way to remove it—physical activity.

> We have many ways to acquire fat but only one good way to remove it—physical activity.

Fat isn't all bad. It is an essential component of cell walls, vital insulation in the nervous system, a precursor for important compounds such as hormones, and a shock absorber for internal organs. And fat can be an efficient fuel for sustained physical activity, especially in muscles that have undergone endurance training. Furthermore, fat enhances the taste of food and helps fill us up. So we don't need to eliminate dietary fat, just limit the intake. Excess dietary fat is a major cause of overweight and obesity and a contributor to heart disease, hypertension, diabetes, some cancers, and other ills. Research indicates that high fat intake is inversely related to physical activity, suggesting a behavioral link between the two (Simoes et al. 1995).

Fat comes in several forms, including triglycerides and cholesterol. Triglyceride fat is composed of three fatty acids and glycerol. The fatty acids can be saturated (with a hydrogen molecule filling each binding site on a carbon molecule) or unsaturated, with one or more double bonds (see figure 11.2).

Monounsaturated fatty acids have one double bond, whereas the polyunsaturated have two or more. The double bonds of unsaturated fatty acids may be more susceptible to oxidation; therefore, unsaturated fats are recommended over saturated fats, which promote cholesterol synthesis. Saturated fats are found in meat and dairy products. Watch out also for the tropical oils, palm and coconut, which are believed to be more atherogenic (likely to clog arteries), as are otherwise health-

The fatty acid may be saturated, meaning they have single bonds, such as stearic acid;

Stearic acid

they may be monounsaturated, meaning they have one double bond, such as oleic acid;

Oleic acid

or they may be polyunsaturated, meaning they have two or more double bonds, such as linoleic acid.

Linoleic acid

Figure 11.2 Fatty acids: saturated, monounsaturated, and polyunsaturated.

Fat Intake

If you eat 2,000 calories a day and get 25 percent of your calories from fat, you'll get 500 fat calories. Divide 500 by 9.3 calories per gram of fat and you get 54 grams, the amount of fat that you can eat each day (far less than the 86 grams you'd eat if fat constituted 40 percent of your caloric intake). Labels on food packages indicate the grams of fat in each serving.

ful oils (e.g., soybean oil) when they are partially hydrogenated. Hydrogenation eliminates double bonds and creates unhealthy trans-fatty acids. These trans-fatty acids are common in snack crackers and other prepared foods, in which, to promote shelf life, otherwise healthy fats are made dangerous. Read labels and watch out for partially hydrogenated fats. The performance diet recommends that 25 percent of daily calories should come from fat, with no more than one-third from saturated fats, and an extremely small intake of hydrogenated or trans-fatty acids. This amount of fat is substantially less than the 30 to 40 percent that many people currently consume.

Protein

When we ingest animal or plant protein, the large molecules are cleaved into amino acids and absorbed. The amino acids are building blocks used to construct cell walls, muscle tissue, hormones, enzymes, and a variety of other molecules. The blood contains several large proteins: globulin for antibody formation, albumin for buffering and osmosis, fibrinogen for clotting, and hemoglobin for oxygen transport. Training builds proteins, aerobic training builds aerobic enzyme proteins for energy production, and strength training builds contractile proteins (actin and myosin) for strength. So it should be no surprise to learn the importance of protein to the active life.

The performance diet recommends 15 percent of daily caloric intake in the form of protein. Moderately active adults can get by with 10 percent, but we recommend more for those who are very active or training. Fifteen percent of 2,000 calories is 300 calories (300 divided by 4.3 kilocalories per gram equals 70 grams, which is 1 gram per kilogram for a person who weighs 70 kilograms, or 154 pounds). More important than quantity, however, is the quality of protein. Quality protein is high in essential amino acids, those that the body cannot synthesize. These essential amino acids are macronutrients, major food sources that must be available for optimal function. When essential amino acids are missing, the body is unable to construct proteins that require them. Although animal protein is a better source of essential amino acids (as well as iron and vitamin B12), proper combinations of plant protein can meet nutritional needs. If you are or plan to become a vegetarian, be ready to eat a variety of grains, beans, and leafy vegetables.

Protein isn't a major source of energy at rest or during exercise—it seldom amounts to more than 5 to 10 percent of energy needs—but when one trains hard while dieting to lose weight, the body senses starvation and begins to use tissue protein for energy. To avoid loss of muscle tissue and achieve the benefits of training, ensure adequate protein and energy intake. The best bet is to lose weight slowly or not at all during vigorous training. Even with adequate protein, rapid weight loss while training risks the loss of the muscle and enzyme proteins that you are trying so hard to increase.

Protein Needs?

A review of protein needs for athletes concludes that endurance athletes will benefit from dietary intakes of 1.2 to 1.4 grams of protein per kilogram of body weight (.56 to .64 gram per pound), and strength athletes need 1.4 to 1.8 grams (.64 to .82 gram per pound) (Lemon 1995). These values are well above the RDA of .8 gram per kilogram (.36 gram per pound) but are attainable with the performance diet recommended in this chapter. If you participate in endurance and strength training, you'll need at least 1.4 grams per kilogram of body weight (.64 gram per pound). Simply multiply that number times your body weight in kilograms (1 kilogram equals 2.2 pounds) to get your daily requirement.

For example, if you weigh 70 kilograms (154 pounds), multiply 70 kilograms times 1.4 grams (154 pounds times .64 gram) to get your daily protein needs (98 grams). Because each gram of protein yields 4.3 calories, you'll need about 420 calories (98 grams times 4.3) of energy from protein.

Athletes usually raise total caloric intake to meet the increased energy needs of training. If your diet fails to meet the energy requirements for your type of training, increase your intake of good-quality protein (lean meats, skinned poultry, fish, beans, nuts) (see table 11.3). Recent evidence regarding protein utilization indicates that the timing of protein ingestion (after exercise) and the adequacy of total energy intake are important factors (Tipton and Wolfe 2004).

Table 11.3   Protein in Common Foods

Food	Portion	Protein (g)
Beans	1/2 cup (118 ml)	6–8
Beef	4 ounces (113 g)	20–28
Cheese	1 ounce (28 g)	7
Chicken	3 1/2 ounces (100 g)	24–30
Chili	1 cup (236 ml)	20
Corn	1/2 cup (118 ml)	3
Fish	4 ounces (113 g)	25–30
Hamburger	4 ounces (113 g)	20
Milk	1 cup (236 ml)	9
Peanut butter	1 tablespoon (14 ml)	4
Pizza	1 slice	10

Excess protein intake accompanied by fat from animal sources (e.g., eggs, meat, fish, poultry, dairy products) leads to storage of fat. By following the performance diet you will have the protein that you need. The recommended carbohydrate intake spares or conserves tissue protein.

Energy Availability

A limited supply of glucose is available in the blood, but glucose is needed for brain and nerve metabolism, for which it is the sole source of energy. Glucose is stored in the liver (about 80 grams) and muscle (15 grams per kilogram of muscle, or 33 grams per pound) as glycogen. If you could use it all for exercise, you would have about 1,200 calories, enough to fuel a 10-mile (16.1-kilometer) run.

Fat is the most abundant source of energy. Young men average 12.5 to 15 percent body fat; young women average 25 to 33 percent. If you weigh 121 pounds (55 kilograms) and have 25 percent fat, you'll have about 30 pounds (13.6 kilograms) of fat. Because each pound of fat yields 3,500 calories, 30 pounds of fat provides 105,000 calories of energy. When you consider that you burn about 100 calories per mile (1.6 kilometers) of jogging, you'll realize that you have enough fat energy to fuel 1,000 miles (1,600 kilometers) of running! Most of us have more fat than we need, so you can benefit from teaching the body how to burn fat during exercise. In so doing, you extend your endurance dramatically, eliminate the problem of excess weight, and improve your overall health.

Nutrients

The macronutrients are carbohydrate, fat, and protein. Vitamins and minerals are called micronutrients because we need only small amounts on a daily basis. They play an essential role in cell metabolism, immune function, clotting, and other important functions.

Vitamins

Why are vitamins, which do not supply energy and are needed only in minute quantities, considered essential for life? In many cases the answer lies in the structure of enzymes that are essential for cellular metabolism. Enzymes are composed of a large protein portion and a coenzyme. The shape of the protein molecule dictates the role of the enzyme, whereas the coenzyme is the active portion that performs a specific task. For example, vitamin B1 is a coenzyme that removes carbon dioxide in a metabolic pathway. Without the vitamin coenzyme the metabolic pathway grinds to a halt, usually with the toxic buildup of intermediary compounds. Lack of vitamin B1 (thiamine) leads to beriberi, a vitamin deficiency disease characterized by weakness, wasting, nerve damage, and even heart failure. Fortunately, the small amount of vitamins needed is readily available from a variety of foods in a well-balanced diet. Doses far in excess of daily requirements (megadoses) do not improve function or performance, and they may be toxic.

> Fortunately, the small amount of vitamins needed is readily available from a variety of foods in a well-balanced diet.

Vitamins are classified according to their solubility. The fat-soluble vitamins A, D, E, and K have widely different functions (see table 11.4 on page 220). These vitamins are ingested with fats in the diet. Amounts in excess of daily needs are stored in body tissue, and megadoses can become toxic (e.g., vitamin A). Because they are stored, deficiencies are less likely, except in diets very low in fat.

The B complex vitamins and vitamin C are water soluble. Excess water-soluble vitamins are flushed away in the urine, making deficiencies more likely. Table 11.4 lists the vitamins along with their reference daily intakes, functions, and good food sources.

Vitamins and Health

Vitamins perform many functions essential for life and health. Recent studies indicate that some vitamins are important to the optimal function of the immune system. To help maintain a healthy immune system, the well-balanced diet should include foods with the following micronutrients:

- Beta-carotene (carrots, sweet potatoes), which stimulates natural killer cells, immune system cells that fight infections
- Vitamin B6 (potatoes, nuts, spinach), which promotes proliferation of white blood cells
- Folate (peas, salmon, romaine lettuce), which increases white blood cell activity
- Vitamin C (citrus fruits, broccoli, peppers), an antioxidant that enhances the immune response
- Vitamin E (whole grains, wheat germ, vegetable oils), an antioxidant that stimulates the immune response

The minerals selenium and zinc also aid the immune response. Selenium (tuna, eggs, whole grains) promotes action against toxic bacteria, and zinc (eggs, whole grains, oysters) promotes wound healing. Regular, moderate physical activity bolsters the immune system, whereas exhaustion and stress impair its function, opening the door to upper respiratory and other infections.

A balanced diet is the best way to achieve your daily vitamin needs.

Beta-carotene and vitamins C and E, the so-called antioxidant vitamins, may reduce muscle damage and even the risk of heart disease, cancer, and eye disease. Intense exercise produces compounds called free radicals. These highly reactive compounds can damage muscle tissue, especially in untrained people who have limited antioxidant capabilities. We have natural antioxidant protection, but the supply is limited. The antioxidant vitamins react with free radicals and reduce their ability to do microscopic damage (Kanter 1995). Regular activity and fitness training increase the body's ability to deal with free radicals.

Concerning heart disease, the antioxidant vitamins may prevent the oxidative deterioration of lipid, a step in the artery-clogging process of atherosclerosis. When oxidized, LDL turns rancid and becomes part of the growing plaque in the wall of the artery. Dietary antioxidants have been associated with lower risk of heart disease. Recent studies suggest that large doses of vitamin E may increase all-cause mortality in adults with chronic diseases (Miller et al. 2005). The American Heart Association, American Cancer Society, and the American Dietetics Association agree that scientific data do not justify the use of vitamin supplements to reduce heart disease, cancer, or other health problems.

So you should begin now to consume a diet rich in natural antioxidants. Vitamin supplements are not as effective as the nutrients in fruits and vegetables. Vitamins in food come with other vitamins, minerals, and trace nutrients that may enhance the effect of the nutrients. Vitamin supplements are not a satisfactory replacement for a well-balanced diet. Dietary reference intake (DRI) supplements of vitamins may offer a margin of safety for those who lose considerable weight during training or will not eat nutritious food. All others should use a variety of nutritious foods as their source for micronutrients.

Vitamins and Performance

Athletes are a gullible bunch, inclined to try anything to improve performance. Plenty of snake-oil salespersons are willing to sell a food or drug guaranteed to enhance performance. Vitamin supplements are frequently marketed to this gullible audience and to millions of others in search of health. Unfortunately, much of the money spent on vitamin megadoses washes away in the urine. Vitamin supplements will not improve the performance or health of those who consume an adequate diet.

Supplementation, however, may sometimes be prudent. Highly active people and athletes need more vitamins when they burn more energy. They should meet this increased need with a larger intake of food to satisfy energy and nutrient needs. But during periods when you combine vigorous training with weight loss, you may want to take a daily vitamin and mineral supplement that does not exceed the recommended daily intake. Because certain vitamins enhance the immune response, some believe that supplements may help reduce the risk of illness that accompanies exhaustion and overtraining (Evans 2000). Recent studies on endurance athletes, however, have not shown a reduction in infections with vitamin C (Nieman, Henson, and McAnulty 2002) or lipid oxidation with vitamin E (Nieman et al. 2004). Antioxidant vitamins may reduce the severity of muscle damage during intense activity. We recommend vitamins in food over those contained in pills. If you decide to take supplements, do not exceed the reference daily intake, or RDI (see table 11.4).

Table 11.4   Vitamins: Daily Intake, Functions, and Sources*

Vitamins	DRI (female/male)	Functions	Sources
FAT SOLUBLE			
Vitamin A (retinal)	700/900 μg	Vision, immune function	Milk products, liver, eggs
Vitamin D	5 μg	Bones, teeth	Sunlight, eggs, fish, milk
Vitamin E	15 mg	Antioxidant	Vegetable oils, nuts, greens
Vitamin K	90/120 μg	Blood clotting	Greens, milk, meats
WATER SOLUBLE			
Beta-carotene	3 mg	Cell growth, antioxidant	Fruits, vegetables
Vitamin B_1 (thiamin)	1.1/1.2 mg	Energy production	Pork, grains, legumes, nuts
Vitamin B_2 (riboflavin)	1.1/1.3 mg	Energy production	Milk, shellfish, meat, greens, grains
Niacin	14/16 mg	Energy production	Nuts, fish, poultry, grains, milk, eggs
Vitamin B_6 (pyridoxine)	1.3 mg	Energy, protein, and metabolism	Meats, grains, vegetables, fruits, fish, poultry
Folate	400 μg	Red and white blood cells, RNA, DNA, amino acids	Vegetables, grains, legumes
Vitamin B_{12}	2.4 μg	Blood cells, RNA, DNA, energy	Meat, fish, poultry, milk, eggs
Biotin	30 μg	Fat and amino acid metabolism, glycogen synthesis	Eggs, soybeans, fish, grains
Vitamin C (ascorbic acid)	75/90 mg	Healing, immune function, antioxidant, connective tissue	Citrus fruits, strawberries, cantaloupe, greens

*DRI = dietary reference intake; μg = micrograms/day; mg = milligrams/day; grains = whole grains; greens = dark leafy greens.

Minerals

Do you ever wonder why the body needs iron, zinc, magnesium, and even chromium, whereas it definitely doesn't need lead? Minerals are important for enzyme and cellular activity, for some hormones, for bones, for muscle and nerve activity, and for acid–base balance. Some are required in small daily amounts (less than 100 milligrams), whereas we need more of others. Minerals are available in many food sources, but concentrations are higher in animal tissues and products (see table 11.5).

Minerals, like vitamins, are readily available in a well-balanced diet, one drawn from a variety of food sources. Problems arise when a person decides to eliminate a major nutrient source, such as meat.

Minerals are essential to health and performance, but supplementation beyond what the RDI calls for is unnecessary and could cause side effects. Excesses of some minerals pose no problems, whereas others can cause diarrhea (magnesium, zinc), high blood pressure (sodium), or cirrhosis (iron). If you are concerned that your diet may be deficient, consider a supplement that provides the recommended daily intake for vitamins and minerals, including trace minerals (see table 11.5). Supplementation

Table 11.5   Minerals: Daily Intake, Functions, and Sources*

Minerals	DRI (female/male)	Functions	Sources
Calcium	1,000 mg	Bones, teeth, blood clotting, muscle–nerve function	Milk, tofu, broccoli, legumes
Chloride	2,300 mg	Digestion, fluid balance	Salt (in foods)
Chromium	25/35 μg	Energy metabolism	Grains, meats, vegetable oils
Copper	900 μg	Iron metabolism	Seafood, nuts, grains
Fluorine	3/4 mg	Bones, teeth	Water, seafood, tea
Iodine	150 μg	Thyroid hormone	Seafood, milk, iodized salt
Iron	18/8 mg	Oxygen transport	Meats, legumes, dried fruit
Magnesium	320/420 mg	Protein synthesis, muscle–nerve function	Grains, nuts, legumes, seafood, chocolate
Manganese	1.8/2.3 mg	Energy metabolism	Nuts, grains, tea, leafy vegetables
Molybdenum	45 μg	Enzymes	Organ meats, legumes, cereals
Phosphorus	700 mg	Bones, teeth, acid–base balance	Milk, meats, poultry, fish, eggs
Potassium	4,700 mg	Nerve–muscle, fluid, and acid–base balance	Meats, milk, fruits, vegetables grains, coffee
Selenium	55 μg	Antioxidant	Seafood, meats, grains
Sodium	1,500 mg	Nerve function, fluid, and acid–base balance	Salt (in food)
Sulfur	—	Liver function, hormones	Dietary protein
Zinc	8/11 mg	Enzyme activity, wound healing	Meat, poultry, fish, milk, grains, vegetables

*DRI = dietary reference intake; μg = micrograms/day; mg = milligrams/day; grains = whole grains; greens = dark leafy greens.

may be important for those who train hard while losing weight in an effort to enhance performance. But remember that supplements are not an adequate substitute for good nutrition.

Iron

Iron is particularly important for active people, both male and female. Much of the iron absorbed in the blood goes into the production of hemoglobin, the compound in red blood cells that carries oxygen from the lungs to the working muscles. Iron is also used in muscle myoglobin to transport and store oxygen, and in important oxidative (aerobic) enzymes. People deficient in iron risk anemia and poor endurance. Because only 10 to 20 percent of the iron in food is absorbed into the bloodstream, athletes must take in 10 times the amount that they need. Lean meat is a rich source of iron, and the iron in meat is more readily absorbed than that from other sources.

Females lose blood and iron during menstruation, and all active people are subject to iron loss and reduced absorption during hard training. Meats, dates, raisins, beans,

Diet and Performance

Rick was a top runner on the university track team, with a mile (1.6 kilometer) time approaching 4 minutes. The coach expected big things from this elite athlete, but that is not what happened. Instead, as his training progressed, Rick's performance began to deteriorate. By midseason he was struggling to approach 4:20, and things got worse from there. Eventually he was forced to rest and seek medical advice. The team physician was perplexed, because Rick wasn't sick or injured. Yet his vitality was gone, and he exhibited signs of chronic fatigue and overtraining. As the coach and the physician continued their search for the problem, they turned to a specialist in sports nutrition. A dietary analysis documented the cause of Rick's problem—his vegetarian diet. Several months before the season Rick had decided to try vegetarianism. Because meat and animal products are important sources of essential amino acids, vitamins, and minerals, his diet was unhealthy, especially for an athlete. A vegetarian diet can contribute to good health but only if you are willing to study and to spend extra time shopping and preparing nutritious meals.

prunes, and apricots are good sources of iron. If you are concerned about your iron status, consult a physician or sports nutrition specialist before you supplement with more than the dietary reference intake (DRI).

Calcium

Calcium is a major component of bones and teeth, and it is involved in muscle contraction, nerve transmission, blood clotting, and enzyme activity. In relation to the active life, calcium is extremely important because of its relationship to osteoporosis, the loss of bone density that predisposes bones to fractures. Bone is a tissue that responds to stress. Weight-bearing exercise builds young bones, helps keep bones strong, and slows the inevitable loss of bone density with age. After menopause, when estrogen levels decline, women lose bone density at a more rapid rate than they do before menopause. Calcium, vitamin D, and weight-bearing exercise are important throughout life.

Young women face a dilemma. Too much strenuous training, combined with weight loss, inadequate calcium intake, and stress, sometimes interferes with the normal menstrual cycle in female athletes. These changes seem to diminish the protective effect of estrogen on bones, leading to reduced bone density and increased risk of stress fractures. Reduced training, weight gain, and increased calcium intake will stop the loss of bone, but it isn't certain that young women ever fully recover from early bone loss.

Fluids

Besides energy and nutrients, the body needs an ample supply of water. Water, found in the cells and in extracellular fluids such as blood, lymph, saliva, tears, and glands and in the gastrointestinal tract, makes up over half of body weight. Water serves to transport energy, gases, waste products, hormones, antibodies, and heat. In the blood, it is involved in the regulation of the acid–base balance. Water lubricates surfaces and membranes and, through perspiration, serves as a main avenue for temperature regulation.

The inactive person needs about 2.5 liters (2.64 quarts) daily to replace water lost in urine, feces, skin, and exhalation from the lungs. During activity in a hot environment, sweat loss can average 1 liter (1.06 quarts) per hour for many hours, and can temporarily exceed a rate of 2 liters (2.1 quarts) per hour. Failure to replace this fluid will lead to impaired performance, dehydration, and heat stress disorders ranging from muscle cramps and heat exhaustion to life-threatening heatstroke.

We'll discuss fluid replacement in chapter 16, where we'll deal with heat stress; fluid intake before, during, and after activity; and carbohydrate–electrolyte drinks and their effect on performance.

Dehydration Weight Loss

Water constitutes 55 to 60 percent of adult body weight. Thirst, activated by excess sodium or water loss, helps us maintain body fluid levels. Several hormones, such as antidiuretic hormone (ADH), assist in the maintenance of fluids and electrolytes (sodium, potassium, calcium, chloride). The kidneys get rid of excess fluid. In other words, the body knows how much water it needs, and you should not attempt to lose water as a means of weight reduction.

Because each liter of fluid weighs about 2 pounds (.91 kilogram), dehydration can lead to impressive, albeit short-term, weight loss. But the loss is water, not fat. You need the water, and the body will do all it can to get it back. Water and electrolyte loss during dehydration causes diminished muscular strength, and loss of blood volume reduces cardiac output and endurance. Responsible health organizations such as the American College of Sports Medicine have long cautioned against dehydration weight loss because it compromises athletic performance and health. The 1997 deaths of three collegiate wrestlers from dehydration weight loss confirmed the life-threatening effects of dehydration.

So don't exercise in a rubber suit, sauna, or steam room to lose weight. Sweat is a crucial part of the temperature-regulating mechanism. You must allow sweat to evaporate to cause evaporative heat loss and help you avoid heat stress. When you do lose weight through sweat loss, you should replace it as soon as possible. For example, if you lose 4 pounds (1.8 kilograms) of weight during a run or bike ride, you'll need to replace it with more than 2 quarts (1.9 liters) of fluid.

Food Choices

The U.S. Departments of Agriculture and Health and Human Services have released *Dietary Guidelines for Americans 2005*. This revised guide to daily food choices provides science-based advice to promote health and reduce the risk for major chronic diseases (www.health.gov/dietaryguidelines/). The revised guidelines are consistent with the recommendations in this book (performance diet, table 11.2, page 213) and emphasize the need to engage in regular, moderate physical activity and weight control. Important recommendations include the following:

- Consume a variety of nutrient-dense foods and beverages within and among the basic food groups while choosing foods that limit the intake of saturated and trans fats, cholesterol, added sugars, salt, and alcohol.
- Keep total fat between 20 and 35 percent of calories with most fats coming from polyunsaturated and monounsaturated fatty acids (fish, nuts, and vegetable oils). Consume less than 10 percent of calories from saturated fatty acids and keep trans-fatty acid consumption as low as possible.

- Choose fiber-rich fruits, vegetables, and whole grains often. Consume 2 cups (480 milliliters) of fruit (four 1/2 cup servings) and 2 1/2 cups (600 milliliters) of vegetables (five servings) per day for a 2,000-calorie intake (more for higher caloric intake).

- Select from all five vegetable groups (dark green, orange [carrots and so on], legumes, starchy vegetables, and others) several times per week.

- Consume 3 or more ounce-equivalents (85 grams) of whole-grain products per day with the rest of recommended grains (three servings) coming from enriched or whole-grain products (more for higher caloric intake).

- Consume 3 cups (720 milliliters) of fat-free or low-fat milk or equivalent milk products.

Regarding physical activity and weight control, the guidelines recommend the following:

- To maintain body weight in a healthy range, balance calories from food and beverages with calories expended (see chapter 12).

- To prevent gradual weight gain over time, make small decreases in food and beverage calories and increase physical activity.

- For weight loss, aim for a slow, steady weight loss by decreasing caloric intake while maintaining adequate nutrient intake and increasing physical activity (see chapter 14).

- Engage in regular physical activity and reduce sedentary activities to promote health, psychological well-being, and healthy body weight.

  - Children and adolescents should engage in 60 minutes of physical activity most days of week.

  - Adults should engage in at least 30 minutes of moderate-intensity activity most days of the week.

  - Older adults should participate in regular physical activity to reduce functional declines associated with aging and to achieve other benefits of activity.

- To sustain weight loss, people should participate in at least 60 to 90 minutes of daily moderate-intensity activity.

Food Portions

Adapted from *Dietary Guidelines for Americans 2005*, Department of Agriculture (USDA), and Department of Health and Human Services (HHS), this section will help you meet your micronutrient needs. The revised guidelines increase the emphasis on the intake of fruits, vegetables, and whole-grain products. A serving is a method of describing food portions. Everyone should eat a minimum of four servings (2 cups, or 480 milliliters) of fruits and five servings (2 1/2 cups, or 600 milliliters) of vegetables. Those involved in hard work or training should increase fruit intake to five servings (2 1/2 cups, or 600 milliliters) and vegetable intake to eight servings (4 cups, or 960 milliliters). Examples are shown in figure 11.3.

Whole-grain products are important as sources of energy, fiber, and micronutrients. Everyone should eat six servings of whole grains, enriched, or whole-grain products daily. When involved in hard work or training, increase the intake of whole-grain foods

Figure 11.3   Fruit and Vegetable Portions

Dietary Guidelines for Americans 2005 increases the emphasis on the intake of fruits, vegetables, and whole-grain products.

Fruits: Choose from a variety of fruits each day.

1 apple	1/3 cup (80 ml) apple juice	1 cup (240 ml) vegetable juice
1 orange	1/2 cup (120 ml) orange juice	3/4 cup (180 ml) blueberries
4 apricots	1 1/4 cup strawberries (300 ml)	1 1/4 cup watermelon (300 ml)
1/2 banana	2 tablespoons (30 ml) raisins	12 cherries
1 nectarine	4 rings, dried apples	15 grapes
3 prunes	1/2 grapefruit	

Vegetables, 1 cup (240 ml) raw or 1/2 cup (120 ml) cooked: Select from all five vegetable subgroups: dark green, orange (e.g., carrots), legumes, starchy vegetables, and other vegetables, several times a week.

Cabbage	Celery	Cucumber	Green onion	Green, red, or hot peppers
Lettuce	Mushrooms	Radishes	Spinach	Carrots Zucchini

Whole grains: Choose from enriched or whole-grain products.

1 slice (1 oz, or 28 g) whole-grain bread	1/2 cup (120 ml) cooked oatmeal
1/3 cup (80 ml) All-Bran	1 cup (240 ml) whole-grain flaked cereal
1/2 12 in. (30 cm) whole-grain tortilla	1/2 whole-wheat English muffin
1/2 whole-grain bagel	1/2 cup (120 ml) shredded wheat
1/2 cup (120 ml) cooked whole-wheat pasta	

to 10 servings or more. Incidentally, a serving of lean meat is several ounces, about the size of a deck of cards. If you are active, one serving may not be a sufficient portion for a meal. To view your personalized food guidelines, go to the revised USDA food pyramid at www.mypyramid.gov.

Walter Willett is one of the most well know and respected nutritionists in the United States. He is the Fredrick John Stare Professor of Epidemiology and Nutrition at the Harvard School of Public Health in the Departments of Nutrition and Epidemiology. He has proposed an eating plan that is associated with daily exercise and weight control. The bottom level of his pyramid includes whole-grain foods at most meals, along with plant oils (olive, canola, soy, peanut). The next level includes vegetables in abundance and fruits two to three times per day. Next come nuts and legumes one to three times per day. The next level contains fish, poultry, and eggs zero to two times per day; then comes dairy or calcium once or twice a day. The top level calls for sparing use of red meat, butter, white rice, white bread, potatoes, and sweets (Willett 2001).

Mediterranean Diet

A study of Mediterranean people with low rates of chronic disease and high life expectancies led researchers to recommend some variations. The Mediterranean diet emphasizes daily intake of complex carbohydrates, fruits, vegetables, olive oil, yogurt, and cheese; reduces intake of fish, poultry, eggs, and sweets to a few times per week; and limits red meat consumption to a few times per month. The diet also calls for regular physical activity and daily but moderate intake of wine. Among subjects 70 to 90 years of age from 11 European countries, adherence to the Mediterranean diet was associated with more than a 50 percent reduction in all-cause and cause-specific mortality (Knoops et al. 2004).

If your health risk is high, consider the Mediterranean diet or Willett's plan. If not, use the revised USDA food guide. If you are very active you'll need to increase your food intake to fuel vigorous or prolonged activity and consume somewhat more protein to meet the needs of aerobic and strength training.

By now it should be clear that your diet is an important part of the active life and, along with regular activity, the key to weight control. But is diet related to health for other reasons? A poor diet has been implicated as a major factor in obesity, heart disease, cancer, diabetes, digestive problems (GERD, diverticulitis), irritable colon, gallstones, and other problems such as dementia, dental caries, hernia, and hemorrhoids. A low-fat diet is prescribed for those at risk for heart disease. But how does diet influence cancer and other problems?

Dietary Fiber

Fiber, roughage, bulk, and bran all refer to the portion of plants that is indigestible. Why consume an indigestible material? Besides its long-standing reputation for maintaining regularity, fiber has other advantages. Insoluble fiber (wheat bran, beans) holds water, increases bulk, and increases the rate at which stool and cancerous toxins are removed. Soluble fiber such as oat bran, apples, and citrus fruits forms a gel that slows absorption of carbohydrate and binds cholesterol for removal from the body. Soluble fiber may also produce a chemical that slows the rate of cholesterol production.

Epidemiologic studies show that those on a low-fiber diet have a higher incidence of heart disease, cancer, and the other problems mentioned

Citrus fruits and other foods rich in soluble fiber can help eliminate cholesterol.

Anticancer Diet

The anticancer diet recently proposed by the National Academy of Sciences endorses the reduction of fat in the diet. The advice includes the following:

- Eat less fat, fatty meats, and dairy products.
- Eat little salt-cured, pickled, or smoked foods.
- Eat more whole-grained products, including fiber-rich foods.
- Eat more fruits and vegetables, including those in the cabbage family and those high in vitamins A and C.
- Drink alcohol in moderation, if at all.
- Keep caloric intake low.

Remember, fat is a factor in cancer, heart disease, and diabetes, and exercise is the best way to eliminate excess fat from the body.

Remember, fat is a factor in cancer, heart disease, and diabetes, and exercise is the best way to eliminate excess fat from the body.

earlier. The average American consumes about one-third of the 25 to 35 grams (.88 to 1.23 ounces) of fiber recommended by the National Cancer Institute, and most regularly ignore fresh fruits and vegetables. If fiber isn't part of your daily regime, begin now to add bran cereals, fruits, vegetables, beans, and whole-grained breads to your diet. Read labels and try to seek a balance between soluble and insoluble fiber. Finally, consider this: When you combine fiber with a low-fat diet and activity, you'll be able to eat freely, with little concern for weight gain. Daily activity contributes to regularity and may lower colon cancer risk by speeding the rate at which stool and toxins pass through the digestive system.

Food Concerns

Companies spend millions to convince us that we can achieve fitness and health by eating their products. Although sound nutrition is essential to health and fitness, nothing you eat will improve your fitness if you are already on an adequate diet. The only way to achieve fitness is through regular exercise. You can't get there just by eating.

Health Foods

Concerns about the quality of our food supply, such as the use of hormones, pesticides, dyes, and other chemicals, has led to wider availability of so-called health foods, also known as natural or organic foods, as an alternative source of nutrition. To the extent that these chemicals may be harmful to health, especially over extended periods, natural food sources could be safer. But the nutritional value of a food or vitamin is not related to the manner of growth. Foods grown with chemical fertilizers seem just as nutritious as those grown with organic fertilizers. What matters is the active amount of the essential ingredient, such as a vitamin, and how that contributes to the recommended daily intake. Buy more expensive health foods if you are concerned about the effects of chemicals on your health, but don't expect to get super nutrition for the extra expense.

Lite Foods

Interest in health and weight control has led to the development of so-called lite foods and beverages. The products are lower-calorie versions of the original, such as lite beer, lite or no-calorie soft drinks, low-fat crackers and meals, and so on. The products should have at least one-third fewer calories than the original. Although eating these products will not make you lose weight, they can help reduce your caloric intake, as long as you don't eat more of them. Because lite foods usually cost as much as or more than the regular versions, their popularity proves that we will pay more for less—fewer calories or less fat, sodium, or caffeine. Sometimes the products use undesirable substitutes, such as coconut, palm, or cottonseed oil or the hydrogenated form of healthy oil, such as soybean. Read the label to be certain that you are getting what you paid for.

A variation of the lite meal is the diet platter at the restaurant. People select these choices because they believe that they are more nutritious and have fewer calories and less fat. A salad isn't particularly high in nutritive value, however, and if gobs of high-fat salad dressing are used, the salad could be a bad food choice (1 tablespoon [15 milliliters] of dressing can contain 100 calories and 8 grams of fat, and the ladle used to pour the dressing usually holds more than 1 tablespoon).

Responsible restaurant owners label meals to indicate better choices for those concerned with heart health and fat intake. Look for food that is nutritious but low in saturated fat. Avoid fried foods, those with cream sauces or butter, and high-calorie desserts. Ask for dressings and other sauces on the side. Request a dry muffin or toast. Eating out is difficult for those on weight-loss or low-fat diets, but the situation is improving as some restaurant owners realize what the customer wants. Of course, many fast-food outlets continue to promote high-calorie, high-fat food choices (see table 11.6). We'll talk about low-carb diets in chapter 13.

Toxic Foods

Some health activists blame the food industry for promoting the sale of toxic foods, those that are demonstrably bad for your health. These foods include tasty, high-fat fast foods that are aggressively marketed to children and teens. Although an occasional burger and fries may be safe for most consumers, a steady diet of them is not. Some schools have turned school lunch programs over to the fast-food industry. Others turn the students loose to roam nearby strip malls in search of tasty toxic foods. Schools even carry advertisements for fast food on their in-school news channel. At home, busy adults eat out, order in, or use prepared meals. Fast-food serving sizes have grown dramatically. Consequently, we have become the fattest nation in the world, and an epidemic of fat-induced adult-onset diabetes has emerged among overweight teens and adults. We eat too much and exercise too little. What can we do?

Some argue for measures similar to those imposed on the tobacco industry, including limits on advertising, no sales near schools, extra taxes, lawsuits to reclaim medical costs, and more. A better approach might involve a return to brown-bag lunches for kids and adults, limiting reliance on fast foods and meals outside the home, and selecting healthy options (when eating out). If we don't do something, the consequence will be a further explosion of disabling diseases such as obesity, diabetes, and heart disease, and enormous health care costs. Of course, regular, moderate physical activity is the other part of the solution.

Table 11.6   Caloric Values for Fast Foods

	Energy (cal)	Protein (g)	Fat (g)	Carbohydrate (g)
McDonald's				
Two hamburgers, fries, shake	1,030	40	37	135
Big Mac, fries, shake	1,100	40	41	143
Big Mac	550	21	32	45
Quarter Pounder	420	25	19	37
Hamburger	260	14	9	30
French fries	180	3	10	20
Chocolate shake	315	9	8	51
Burger King				
Whopper, fries, shake	1,200	40	47	147
Whopper	630	29	35	50
Whopper Jr.	285	16	15	21
Double hamburger	325	24	15	24
Hamburger	230	14	10	21
French fries	220	2	12	10
Chocolate shake	365	8	8	65
Hardees				
2/3 lb bacon cheese Thickboy	1,340	56	96	60
Large fries	480	5	19	72
Pizza Hut				
10 in. Supreme (cheese, tomato sauce, sausage, pepperoni, mushrooms, and so on)	1,200	72	35	152
10 in. pizza (cheese)	1,025	65	23	140
Kentucky Fried Chicken				
Three-piece dinner (chicken, potatoes, roll, slaw)	1,000	55	55	71
Dairy Queen				
4 oz serving soft ice cream	180	5	6	27
Arby's				
Sliced beef sandwich, two potato patties, slaw, shake	1,200	27	40	166

To convert grams to calories, multiply protein (g) by 4.3, fat (g) by 9.3, and carbohydrate (g) by 4.1.

Summary

This chapter provided a thumbnail sketch of nutrition as well as suggestions for improving health and performance. Although we could write much more on the subject, the basics provided here form the framework for a safe and sensible eating plan. Minor dietary adjustments will lower your daily intake of fat. Reduce fat further if your family history or risk factors indicate the need. Select foods from a variety of sources to ensure the availability of essential amino acids, vitamins, and minerals. Use a daily vitamin and mineral supplement with the recommended dietary intake (RDI) during heavy training or weight loss, or if you are concerned about your diet. It's that simple.

Before we move on, we want to make a confession. We've been using a daily vitamin and mineral supplement for many years. We exercise regularly, train often, and strive to maintain or even lose weight, in spite of prodigious appetites. At times we engage in strenuous or even exhausting activities, such as long-duration hiking, biking, or cross-country ski trips, for which we may be inadequately prepared. The RDI supplement is a hedge against less-than-perfect nutrition. For several years one of us also supplemented his diet with modest amounts of antioxidant vitamins C, E, and beta-carotene. He added these in response to studies suggesting that antioxidants contributed to lower risk of heart, eye, and other problems, and reduced muscle damage from oxidative stress. Our physician friends did the same, until recent studies cast doubt on their effectiveness.

So now we say eat a variety of foods, fruits and vegetables, and whole-grain products. Take steps to minimize inherited risks of heart disease or other potential problems and engage in regular, moderate physical activity. One bonus of this behavior is a healthy immune system. Over the years we have enjoyed consistent good health and effortless weight control. In the next chapters you'll learn how to gain lasting control of your weight.

Energy Balance

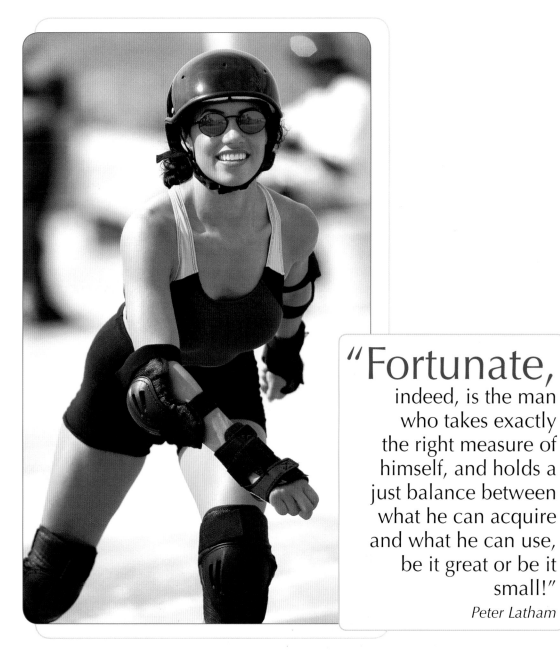

"**Fortunate,** indeed, is the man who takes exactly the right measure of himself, and holds a just balance between what he can acquire and what he can use, be it great or be it small!"

Peter Latham

Ages ago, when the food supply was not so predictable and humans couldn't count on three meals a day plus snacks, their bodies learned how to store energy in the form of fat. Our bodies still store energy, even though the food supply now makes the practice unnecessary for most of us. This ability to store energy, coupled with a plentiful food supply, has created a problem for two-thirds of the population. We put calories in the energy account but seldom draw enough out, so our energy balance grows and grows. This chapter is about energy intake, energy expenditure, and the consequences of eating more than we expend—overweight and obesity.

This chapter will help you

- calculate your energy balance, that is, your caloric intake versus caloric expenditure,
- understand the causes and consequences of overweight and obesity, and
- establish sensible body weight and body fat goals.

Energy Intake

In chapter 11 we explained how you consume energy in the form of carbohydrate, fat, and protein. After you ingest and store it, energy remains until you use it. Carbohydrate is stored in the liver and muscles in clumps of glucose molecules known as glycogen. The liver supply is a reserve that helps maintain the blood glucose level, which is the essential energy source for the brain and nervous tissue. Muscle glycogen is the major fuel that you use to power high-intensity contractions. When you deplete the supply, you are unable to sustain those contractions. Fat is stored in adipose tissue, around organs (visceral fat), and in the muscles. You use intramuscular fat as energy for contractions, especially in lower-intensity, long-duration effort. Moreover, fat can be mobilized from adipose tissue storage and transported through the circulation to fuel working muscles. The amino acids from the protein that you eat are used to construct proteins in your body. A small portion of the energy used for activity (5 to 10 percent) comes from tissue protein.

How is the energy or caloric value of food determined? Nutrition researchers use a calorimeter to measure the energy content of foods. A small amount of food is placed in a chamber and burned in the presence of oxygen. The heat liberated in the process indicates the energy content of the food (1 kilocalorie is the heat required to raise 1 kilogram of water 1 degree Celsius). When a gram of carbohydrate is ignited, the energy yield is 4.1 kilocalories, and when protein is burned the energy yield is 4.3 kilocalories per gram. When fat is tested, more than twice as much energy is released, 9.3 kilocalories per gram (see table 12.1). Notice that it takes more oxygen to burn a gram of fat, yielding less energy per liter of oxygen consumed.

Energy Expenditure

You always expend some energy, even when you are asleep. But when you begin to move, energy needs increase dramatically. Energy expenditure can go from 1.2 calories per minute during rest to more than 20 calories per minute during vigorous activity. You also need energy when you eat to power the processes of digestion and absorption. But physical activity has the greatest effect on energy expenditure. Walking involves an

Table 12.1   Caloric Equivalents of Foods

Food	Energy (cal/g)*	Oxygen (L/g)**	Caloric equivalent (cal/L)***
Fat	9.3	1.98	4.696
Carbohydrate	4.1	0.81	5.061
Protein	4.3	0.97	4.432

The alcohol in alcoholic beverages has a high caloric value, 7.1 cal/g. The calories are "empty," providing little nutritional value. Moreover, because alcohol diminishes appetite and interferes with digestion by inflammation of the stomach, pancreas, and intestine, alcohol often leads to malnutrition. Alcohol also interferes with vitamin activation by the liver and causes liver damage (Lieber 1976).

*Cal (kilocalories) released when 1 gram of this food is oxidized.

**Liters of oxygen required to oxidize 1 gram of this food.

***The calories produced per liter of oxygen when this food is burned.

Reprinted from Sharkey, 1974.

expenditure of about 5 calories per minute, jogging burns 10 or more, and running can expend 15 to 20 calories per minute. Figure 12.1 illustrates the sources of energy at three levels of exercise.

In the fasted state (12 hours after last meal), fat, including plasma free fatty acids (plasma FFA) and muscle triglyceride, is the predominant source of energy for light and moderate levels of exercise intensity. At higher

Figure 12.1 Sources of energy. Approximate contribution of energy sources at three levels of exercise. Plasma free fatty acids (FFA) are transported by the blood to the muscles.

levels, carbohydrate, in the form of muscle glycogen and blood glucose, becomes the major fuel. The contribution of carbohydrate would be somewhat higher during moderate exercise following a high-carbohydrate meal. The relative contribution of each fuel changes throughout several hours of continuous exercise. For example, at 75 percent of $\dot{V}O_2$max, the contribution of muscle glycogen drops from 45 percent to near zero upon depletion of the supply, while energy derived from muscle triglyceride declines from 25 to 10 percent. The role of blood glucose increases from 5 to 40 percent as muscle glycogen is depleted. But when the liver glycogen supply declines, blood glucose falls precipitously. The contribution of fat from adipose tissue (plasma FFA) increases throughout prolonged exercise, rising from 25 to 50 percent after several hours (Coyle 1995).

Your energy expenditure depends on the size of your body. The greater your body weight, the higher your caloric expenditure. The caloric expenditure tables in this book are based on a body weight of about 70 kilograms (154 pounds). If you weigh 7 kilograms (about 15 pounds) more, add 10 percent. If you weigh 7 kilograms less, subtract 10 percent; and so forth. For example, if you weigh 124 pounds (56.2 kilograms) and the caloric cost of slow jogging is listed at 10 calories per minute, subtract 20 percent, or 2 calories, to find the calories burned when you jog (8 calories per minute).

> Your energy expenditure depends on the size of your body.

Exercise and Weight Control

Some types of exercise are better than others for weight control. As you know, we gradually shift from fat to carbohydrate metabolism as exercise becomes more vigorous. If you want to burn excess fat, consider light to moderate exercise (see table 12.2). Because you cannot sustain extremely vigorous activity for long, total caloric expenditure may not be great. In addition, fat utilization increases over time, with more fat being burned after 30 minutes of exercise. You can continue light to moderate activity for hours without undue fatigue, thereby allowing significant fat metabolism and caloric expenditure.

Incidentally, while we are on the subject of fat metabolism, the best time to exercise for weight control may be in the morning, before breakfast, when you are more likely to burn fat after an overnight fast. So if you are interested in fat metabolism and weight control, try morning exercise. If that approach doesn't suit your biological clock, don't despair. Exercise always burns calories, so it always contributes to weight control.

Table 12.2   Physical Activity and Caloric Expenditure

Work intensity	Pulse rate	Expenditure (cal/min)	Examples
Light*	Below 120	Up to 5	Golf, bowling, walking, volleyball, most work
Moderate*	120–150	5 to 10	Jogging, tennis, bike riding, basketball, racquetball, strenuous work
Heavy	Above 150	Above 10	Running; fast swimming; other brief, intense efforts

*Light to moderate activity is preferred for weight control, so long as it is continued for a sufficient time (e.g., 300 calories).
Adapted from Sharkey, 1974.

Measuring Energy Expenditure

In the early 1900s, scientists found a way to measure human energy expenditure. They placed subjects in a double-walled chamber very much like a food calorimeter. Heat generated in physical activity eventually increased the temperature of the water layer surrounding the chamber, indicating the caloric (heat) expenditure. But this method was far too expensive, time consuming, and cumbersome for measurement of vigorous activity. Drawing on their knowledge about the oxygen requirements of metabolism, researchers developed indirect methods of calorimetry. Because each liter of oxygen consumed is equivalent to about 5 calories, they simply measured the oxygen used during exercise. The closed-circuit method of indirect calorimetry still is used in hospitals, usually for resting or basal metabolic studies. The amount of oxygen taken from a large tank is measured directly.

The open-circuit method is best suited for vigorous exercise. The subject breathes readily available atmospheric air, and researchers collect the exhaled air for analysis. The oxygen consumed and carbon dioxide produced during the activity are analyzed, along with the total volume of exhaled air. Oxygen consumption per minute is simply

(atmospheric oxygen – exhaled oxygen) $\times$ volume exhaled air

For moderate exercise, values look like this:

$(20.93\% - 17.93\%) \times 33.3$ liters exhaled = 1.0 liter oxygen per minute

One liter of oxygen equals about 5 calories per minute, the energy cost of a brisk walk. Jogging requires about 2 liters per minute, or about 10 calories. It is easy to do metabolic conversions. Figure 12.2 can help you convert values among several units of measure, including total calories, calories per minute, oxygen use in liters and adjusted for body weight, and metabolic equivalents (METS) of resting energy use.

Energy Intake and Expenditure

Energy intake and expenditure refer to a comparison between the calories consumed in the diet and the calories burned in the course of all daily activities (see figure 12.3). If intake exceeds expenditure, the excess will be stored as fat. Since the 1960s Americans have reduced total dietary fat intake from 40 percent to about 35 percent of daily calories. Unfortunately, we've increased total caloric intake by about 250 calories each day and decreased physical activity. We Americans eat about the same number of calories per day as we did in 1900, but we burn far fewer calories in physical activity, at work or play (Booth et al. 2000). The result is an epidemic of overweight and obesity, and a host of health and economic consequences (Thompson et al. 1999).

One pound (.45 kilogram) of body fat has the energy equivalent of 3,500 calories. Therefore, a person must expend (oxidize or burn) about 3,500 calories to remove 1 pound of stored fat. Conversely, 3,500 calories of excess dietary intake will lead to an additional pound of body weight. For example, suppose that the daily activity of a young man whose body weight is around 70 kilograms (154 pounds) consists of light office work. He does not engage in any physical activity, so his daily caloric needs are about 2,400 calories. If he eats a donut for an additional 250 calories each day, what will happen to him over the course of a year?

250 calories × 30 days per month = 7,500 calories × 12 = 90,000 calories per year

The 90,000 calories he has gained, divided by 3,500 calories per pound, equates to 25.7 pounds (11.7 kilograms) of added weight. No wonder that 66 percent of the population is overweight or obese. Our friend has upset his energy balance to the tune of more than 2 pounds (.9 kilogram) per month, or 25.7 pounds per year. If he does

Figure 12.2 Metabolic conversions. To convert from one unit to another, simply carry out the calculation in the direction indicated by the arrow. For example, if you use 1 liter of oxygen per minute (1 L/min) in a brisk walk, you'll burn 5 calories per minute (1 L times 5 equals 5 calories per minute), or 300 calories per hour (5 times 60).

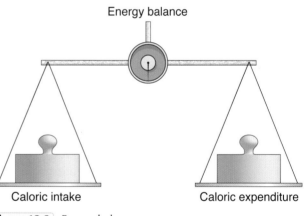

Figure 12.3 Energy balance.

nothing about his diet or exercise, he could gain 257 pounds (116.5 kilograms) in 10 years! Of course, the reverse is also true. If he gives up (or burns) 250 calories each day, he could lose more than 25 pounds a year. One purpose of this book is to teach you how to have your cake and eat it too—how to use diet and exercise to achieve control of your weight.

Caloric Intake

Determining your caloric intake is the first step in calculating your energy balance. Table 12.6, located at the end of this chapter, includes comprehensive calorie charts organized according to general categories (e.g., vegetables, meat). The table lists the number of calories contained in each portion. Remember these conversions (English to metric conversions are listed after the English conversions):

- 3 teaspoons = 1 tablespoon
- 2 tablespoons = 1 fluid ounce
- 16 tablespoons = 1 cup
- 1 cup = 8 fluid ounces, or 1/2 pint
- 4 cups = 1 quart
- 1 pound = 16 ounces
- 1 tablespoon = 14.8 milliliters
- 1 fluid ounce = 29.6 milliliters
- 1 cup = 237 milliliters, or .24 liter
- 1 quart = .95 liter
- 1 pound = 453.6 grams, or .45 kilogram

Determine your daily caloric intake by keeping an accurate account of everything that you eat and drink. The most accurate picture comes when you keep records for several days. Record the food or drink and the amount that you actually consume. Then use figure 12.4 to determine your caloric intake. For example, breakfast consists of 1 cup of cornflakes (100 calories) with 1/2 cup skim milk (40), sugar (25), and a sliced banana (94), plus two pieces of toast (110) with butter (20) and jelly (50), and black coffee (1). Total caloric intake is 440 calories. Do the same for all meals, snacks, beverages—everything. Add up the total for the day, and that is your caloric intake. If it regularly exceeds your daily caloric expenditure, you will gain weight. See figure 12.4 for a sample worksheet.

Carry a small notepad with you so that you can jot down any food, drink, or snack that you consume. At the end of the day sit down with the calorie charts and figure your daily intake. Computer programs are available to simplify the calculations and provide information on the nutritional value of your diet. You should attempt to assess your caloric intake for several typical days. Go to www.mypyramid.gov to calculate your energy balance.

Table 12.6 also includes the grams of fat contained in each portion of food or beverage. This listing should help you avoid high-fat foods if you decide to pursue a low-fat diet, which helps to reduce body weight and blood lipids. Each gram of fat contains 9.3 calories. If your goal is to reduce fat intake from the typical 40 percent of calories, try to stay within the following targets.

Figure 12.4   Caloric Intake Record

(Use calorie charts in table 12.6 on page 256.)

Date_____ Weight _____

	Food	Portion	Intake (cal)
Breakfast			
Lunch			
Dinner			
Desserts			
Snacks			
Drinks			
Other			

Total caloric intake   _____

Total caloric expenditure (figure 12.5)   _____

Energy balance (+ or -)   _____ Cal/day

From *Fitness and Health, Sixth Edition* by Brian J. Sharkey and Steven E. Gaskill, 2007, Champaign, IL: Human Kinetics.

For a daily caloric intake of 2,000 calories:

40% fat = 86 g of fat

(40% × 2,000 cal = 800 cal ÷ 9.3 cal/g = 86 g of fat)

30% fat = 65 g

20% fat = 43 g

10% fat = 22 g

Caloric Expenditure

For the next few days, keep an inventory of your physical activity. Simply list your activity (exercise, work, household chores) and the time spent for each (see figure 12.5). Don't omit anything, even sleeping. This activity inventory is educational, because it shows you when you burn calories and provides insight about how you can increase caloric expenditures in your normal routine.

Then use the caloric expenditure tables (table 12.7 at end of the chapter on page 261) to estimate your expenditures on the caloric expenditure log (figure 12.5). The method requires that you keep records of your daily activities: sleep, dressing, cooking, work, and all physical activity, including walking, stair climbing, fitness, and recreation.

Begin by making a list of your daily activities and the time spent in each. Then determine the cost of each activity in calories per minute. Finally, get the total for each activity and the total for the day. Figure 12.6 shows how to do this.

Figure 12.5 Caloric Expenditure Log

(Use energy expenditure tables in this chapter.)

Activity	Time (min)	Expenditure rate (cal/min)	Total expenditure (cal)
Sleep	_____	_____	_____
Nonwork and household			
_____	_____	_____	_____
_____	_____	_____	_____
_____	_____	_____	_____
Work			
_____	_____	_____	_____
_____	_____	_____	_____
_____	_____	_____	_____
Recreation and sport			
_____	_____	_____	_____
_____	_____	_____	_____
_____	_____	_____	_____
	24 hr	Total for day = _____	

Example	Time (min)	Expenditure rate (cal/min)	Total expenditure (cal)
Sleep	480	1.2	576
Nonwork			
Personal toilet	10	2.0	20
Cook breakfast	10	1.5	15
Cook dinner	60	1.5	90
Watch TV or read	210	1.5	315
Visit	60	2.0	120
Shop	50	3.0	150
Work			
Walk to work and return	20	5.0	100
Work (standard activity)	400	2.6	1,040
Rest breaks	80	1.5	120
Lunch	30	1.5	45
Jogging	30	10.0	300
			Total 2,891

From *Fitness and Health, Sixth Edition* by Brian J. Sharkey and Steven E. Gaskill, 2007, Champaign, IL: Human Kinetics.

Figure 12.6 Form for Assessment of Energy Expenditure

Activity	Kcal/min		Min		Totals
Sleeping	_____	×	_____	=	_____
Working	_____	×	_____	=	_____
Eating	_____	×	_____	=	_____
Personal	_____	×	_____	=	_____
Play or sport	_____	×	_____	=	_____
Relaxation (e.g., TV)	_____	×	_____	=	_____
_____	_____	×	_____	=	_____
_____	_____	×	_____	=	_____
_____	_____	×	_____	=	_____
_____	_____	×	_____	=	
			1,440 min (24 hr)	=	_____ cal/day

Now: Adjust your total calories per day for your body weight:

_____ cal/day × _____ lb (your weight) ÷ 150 = _____ cal/day

or

_____ cal/day × _____ kg (your weight) ÷ 68 = _____ cal/day

Activity	Kcal/min		Min		Totals
Sleeping	1.2	×	480	=	576
Working	2.6	×	480	=	1,248
Reading	1.3	×	120	=	156
Writing	2.6	×	60	=	156
Eating	1.5	×	60	=	90
Personal	2.5	×	60	=	150
Walking, moderate pace	5.0	×	60	=	300
Talking	1.3	×	60	=	78
Tennis	7.0	×	60	=	420
			1,440 min (24 hr)	=	3,174 cal/day

Now: Adjust your total calories per day for your body weight:

__3,174__ cal/day × __175__ lb (your weight) ÷ 150 = __3,703__ cal/day

or

__3,174__ cal/day × __79.4__ kg (your weight) ÷ 68 = __3,706__ cal/day

From *Fitness and Health, Sixth Edition* by Brian J. Sharkey and Steven E. Gaskill, 2007, Champaign, IL: Human Kinetics.

Table 12.7, which shows caloric expenditure, is a guide to exercise intensity because intensity is directly related to calories expended per minute. The caloric expenditure charts can guide you to appropriate weight-control activities. You can readily see that walking burns more calories than recreational volleyball and that running burns more calories than doing calisthenics. The charts will tell you how long you should exercise to burn a specific number of calories (e.g., 10 calories per minute for 10 minutes will burn 100 calories) (www.mypyramid.gov).

Be sure to adjust the totals for your body weight: Add 10 percent for each 15 pounds (6.8 kilograms) above 150 pounds (68 kilograms), and subtract 10 percent for each 15 pounds below 150 pounds.

You can now calculate your energy balance as follows:

caloric intake (___ calories) – caloric expenditure (___ calories) = ___ calories

If intake regularly exceeds expenditure, you have a positive energy balance, and the excess energy will be stored as fat. If caloric intake regularly falls short of expenditure, you will lose weight.

When you know your energy balance, you'll have a clear idea of what you can do to reduce caloric intake and increase caloric expenditure. Table 12.3 indicates basal energy needs for 24 hours of complete bed rest, approximately 1.2 calories per minute. Recent evidence shows that the sleeping metabolic rate is lower than the resting metabolic rate (RMR) in metabolically efficient obese individuals, and higher than RMR in nonobese subjects (Zhang et al. 2002). Table 12.4 shows approximate increases in caloric expenditure for selected daily activities. You can see that physical activity is the only way to increase caloric expenditure.

Table 12.3 Basal Energy Expenditure for Men and Women

MEN		WOMEN	
Weight	Energy expenditure* (cal)	Weight	Energy expenditure** (cal)
140 lb (64 kg)	1,550	100 lb (45 kg)	1,225
160 lb (73 kg)	1,640	120 lb (54 kg)	1,320
180 lb (82 kg)	1,730	160 lb (73 kg)	1,485
220 lb (100 kg)	1,900	180 lb (82 kg)	1,575

*5 ft 10 in. (180 cm) tall (add 20 cal for each inch taller; if shorter subtract 20 cal for each inch).
**5 ft 6 in. (170 cm) tall (add 20 cal for each inch taller; if shorter subtract 20 cal for each inch).
Basal energy = calories expended in 24 hr of complete bed rest.

Table 12.4 Approximate Increases in Caloric Expenditure for Selected Activities

Activity	Percent above basal
Bed rest (eating and reading)	10%
Quiet sitting (reading, knitting)	30%
Light activity (office work)	40–60%
Moderate activity (housekeeping)	60–80%
Heavy occupational activity (construction)	100%

Alternative Method

Here is another way to calculate energy expenditure that illustrates the effects of body size and age on energy expenditure. Follow steps 1 through 4:

1. Calculate basal energy expenditure using table 12.3.
2. Add increases in caloric expenditure using table 12.4.
3. Adjust total for age: Subtract 4 percent of caloric expenditure for each decade (10 years) over 25 years of age.
4. Add calories expended in nonwork (recreational) activities.

Use the caloric expenditure charts in tables 12.3 and 12.7 to calculate minutes of activity and cost in calories per minute. For example, consider a 45-year-old construction worker, 5 feet 10 inches tall (213 centimeters), weighing 200 pounds (.91 kilogram):

$$basal = 1,815 \text{ cal} + 100\%$$

$$= 3,630 \text{ cal} - 8\% \text{ (age)}$$

$$= 3,340 \text{ cal} + 30 \text{ min of table tennis with son (30 min} \times 5 \text{ cal per min)}$$

$$= 150 \text{ calories}$$

$$Total = 3,490 \text{ cal per day}$$

Overweight and Obesity

In horse racing, the favorite often is handicapped to provide a better contest. If a few pounds are added, the favorite may become an also-ran. Excess weight can affect performance in humans as well; few of us realize how much. Excess weight proves a burden physically, socially, psychologically, and economically. It may be the most significant health problem for most people. Yet it is a symptom, not a disease, and it is among the least complicated of all health problems.

What are the medical consequences of overweight and obesity? Disease risks and costs increase substantially with increased body mass index. Body mass index (BMI) relates weight to height, and is calculated as weight in kilograms divided by the square of height in meters. The death rate rises as BMI increases above 30, especially in the younger age groups. Those with a high BMI have a higher incidence of atherosclerotic heart disease, hypertension, some cancers, diabetes, and cirrhosis of the liver. Accidents and surgical complications are more prevalent, as are complications of pregnancy. When a person removes the excess weight through diet and exercise, these problems diminish or disappear. The body mass index provides a simple way for you to assess body composition. All you need is your body weight in pounds (or kilograms) and your height in inches (or centimeters). Then use figure 12.7 to get your score.

You should strive to remain in the desirable category because heavier men and women in all age groups have increased risk of death from all causes (Calle et al. 1999). You should also realize that low fitness is an independent predictor of mortality in all body mass index groups, and the risk of death for being

> You should strive to remain in the desirable category because heavier men and women in all age groups have an increased risk of death from all causes.

Height (in) Weight (lb)	49	51	53	55	57	59	61	63	65	67	69	71	73	75	77	79	81	83
66	19	18	16	15	14	13	12	12	11	10	10	9	9	8	8	8	7	7
70	20	19	18	16	15	14	13	13	12	11	10	10	9	9	9	8	8	7
75	22	20	19	17	16	15	14	13	12	12	11	10	10	9	9	9	8	8
79	23	21	20	18	17	16	15	14	13	12	12	11	11	10	9	9	9	8
84	24	22	21	19	18	17	16	15	14	13	12	12	11	11	10	10	9	9
88	26	24	22	20	19	18	17	16	15	14	13	12	12	11	11	10	10	9
92	27	25	23	21	20	19	17	16	15	15	14	13	12	12	11	11	10	10
97	28	26	24	22	21	20	18	17	16	15	14	14	13	12	12	11	10	10
101	29	27	25	23	22	20	19	18	17	16	15	14	13	13	12	12	11	10
106	31	28	26	24	23	21	20	19	18	17	16	15	14	13	13	12	11	11
110	32	30	27	26	24	22	21	20	18	17	16	15	15	14	13	13	11	11
114	33	31	29	27	25	23	22	20	19	18	17	16	15	14	14	13	12	12
119	35	32	30	28	26	24	22	21	20	19	18	17	16	15	14	14	13	12
123	36	33	31	29	27	25	23	22	21	19	18	18	17	16	16	15	14	13
128	37	34	32	30	28	26	24	23	21	20	19	18	17	16	15	15	14	13
132	38	36	33	31	29	27	25	23	22	21	20	19	18	17	16	15	14	14
136	40	37	34	32	29	28	26	24	23	21	20	19	18	17	16	16	15	14
141	41	38	35	33	30	28	27	25	24	22	21	20	19	18	17	16	15	15
145	42	39	36	34	31	29	27	26	24	23	22	20	19	18	17	17	16	15
150	44	40	37	35	32	30	28	27	25	24	22	21	20	19	18	17	16	15
154	45	41	38	36	33	31	29	27	26	24	23	22	20	19	18	18	17	16
158	46	43	40	37	34	32	30	28	26	25	24	22	21	20	19	18	17	16
163	47	44	41	38	35	33	31	29	27	26	24	23	22	20	19	19	18	17
167	49	45	42	39	36	34	32	30	28	26	25	23	22	21	20	19	18	17
172	50	46	43	40	37	35	32	30	29	27	25	24	23	22	21	20	19	18
176	51	47	44	41	38	36	33	31	29	28	26	25	23	22	21	20	19	18
180	52	49	45	42	39	36	34	32	30	28	27	25	24	23	22	21	20	19
185	54	50	46	43	40	37	35	33	31	29	27	26	25	23	22	21	20	19
189	55	51	47	44	41	38	36	34	32	30	28	27	25	24	23	22	20	20
194	56	52	48	45	42	39	37	34	32	30	29	27	26	24	23	22	21	20
198	58	53	49	46	43	40	37	35	33	31	29	28	26	25	24	23	21	20
202	59	54	50	47	44	41	38	36	34	32	30	28	27	25	24	23	22	21
207	60	56	52	48	45	42	39	37	35	33	31	29	27	26	25	24	22	21
211	61	57	53	49	46	43	40	38	35	33	31	30	28	27	25	24	23	22
216	63	58	54	50	47	44	41	38	36	34	32	30	29	27	26	25	23	22
220	64	59	55	51	48	44	42	39	37	35	33	31	29	28	26	25	24	23
224	65	60	56	52	49	45	42	40	37	35	33	31	30	28	27	26	24	23
229	67	62	57	53	49	46	43	41	38	36	34	32	30	29	27	26	25	24
233	68	63	58	54	50	47	44	41	39	37	35	33	31	29	28	27	25	24
238	69	64	59	55	51	48	45	42	40	37	35	33	32	30	28	27	26	24
242	70	65	60	56	52	49	46	43	40	38	36	34	32	30	29	28	26	25
246	72	66	61	57	53	50	47	44	41	39	37	35	33	31	29	28	27	25
251	73	67	63	58	54	51	47	45	42	39	37	35	33	32	30	29	27	26
255	74	69	64	59	55	52	48	45	43	40	38	36	34	32	31	29	28	26
260	76	70	65	60	56	52	49	46	43	41	39	36	34	33	31	30	28	27
264	77	71	66	61	57	53	50	47	44	42	39	37	35	33	32	30	29	27
268	78	72	67	62	58	54	51	48	45	42	40	38	36	34	32	31	29	28
273	79	73	68	63	59	55	52	48	46	43	40	38	36	34	33	31	30	28
277	81	75	69	64	60	56	52	49	46	44	41	39	37	35	33	32	30	29
282	82	76	70	65	61	57	53	50	47	44	42	40	37	35	34	32	30	29
286	83	77	71	66	62	58	54	51	48	45	42	40	38	36	34	33	31	29
290	84	78	72	67	63	59	55	52	48	46	43	41	39	37	35	33	31	30
295	86	79	74	68	64	60	56	52	49	46	44	41	39	37	35	34	32	30
299	87	80	75	69	65	60	57	53	50	47	44	42	40	38	36	34	32	31
304	88	82	76	70	66	61	57	54	51	48	45	43	40	38	36	35	33	31
308	90	83	77	71	67	62	58	55	51	48	46	43	41	39	37	35	33	32
312	91	84	78	72	68	63	59	55	52	49	46	44	41	39	37	36	34	32

Underweight (<19)

Desirable (19-25)

Increased health risks (25-30)

Obese (30-40)

Extremely obese (>40)

Figure 12.7 Body mass index chart.
Executive summary of the clinical guidelines on the identification, evaluation, and treatment of overweight and obesity in adults, 1998.

overweight are much lower in those who maintain a higher level of aerobic fitness (Wei et al. 1999). Incidentally, the risks of having a BMI above 25 are somewhat lower if waist measurement is less than 40 inches (101.6 centimeters), a condition common in athletes who engage in significant training.

You may say, "I'm not overweight; I weigh the same as I did in my senior year of high school." True, your weight may be the same, but what about your ratio of lean to fat tissue? Isn't it possible that you have lost muscle and gained fat? Has your waist measurement remained the same? Overweight is defined as a BMI of 25 to 29. An alternative to the BMI for determining overweight is comparison with desirable body weight (see table 12.5). Desirable weights are associated with the longest life span for people of a certain skeleton size. Recent evidence suggests that fitness reduces the risks of being overweight and that fit but overweight men have lower all-cause mortality than do unfit men of normal weight (Lee, Jackson, and Blair 1998). Incidentally, because overweight and low fitness are associated with heart disease, diabetes, and hypertension, some insurance companies charge a higher premium for people judged to be 20 percent or more above desirable weight, or physically inactive, or both.

Excess fat or muscle can make you overweight, although extra fat poses more of a burden because the muscles can do useful work and take less space for equal weight (muscle is denser than fat). But even excess muscle seems unnecessary for adults, unless they need it for sport or occupational reasons. Muscular men with excess fat,

Table 12.5   Desirable Weights for Men and Women[*]

Height (without shoes) in ft and in. (cm)	Weight (without clothes) in lb (kg)	
	WOMEN	MEN
5 ft 0 in. (152.4)	103–115 (46.7–52.2)	—
5 ft 1 in. (154.9)	106–118 (48.0–53.5)	111–122 (50.3–55.3)
5 ft 2 in. (157.5)	109–122 (49.4–55.3)	114–126 (51.7–57.2)
5 ft 3 in. (160.0)	112–126 (50.8–57.2)	117–129 (53.1–58.5)
5 ft 4 in. (162.4)	116–131 (52.6–59.4)	120–132 (54.4–59.9)
5 ft 5 in. (165.1)	120–135 (54.4–61.2)	123–136 (55.8–61.7)
5 ft 6 in. (167.6)	124–139 (56.2–63.0)	127–140 (57.6–63.5)
5 ft 7 in. (170.2)	128–143 (58.0–64.9)	131–145 (59.4–65.8)
5 ft 8 in. (172.7)	132–147 (59.9–66.7)	135–149 (61.2–67.6)
5 ft 9 in. (175.3)	136–151 (61.7–68.5)	139–153 (63.0–69.4)
5 ft 10 in. (177.8)	140–155 (63.5–70.3)	143–158 (64.9–71.7)
5 ft 11 in. (180.3)	—	147–163 (66.7–73.9)
6 ft 0 in. (182.9)	—	151–168 (68.5–76.2)
6 ft 1 in. (185.4)	—	155–173 (70.3–78.5)
6 ft 2 in. (188.0)	—	160–178 (72.6–80.7)
6 ft 3 in. (190.5)	—	165–183 (74.8–83.0)

[*]Age 25 and above.

These guidelines, issued by the Metropolitan Life Insurance Company in 1959, are recommended over more recent editions, which provide false reassurance to a large fraction of people who are not defined as overweight but who are at substantially increased risk of heart disease.

Reprinted with permission of the Metropolitan Life Insurance Company.

such as inactive former football players, seem to have increased risk of high blood pressure and heart disease.

Obesity is defined as an excessive accumulation of fat beyond what is considered normal for one's age, sex, and body type. Obesity is a case of being overfat, not just overweight. A person can be underweight and still be obese, by having excess fat along with poorly developed muscles. Obesity is defined as being more than 20 percent above desirable weight, or as having more than 20 percent fat for men or more than 30 percent fat for women (or having a BMI of 30 or greater). These levels are arbitrary, and some experts prefer lower or higher levels, but by this BMI standard one-third of the adult population is obese. Sadly, we note that we now have a new category, morbid obesity, defined as a percent body fat or BMI score of 40 or more.

Measuring Body Fat

College-aged men average 12.5 to 15 percent fat; college women average about 25 percent. The standard method for determining percentage of body fat is underwater, or hydrostatic, weighing. The subject is weighed both in air and while submerged in water. After making appropriate adjustments for air in the lungs and gas in the gastrointestinal tract, body density is determined.

$$\frac{\text{weight in air}}{\text{weight in air} - \text{weight in water}}$$

Because fat is less dense than bone or muscle, we can calculate the percentage of body fat. As the percentage of body fat goes up, the weight in water goes down, and vice versa. Thus, lean people sink and fat people float because fat weighs less than muscle per unit of volume.

A less accurate but serviceable method for the estimation of percentage body fat uses skinfold calipers. The skinfold calculation of body fat is based on the relationship of subcutaneous (under the skin) fat to total body fat. One-third of the fat in the body may be located just under the skin, and the rest is around internal organs, around nerves as insulation, and in all cells, including muscle. To perform the skinfold measurements, grasp skinfolds between the thumb and forefinger and then apply calipers about .5 inch (1.3 centimeters) from the fingers. The calipers go in about as deep as the fold is wide (e.g., if the fold is .5 inch, go in .5 inch with the calipers). Take the measurement, release, repeat the measurement, and continue until your measurement is consistent. Use chest, abdomen, and thigh skinfolds for males and use triceps, thigh, and suprailium for females (see figure 12.8). Several carefully selected skinfold sites provide an estimate of body fat (use figure 12.9 to calculate the percentage of fat). Inexpensive but accurate skinfold calipers are available from several sources (e.g., www.fitnessmart.com, www.morleyathletics. com, and others).

Other methods used to determine body fat range from girth or other body measurements to expensive laboratory techniques. Many health clubs use a bioelectric

a   *b*

c   *d*   *e*

Figure 12.8   Sites for estimation of body fat: *(a)* chest: a diagonal fold taken halfway between the shoulder crease and the nipple, *(b)* abdomen: a vertical fold taken 1 inch (2.5 centimeters) to the right of the umbilicus, *(c)* thigh: a vertical fold taken on the front of the thigh half way between the knee and the hip crease, *(d)* triceps: a vertical fold taken on the back medial aspect of the triceps (back of the upper arm) midway between the shoulder and the elbow, *(e)* suprailium: a diagonal fold measured above the crest of the illium on the side of the hip. Males use *a*, *b*, and *c*. Females use *c*, *d*, and *e*.

Figure 12.9 A nomogram for the estimate of percent body fat for both male and female populations, using age and the sum of three skinfolds. Use a straight edge to draw a line from your age to the sum of the three skinfolds, and read your percent fat from the appropriate scale.
Recreated from American Alliance for Health, Physical Education, Recreation and Dance, 1981.

impedance technique that estimates fat from body water content. The technique, based on the fixed amount of water in fat, requires strict adherence to hydration standards to achieve acceptable accuracy. Some labs now use an air displacement technique to determine body fat. Scientists use the potassium-40 emitted from lean tissue, or sophisticated imaging techniques to measure fat. New methods of estimating fat are often compared with underwater weighing to see whether they are accurate. Studies indicate, however, that underwater weighing itself is subject to errors, especially with younger and older subjects and those at the extremes of leanness and fatness (Going 1996). Age-related differences in body water and bone density can throw off this method, as can dehydration. Therefore, studies are under way to

Getting Fat

Excess caloric intake starts the process. Fat intake poses more of a problem, though, because it has 9.3 calories per gram, whereas carbohydrate and protein have 4.1 and 4.3 calories per gram, respectively. Moreover, fat is similar to the composition of our adipose tissue and easier to store. Obese people eat more fat and engage in less physical activity (Rising et al. 1994), thereby contributing to the problem. Some researchers believe fat cells may continue to increase in size and number in severely obese individuals with increasing food intake, creating an even greater urge to eat. Rising obesity increases levels of the enzyme lipoprotein lipase (LPL), which helps fat cells take on more fat. Excess fat seems to inhibit the action of insulin, the hormone that helps glucose get into cells, leading to feelings of weakness and hunger that cause one to eat more. And the cycle continues.

improve the equations used to calculate body fat from underwater weighing. Until then, BMI, skinfolds, or the mirror can guide your weight-control efforts.

Causes of Overweight and Obesity

Why are over 80 million Americans overweight to the point of obesity? Is it merely because their caloric intake exceeds expenditure? To a large extent, the answer is yes! Although Americans have lowered the proportion of fat in their diet, they have simultaneously increased carbohydrate and caloric intake and decreased their level of physical activity. Even so, scientists continue to study other possible contributions to the epidemic of obesity.

Heredity Versus Environment

When we see obese parents with obese offspring, we are likely to think that the problem runs in the family. When both parents are obese, a child has an 80 percent risk of obesity. Studies of identical twins reared in different environments also indicate that obesity has a genetic root. But the pattern and extent of that relationship have not been well defined.

Much of the obesity that we see in families could be due as much to the environment as to a genetic cause. Overweight people eat more and exercise less, and the same may be true of their children. But in a study of identical and fraternal twins (Stunkard, Foch, and Hrubec 1986), the authors found a high heritability for weight and body mass index and concluded that body weight and obesity are under strong genetic control and that childhood family environment by itself has little effect. The discovery of genes partially responsible for obesity supports this reasoning.

Leptin, a genetically influenced hormone that governs how efficiently we burn fat, is released by fat cells. Higher levels of fat reduce the sensitivity of the body to leptin, making it possible to gain more weight. Conversely, leptin levels have been found to be low in restrained eaters, those with the eating disorder anorexia nervosa (Matejek et al. 1999). Clearly, behavior modulates genetic expression.

Genetics?

To see whether physical activity protects susceptible populations from developing obesity and type 2, or adult-onset, diabetes, a study compared physical activity levels of two groups of genetically similar Pima Indians, one group living in Arizona and the other in Mexico. The U.S. Pima Indians had a high incidence of obesity and diabetes, whereas the Mexican Indians did not. Physical activity was higher in the Mexican Pimas, with an average total energy expenditure of 3,289 calories per day versus 2,671 for the Arizona Indians. The authors concluded that physical activity played a significant role in the prevention of obesity in a genetically susceptible population (Esparza et al. 2000). The authors also noted the contribution of high-fat fast-food diets on the development of obesity and diabetes in the U.S. Pimas.

Do genetic influences on body weight mean that energy balance doesn't apply? No, it doesn't. In spite of genetic influence, the basic cause of overweight and obesity remains a positive energy balance because of excess caloric intake, inadequate caloric expenditure, or both. Further proof is the fact that our current epidemic of overweight and obesity has emerged in the last several decades, far faster than it could occur because of the influence of heredity. What else influences this tendency to store fat?

Glandular Causes

One authority has said, "With the exception of diabetes, glandular disease is associated with obesity in less than one case out of a thousand. Even in the presence of the disease, the individual is obese because energy acquisition has exceeded energy expenditure" (Gwinup 1970). Obese people have a significantly higher incidence of diabetes than do people of normal or desirable weight, but it is not clear whether obesity is a cause or a result of diabetes. After weight reduction, the diabetes may improve tremendously. In fact, it seems that overeating, particularly on a high-fat diet, may lead to obesity and non-insulin-dependent diabetes (Ivy, Zderic, and Fogt 1999).

> "With the exception of diabetes, glandular disease is associated with obesity in less than one case out of a thousand. Even in the presence of the disease, the individual is obese because energy acquisition has exceeded energy expenditure."

Diabetes is characterized by problems associated with the hormone insulin, which is needed to get blood sugar into cells, including fat cells. When sugar doesn't reach the cells, energy is low and the appetite is stimulated, so the person with diabetes eats more. We are becoming aware that a high-fat diet may increase insulin resistance, thereby requiring more insulin to do the same job. After a while, years perhaps, the pancreatic cells responsible for the production of insulin may fatigue, thereby producing a bona fide case of diabetes.

Before the discovery of insulin in 1921, diet and exercise were the only treatments available to people with diabetes. Nowadays, diet, insulin, and other drugs are used to control this metabolic malfunction of insulin production and sugar utilization. Because muscular activity increases the transport of glucose into muscle cells, even in the absence of insulin or failure of insulin to stimulate glucose uptake, and because muscular activity is effective in the reduction of body weight and the risk of heart disease (diabetes and heart disease frequently are associated), attention has turned again to the use of exercise in the treatment and control of diabetes. Moderate physical activity reduces insulin resistance and insulin requirements for all people, including those with diabetes. Regular participation in aerobic activity often reduces reliance on insulin. When coupled with a low-fat diet and significant weight loss, physical activity can further reduce the need for insulin.

Fat Cells

Researchers have studied the growth and development of fat cells. Excess calories are stored in fat cells in the form of triglycerides. Some people have more fat cells, causing them to store fat more readily. With the development of methods to determine fat cell size and number, researchers have been able to follow the development of obesity. Fat cells are apparently able to increase in size or number, and overfeeding can stimulate the increase. Traditionally, a chubby baby has been considered a healthy baby, but overfeeding during the first few years of life will stimulate the development of larger and more numerous fat cells (three times more). These cells remain for life and may influence the appetite when they are not filled. This early onset of hypercellularity generally leads to the most severe form of obesity. Another period of intense concern comes at or around the time of puberty, when overfeeding can lead to increases in the number and size of fat cells (Malina and Bouchard 1991).

Waist to Hip Ratio

Figure 12.10 Waist to hip ratio (e.g., 32/37 = .86).

Unfortunately, the fat located around visceral organs can't be measured with skinfold calipers because it lies below abdominal muscles. Researchers are looking at the waist to hip girth ratio (WHR) to determine why one fat storage location carries a greater risk of heart disease, hypertension, stroke, diabetes, and some cancers. To calculate your ratio, simply measure the waist at the level of the navel and the hips at the greatest circumference of the buttocks (measure to the nearest .25 inch, or .5 centimeter) and divide the waist measurement by the hip measurement. Results suggest that WHR values above .85 to .9 for men or .75 to .8 for women exceed safe limits (see figure 12.10).

Why is visceral fat a risk? Abdominal fat, fat stored in and around the viscera, has a direct circulatory route to the liver. Fat cells in that region are likely to send free fatty acids directly to the liver, where they can be used to synthesize cholesterol. Whatever the reason, visceral fat is a risk, and we know that exercise is an effective way to reduce the amount of metabolically active visceral fat, especially in men (Trichopoulou et al. 2001). In the normal, overweight, and obese BMI categories, those with higher waist circumference measurements are increasingly likely to have hypertension, diabetes, lipid problems, and the metabolic syndrome when compared with those with normal waist circumference values (Janssen, Katzmarzyk, and Ross 2002).

Enlarged fat cells characterize adult-onset obesity. The number of fat cells, however, does not seem subject to significant change. The pattern of obesity is a significant factor in determining health risk. Obesity that begins in childhood and continues into the adult years is a greater risk than adult-onset obesity. The location of stored fat also predicts health risk; potbellies are associated with a higher risk of heart disease, whereas pear shapes are not. The tendency of men to accumulate fat in their abdomens may be a factor in their higher risk of heart disease. Studies are now under way to determine why some cells take in more fat and why that is related to heart disease.

Metabolic Rate

Studies on obese infants, adolescents, and adults agree that fat people are more fuel efficient; their bodies burn calories more sparingly than the bodies of normal-weight subjects do. Their lower metabolic rate or energy expenditure makes weight loss more difficult. This finding may explain how heredity influences overweight and obesity. Why is the metabolic rate lower? One line of reasoning points to a lethargic or less active sympathetic nervous system. This portion of the autonomic nervous system secretes epinephrine (adrenaline) to speed up the heart rate and other responses during stress or exercise. Epinephrine also prompts the release of fatty acids from fat cells. Less sympathetic activity means less epinephrine, and less epinephrine means a lower metabolic rate and less fat utilization.

Some other lines of research tend to lift some of the blame for excess fat from the shoulders of the obese.

- **Brown fat thermogenesis.** Brown fat, a form of fat that uses excess food to make heat, may be deficient in some obese people. Normally, brown fat serves to keep extra calories from being stored as fat. Studies on lean and obese humans will shed more light on this potential contributor to obesity.

- **Lipoprotein lipase.** Lipoprotein lipase (LPL) is an enzyme in adipose tissue (also found in muscle). Its activity has been found to increase in the fat cells of obese people who lose weight, leading researchers to wonder if it might be a reason why previously overfat people usually regain lost weight. The effect of exercise on muscle LPL will be discussed in chapter 13.

If one or both of these lines of research are confirmed on human subjects, we will be better able to understand why so many millions are overweight or obese. We don't yet know whether metabolic problems cause obesity or whether overeating is the cause (Bray 1983). We have evidence that Americans eat a similar number of calories as our ancestors did in 1900 but that we are far less active than they were. Clearly, weight loss through dieting is associated with a reduction in 24-hour energy expenditure, and this reduction makes it more difficult to maintain a body weight that is different from the usual weight (Leibel, Rosenbaum, and Hirsch 1995). We will deal with the implications of this finding in chapter 13. Just remember that regardless of genetic, glandular, psychological, or other complications or causes, overweight and obesity are problems of energy balance. We take in too many calories, or expend too few, or both.

> We don't yet know whether metabolic problems cause obesity or whether overeating is the cause.

Contributors to Obesity

A few other factors contribute to overweight and obesity, including psychological causes, physical inactivity, and, of all things, dieting! Our environment, culture, genetics, and history may blend together such that obesity seems to quietly sneak up on us. Many of the factors leading to obesity may be connected to denial—food becomes a coping strategy for other problems not being addressed. We eat without being conscious of energy balance and of the calories that we actually need for daily activity. We buy into schemes that promise quick and easy results.

Psychological Causes

Overweight can stem from an underlying emotional problem. Eating may be a defense mechanism, a retreat from reality, or a defiant gesture used to get attention or sympathy. All of us have used food as a crutch when we were bored or lonely, and all of us have eating habits that border on overfeeding—doughnuts during coffee break, chips with TV, or late-night snacks. Eating and drinking are complex social behaviors, and others may view failure to participate as a social rebuff. The psychological and social causes of overeating are beyond the scope of this book, but eating behaviors are not. We will deal with ways to alter eating behavior in chapter 14.

Although some obese people suffer anxiety and depression, it isn't clear whether these reactions are a consequence of excess weight, of social and psychological treatment by others, or of problems related to dieting. In other words, emotional problems associated with obesity may be a cause or a result of excess weight, and some may be a consequence of the treatment, dieting.

Lack of Activity

At a symposium devoted to the causes and treatment of obesity, researchers concluded that the most likely factor contributing to the current epidemic of obesity is a continued decline in daily energy expenditure that has not been matched by an equivalent reduction in energy intake. Because daily energy expenditure is decreasing and most people do not restrict intake to meet lower energy requirements, more people are becoming obese (Hill and Melanson 1999). This outcome is true for adults and children.

Previously, researchers found that overweight children are less active than their thinner counterparts. Trained observers plotted the movements of fat and thin children while they engaged in games such as volleyball. The thin children ranged all over the court, whereas the heavyweights literally held down their positions (Mayer and Bullen 1974).

You may be wondering, "What comes first, inactivity or fat?" The earlier section on fat cells answers part of that question (overfeeding), but we do know that people reduce their activity and range of movement as they become larger, not wishing to call attention to their size. When adult-onset obesity follows an active childhood, the overweight person is likely to be less inhibited and more active than one who became obese as a child. But inactivity leads to weight gain, which leads to further inactivity, which leads to more weight gain, and so on. The problem is to break this painful cycle and restore normal levels of activity and food intake.

We talked about energy balance, caloric intake versus caloric expenditure. Some research suggests we may need to refine that equation and focus specifically on fat balance. Unlike carbohydrate and protein stores, fat stores are not controlled, and their capacity for expansion is enormous (Swinburn and Ravussin 1993). We can view obesity as a long-standing positive fat balance, often the consequence of a high-fat diet. The message is clear. Lower your dietary intake of saturated fat and trans-fatty acids (hydrogenated oils), and use physical activity to burn excess calories.

Dieting

Are you surprised that we list dieting as a contributor to obesity? How can dieting lead to overweight or obesity? When animals or humans gain weight, go on a diet, gain weight, diet, and so on—a process called weight cycling—the body becomes more fuel efficient and the metabolic rate declines. Thereafter, the body needs more dieting or exercise to reduce excess weight. Weight loss slows, and weight is regained three times faster during the second cycle. Eventually, the body maintains weight on a reduced caloric intake that inhibits weight loss and promotes regaining (Brownell et al. 1986). In other words, the weight cycling, or yo-yo approach to weight control, leads to weight gain, not loss.

> Every time you diet to lose weight, you lose lean tissue; therefore, you must decrease caloric intake to avoid subsequent weight gain.

The reason for this weight gain is the loss of muscle protein with each cycle of dieting. Muscle is metabolically active; it is the furnace that burns excess calories. If you lose muscle, you have less ability to burn calories, at rest or during exercise. When you diet, the body turns to protein as an energy source, thereby reducing muscle mass. Every time you diet to lose weight, you lose lean tissue; therefore, you must decrease caloric intake to avoid subsequent weight gain. If you return to past eating habits, you increase weight and fat above previous levels. Exercise is the only way to minimize the loss of lean tissue while dieting. In fact, if you do enough exercise, you can reverse the drop in metabolic rate and increase lean tissue, thereby easing the problem of weight control.

Oprah!

When popular television personality Oprah Winfrey used a commercial diet program to lose weight, her story was big news. But it was even bigger news when she gained it all back within a few months. Today, Oprah strives to maintain her weight the sensible way: with wise food choices and regular activity. She runs regularly, works out with a personal trainer, and has completed the Chicago Marathon!

Set Point

We'll close this discussion of overweight and obesity with a brief mention of the set point theory, which has been around for many years. Some believe that the body has a preferred weight range that it tries to maintain. The body's effort to maintain the set point counters any attempt to gain or lose weight. For example, if you eat less, the body lowers your metabolism, making weight hard to lose and easy to regain. The set point seems to change slowly, and that may explain why gradual weight-loss programs are more successful than rapid weight-loss programs are in keeping weight off. Although this theory makes some sense and seems to fit certain people, others are able to lose weight and keep it off. Moreover, alternative explanations can account for the lower metabolic rate associated with weight loss because of caloric restriction. As we have said, a low-calorie diet causes loss of muscle, and muscle is needed to metabolize fat. The set point theory may discourage people from embarking on a weight-loss program or give them an excuse to quit. It shouldn't. The set point, if it exists, may make weight loss more difficult for some, but it still can be done.

Ideal Body Weight

Is there such a thing as an ideal body weight or an ideal amount of body fat? Should one strive to reduce body fat to the minimum? The minimum amount of fat consistent with good health and nutrition is around 5 to 7 percent for young men and 11 to 12 percent for young women. Healthy high school wrestlers and male distance runners may have a bit less than 5 percent, but only during a few days of competition. Female distance runners have had a temporary low of 7 percent. These figures do not suggest, however, that all men and women should attempt to achieve those levels. We offer them only to indicate the minimum level consistent with health and performance. Studies show that weight shouldn't regularly fall more than 10 percent below the desirable weight. The upper limit consistent with good health probably approaches 20 percent above the desirable weight.

Somewhere between the extremes (minus 10 percent to plus 20 percent of desirable weight) lies a level that is best for you. The level you choose will relate to your current activity and interests. If you are training for a long-distance race, you'll want to minimize your weight handicap. If you've been burdened with a large number of fat cells, you may be doing well to keep the level below 20 percent. Data indicate that those who weigh less than the desirable body weight for their height and frame live longer than those who weigh more. Because desirable weights are based on average values of body fat, maintaining body weight and body fat at or below desirable weight or average fat levels seem advisable. But in the absence of heart disease, hypertension, or diabetes, little health difference occurs between the extremes of 5 percent and 20 percent body fat for men, or between 12 percent and 30 percent body fat for women. Suggested desirable weights are shown in table 12.5 on page 243.

Optimal Weight

Some believe that U.S. weight guidelines are too lax, encouraging obesity in both men and women. The researchers found that 40 percent of all heart attacks in middle-aged women were due to overweight, a figure similar to that found in men. Women of average (not desirable) weight had a 50 percent higher risk of heart attack than those 15 percent below the average U.S. weight. Also, gaining more than 10 pounds (4.5 kilograms) in early to middle adult life increased the risk (Manson et al. 1995). Based on this study, we can estimate optimal weight as follows:

- Women—100 pounds (45.4 kilograms) for 5 feet (60 inches, or 152.4 centimeters) plus 5 pounds (2.3 kilograms) for each additional inch (or every 2.5 centimeters). For example, optimal weight for a woman 5 feet, 6 inches (165.1 centimeters) tall is 100 + (5 × 6), or 130 pounds (59.0 kilograms).

- Men—106 pounds (48.1 kilograms) for 5 feet, plus 6 pounds (2.7 kilograms) for each additional inch (2.54 centimeters). For example, optimal weight for a man 5 feet, 10 inches (177.8 centimeters) tall is 106 + (6 × 10), or 166 pounds (75.3 kilograms).

Estimated weights are plus or minus 10 percent.

Gender-Specific Fat

Some of the fat differences between males and females are due to gender-specific fat. Female hormones dictate different patterns of fat deposition, including breasts, which are largely fat. But only a portion of the difference, perhaps an extra 6 percent, is due to gender-specific fat. The rest is probably because of lack of activity or excess caloric intake or both. That circumstance is changing, however, as more women undertake the active life. Active college-age women average 18 to 22 percent fat, and female endurance athletes are often in the range of 12 to 17 percent fat (Sharkey 1984).

Age and Body Fat

With each decade above age 25, the body loses about 4 percent of its metabolically active cells. If diet remains relatively unchanged during a 10-year period, a person will gain weight because total energy expenditure declines. To maintain a desirable weight, the adult should either exercise more or eat less. People who can claim that their weight has not changed since college deserve congratulations. But they should also know that the loss of metabolically active cells with age usually means a decline in lean body weight, including muscle (Piers et al. 1998). Therefore, maintenance of body weight usually indicates an increase in the percentage of body fat.

Regular activity can counteract a slowing metabolism and maintain lean tissue as you age.

Seasonal Fluctuation

Body weight and body fat fluctuate from season to season and year to year. Typically, lean body weight (body weight minus fat weight) does not change as rapidly. Lean body weight consists mainly of muscles, bones, and organs. Thus, seasonal changes in body weight result from differences in the amount of fat being stored in adipose tissue. Total body fat storage often is higher during winter months, when subcutaneous fat serves as insulation against the cold. In summer, weight and fat often decline in response to an increase in energy expenditure and a decrease in appetite (stimulated in part by the increase in daylight).

Summary

Overweight and obesity clearly have a genetic link, and people who inherit the tendency are more metabolically efficient (they use less energy), even when sleeping. One can become overweight even though he or she eats little more than those who remain thin. But how much of the problem of obesity and overweight can we attribute to heredity and how much can we attribute to a positive energy balance, to intake of calories exceeding expenditure? Obesity researcher Claude Bouchard has estimated that 40 percent of the variance in body weight among people of similar stature can be attributed to genetic causes, leaving 60 percent as one's personal responsibility (Malina and Bouchard 1991). Immigrants come to the United States with a low rate of obesity, but after 15 years, they resemble U.S. born adults in BMI and obesity (Sanghavi et al. 2004).

According to the National Health and Nutrition Examination Surveys (NHANES), between 1971 and 2000 U.S. men increased caloric intake 168 calories per day while women increased their intake 335 calories per day. With that positive energy balance a man could gain 17.5 pounds (7.9 kilograms) in one year while a woman could gain 34.8 pounds (15.8 kilograms)! The percentage of calories from fat decreased although absolute fat consumption increased. The percentage of daily calories from carbohydrate increased 277.6 calories for men and 255.8 calories for women (Wright et al. 2004). Apparently, we are eating more calories while burning far fewer in work or recreational activity.

Overweight and obesity increase health care and human costs. Median health costs for obese people were 75 percent higher than they were for nonobese subjects (Raebel et al. 2004). The years of life lost because of severe obesity (BMI greater than 45) for 20- to 30-year-old men and women were 13 years and 8 years, respectively (Fontaine et al. 2003). In another study, a 40-year-old male nonsmoker lost 3.1 years to overweight and 5.8 years to obesity, and a female lost 3.3 years to overweight and 7.1 years to obesity. The picture was far worse for smokers, with losses of 13.7 and 13.3 years for obese male and female smokers compared with normal-weight nonsmokers (Peeters et al. 2003).

Calorie-burning exercise is the positive side of the fat balance equation. Moderate-intensity exercise burns fat while preserving lean tissue, something that dieting alone cannot do. Chapter 13 will tell you how to incorporate activity into a sensible program of weight control and show you how improved aerobic and muscular fitness magnify the benefits of regular, moderate activity.

Table 12.6 Caloric Content of Foods

Food	Portion	Fat* (grams)	Cal
Beverages, alcoholic			
Beer	12 oz (355 ml)	0	150
Beer, light	12 oz (355 ml)	0	100
Brandy	1 oz (30 ml)	0	70
Eggnog	8 oz (240 ml)	19	335
Highball	8 oz (240 ml)	0	165
Port, vermouth, muscatel	4 oz (120 ml)	0	155
Rum	1 jigger (1.5 oz) (44 ml)	0	140
Whiskey	1 jigger (1.5 oz) (44 ml)	0	130
Wine, white, rosé	4 oz (120 ml)	0	85–105
Beverages, nonalcoholic			
Carbonated soft drinks	8 oz (240 ml)	0	80
Chocolate milk	8 oz (240 ml)	10.5	200
Cocoa	8 oz (240 ml)	11	75
Coffee, black	8 oz (240 ml)	0	1
Coffee with cream and sugar (1 tsp each)	8 oz (240 ml)	3	45
Tea	8 oz (240 ml)	0	1
Cereals, cereal products			
Boston bread, enriched, brown	2 large slices	1.2	200
Cornbread or muffins, enriched	2	6	220
Raisin bread, enriched	2 slices	1.5	130
Rye bread, American	2 slices	0.6	110
White bread, enriched	2 slices	1.5	120
Whole-wheat bread	2 slices	1.5	110
Bread, rolls, sweet, unenriched	1	3	320
Cornflakes	1 cup (240 ml)	0.1	100
Crackers, graham	2	1.0	60
Saltines	2	1.5	50
Soda crackers	10 oyster	1.3	40
Macaroni, cooked	1/2 cup (120 ml)	0.3	70
Noodles, cooked	1 cup (240 ml)	2.0	150
Oat flakes, cooked	1 cup (240 ml)	1.0	75
Pancakes, wheat	2 cakes	6.0	150
Popcorn, popped	1 cup (240 ml)	0.8	60
Pretzels	Handful	1.0	110
Rice, cooked	1/2 cup (120 ml)	0.1	100
Spaghetti with tomato sauce	1 cup (240 ml)	7.0	220
Tapioca, cooked	1/2 cup (120 ml)	4.0	130
Waffles, baked (frozen or mix)	1 waffle	4–8	225
Wheat germ	1 oz (28 g)	3.5	120
Confections			
Chocolate	1 oz (28 g)	16	150
Fudge	1 piece	5	120
Honey	1 tbsp (15 ml)	0	65
Jams	1 tbsp (15 ml)	0	55
Jellies	1 tbsp (15 ml)	0	50
Molasses	1 tbsp (15 ml)	0	50

Food	Portion	Fat* (grams)	Cal
Syrup (chiefly corn syrup)	1 tbsp (15 ml)	0	60
Sugar, maple	1 tbsp (15 ml)	0	55
Sugar, cane or beet	1 tbsp (15 ml)	0	50
Dairy products, eggs			
Cheese, cheddar	1 oz (28 g)	9.5	115
Cheese, cottage	4 oz (120 ml)	5	100
Cheese, cream	2 tbsp (30 ml)	10	100
Cheese, Limburger	1 oz (28 g)	8	100
Cheese, Parmesan	1 oz (28 g)	8.5	110
Cheese, Roquefort	1 oz (28 g)	8	105
Cheese, Swiss	1 oz (28 g)	8	105
Cream, light	1 tbsp (15 ml)	3	30
Cream, heavy or whipping	1 tbsp (15 ml)	5.5	50
Eggs, whole	1 medium	5	75
Egg white, raw	1 medium	0	15
Egg yolk, raw	1 medium	5	60
Milk, pasteurized, whole	8 oz (240 ml)	8.5	165
Buttermilk, cultured	8 oz (240 ml)	0.4	80
Milk, canned, evaporated, unsweetened	4 oz (120 ml)	10.0	140
Milk, condensed, sweetened	4 oz (120 ml)	14	480
Milk, nonfat	8 oz (240 ml)	0.4	80
Ice cream	4 oz (120 ml)	9–13	155–225
Sherbet	4 oz (120 ml)	2–3	135
Yogurt, low fat	8 oz (240 ml)	2.0	61
Yogurt, regular	8 oz (240 ml)	8.5	152
Fats, oils			
Butter	1 tbsp (15 ml)	4.0	35
Mayonnaise	1 tbsp (15 ml)	11.0	100
Olive oil	1 tbsp (15 ml)	12.0	125
Peanut butter	1 tbsp (15 ml)	8.0	85
Fruit, fruit juices			
Apples	1	0.8	60–90
Apple juice, fresh	8 oz (240 ml)	0	120
Applesauce, sweetened	4 oz (120 ml)	0	80
Apricots	1 medium	0	18
Avocados, fresh	1/2	18	190
Bananas	1 (about 6 in., or 15 cm)	0	94
Blackberries, fresh	1/2 cup (120 ml)	0.6	40
Blueberries, fresh	1/2 cup (120 ml)	0.4	45
Cantaloupe, fresh	1/2	0.2	40
Cherries, canned, sweetened	1/2 cup (120 ml)	0.2	100
Cranberry sauce	2 tbsp (30 ml)	0	60
Dates, dried, pitted	5	0.2	100
Fruit cocktail, canned	4 oz (120 ml)	0.2	90
Grapes, fresh	20	0.8	45
Grape juice	4 oz (120 ml)	0	80
Grapefruit	1/2 (4 1/4 in., or 11 cm)	0.1	75
Grapefruit juice, fresh	4 oz (120 ml)	0.2	45

(continued)

(continued)

Food	Portion	Fat* (grams)	Cal
Lemons, fresh	1 (2 in., or 5 cm)	0	30
Olives, green or ripe	5 large	2.5/4.0	20/35
Oranges, fresh	1 (3 in., or 7.6 cm)	0.1	70
Orange juice, fresh	4 oz (120 ml)	0.3	55
Peaches, fresh	1 (2 1/2 in., or 6 cm)	0.1	45
Peaches, canned, sweetened	2 halves	0.2	85
Pears	1 (2 1/2 in., or 6 cm)	0.7	95
Pineapple, canned, sweetened	1/2 cup (120 ml)	0.2	100
Pineapple juice, canned	4 oz (120 ml)	0.1	60
Plums	1 (2 in., or 5 cm)	0.1	30
Prunes, dried, uncooked	4 large	0.3	110
Raisins, dried	1/4 cup (60 ml)	0.1	100
Raspberries, fresh	1/2 cup (120 ml)	0.5	50
Strawberries, fresh	10 large	0.5	35
Strawberries, frozen, sweetened	1/2 cup (120 ml)	0.2	125
Sorbet	1/2 cup (120 ml)	0.2	110
Meat, poultry (raw unless otherwise stated)			
Bacon, medium fat, cooked	2 strips	9.0	100
Beef (medium fat), hamburger, cooked .	4 oz (114 g)	15	225
Beef, rib roast, cooked	3 oz (85 g)	33	335
Beef, sirloin, cooked	3 oz (85 g)	27	330
Beef, canned, corned	4 oz (114 g)	11	240
Beef, liver, fried	3 oz (85 g)	9.0	200
Chicken, fried	4 oz (114 g)	9.0	275
Chicken, roasted	4 oz (114 g)	3.0	170
Chicken, liver	3 oz (85 g)	15.0	235
Ham, baked	3 oz (85 g)	19	250
Ham, canned, spiced	3 oz (85 g)	21	245
Lamb (medium fat), leg roast	3 oz (85 g)	6.0	160
Lamb, rib chop	1	15.0	230
Pork (see also bacon and ham), medium fat	3 oz (85 g)	24	310
Pork, loin or chops	1	24.5	300
Turkey, light and dark	3 oz (85 g)	3.5/7.0	150/170
Veal	3 oz (85 g)	9.5	180
Venison	3 oz (85 g)	2.5	120
Nuts			
Almonds	15	8.0	100
Brazil nuts	5	12.0	100
Cashews, roasted or cooked	10	14.0	200
Peanuts, roasted	30	14.0	165
Pecans	1 tbsp (15 ml)	5	52
Walnuts	2 tbsp (30 ml)	10	95
Seafood (raw unless otherwise stated)			
Clams	4 oz (114 g)	0.8	80
Cod	4 oz (114 g)	6.0	180
Crab, canned or cooked	4 oz (114 g)	2.0	100
Flounder	4 oz (114 g)	7.0	180
Frog legs, fried	4 legs	28.0	418

Food	Portion	Fat* (grams)	Cal
Haddock	4 oz (114 g)	7.0	180
Halibut	4 oz (114 g)	8.0	200
Lobster	12 oz (340 g)	5.0	300
Oysters	5–8 medium	2.0	80
Salmon, Pacific, cooked	4 oz (114 g)	7.0	180
Salmon, canned	4 oz (114 g)	7.0	190
Sardines, canned in oil	5 medium	9.0	180
Scallops, fried	4 oz (114 g)	10.0	200
Shrimp, canned	3 oz (85 g)	0.9	100
Shrimp, fried	3 oz (85 g)	9.5	190
Trout (brook/lake)	4 oz (114 g)	10–13	210–290
Soup			
Broth	8 oz (240 ml)	0	25
Bean	8 oz (240 ml)	6.0	170
Beef	8 oz (240 ml)	4.0	115
Beef with vegetables	8 oz (240 ml)	2.0	90
Chicken noodle	8 oz (240 ml)	2.0	68
Pea	8 oz (240 ml)	3.0	140
Tomato	8 oz (240 ml)	2.5	100
Vegetable	8 oz (240 ml)	2.0	90
Vegetables			
Asparagus, canned	1/2 cup (120 ml)	0.4	25
Beans, kidney	1/2 cup (120 ml)	0.5	120
Beans, lima, fresh	1/2 cup (120 ml)	0.4	90
Beans, snap, fresh	1/2 cup (120 ml)	0.4	35
Beans, wax, canned	1/2 cup (120 ml)	0.2	20
Beets (beetroots), peeled, fresh	1/2 cup (120 ml)	0.1	35
Broccoli, fresh	1/2 cup (120 ml)	0.2	30
Brussels sprouts, fresh	1/2 cup (120 ml)	0.3	30
Cabbage, fresh	Wedge	0.2	25
Carrots, canned	1/2 cup (120 ml)	0.2	30
Carrots, fresh	1 carrot (6 in., or 15 cm)	0.1	20
Cauliflower, fresh	1 cup (240 ml)	0.2	25
Celery	2 stalks	0.1	17
Corn, fresh, with butter	1 ear	2.0	90
Corn, canned	1/2 cup (120 ml)	0.6	70
Cucumbers	1 (7 1/2 in., or 19 cm)	0.2	20
Eggplant, fresh	1/2 cup (120 ml)	0.2	25
Kale, fresh	1/2 cup (120 ml)	0.4	20
Lentils	1/2 cup (120 ml)	—	110
Lettuce, headed, fresh	1/4 head	0.1	15
Mushrooms	1/2 cup (120 ml)	0.1	10
Onions	1 (2 1/2 in., or 6 cm)	0.1	40
Peas, green, fresh	1/2 cup (120 ml)	0.2	55
Peas, canned	1/2 cup (120 ml)	0.4	70
Peppers, green, fresh	1 large	0.1	24
Potatoes, raw	1 medium	0.2	90
French fried	20 pieces	12	220

(continued)

(continued)

Food	Portion	Fat* (grams)	Cal
Radishes, fresh	4 small	—	10
Rhubarb, fresh	1/2 cup (120 ml)	—	10
Spinach, canned	1/2 cup (120 ml)	0.2	25
Sweet potatoes, fresh	1 small	0.6	150
Sweet potatoes, candied	1 medium	3.5	180
Tomatoes, fresh	1 medium	0.2	25
Tomatoes, canned	1/2 cup (120 ml)	0.2	25
Tomato juice, canned	4 oz (114 g)	0.2	35
Miscellaneous			
Gelatin dessert	4 oz (114 g)	0	60
Pie	1 slice	16–18	300–400
Pecan pie	1 slice	31.5	580
Potato chips	7–10	8.0	110
Salad dressing (French, Thousand Island)	1 tbsp (15 ml)	6–8	60–100
Tomato catsup	2 tbsp (30 ml)	0.1	40
Yeast, compressed, baker's	1 cake	0.1	20

*1 g of fat contains 9.3 calories.

Table 12.7 Caloric Expenditure During Various Activities

Activity	Cal/min*
Sleeping	1.2
Resting in bed	1.3
Sitting, normally	1.3
Sitting, reading	1.3
Lying, quietly	1.3
Sitting, eating	1.5
Sitting, playing cards	1.5
Standing, normally	1.5
Class work, lecture (listening)	1.7
Conversing	1.8
Personal toilet	2.0
Sitting, writing	2.6
Standing, light activity	2.6
Washing and dressing	2.6
Washing and shaving	2.6
Driving a car	2.8
Washing clothes	3.1
Walking indoors	3.1
Shining shoes	3.2
Making bed	3.4
Dressing	3.4
Showering	3.4
Driving motorcycle	3.4
Metalworking	3.5
House painting	3.5
Cleaning windows	3.7
Carpentry	3.8
Farming chores	3.8
Sweeping floors	3.9
Plastering walls	4.1
Repairing trucks and automobiles	4.2
Ironing clothes	4.2
Farming, planting, hoeing, raking	4.7
Mixing cement	4.7
Mopping floors	4.9
Repaving roads	5.0
Gardening, weeding	5.6
Stacking lumber	5.8
Sawing with chain saw	6.2
Working with stone, masonry	6.3

(continued)

(continued)

Activity	Cal/min*
Working with pick and shovel	6.7
Farming, haying, plowing with horse	6.7
Shoveling (miners)	6.8
Walking down stairs	7.1
Shoveling snow	7.5
Chopping wood	7.5
Sawing with crosscut saw	7.5–10.5
Tree felling (ax)	8.4–12.7
Gardening, digging	8.6
Walking up stairs	10.0–18.0
Playing pool or billiards	1.8
Canoeing (2.5–4.0 mph, or 4.0–6.4 kph)	3.0–7.0
Playing volleyball, recreational to competitive	3.5–8.0
Golfing, foursome to twosome	3.7–5.0
Pitching horseshoes	3.8
Playing baseball (except pitcher)	4.7
Playing table tennis	4.9–7.0
Practicing calisthenics	5.0
Rowing, pleasure to vigorous	5.0–15.0
Cycling, easy to hard	5.0–15.0
Skating, recreational to vigorous	5.0–15.0
Practicing archery	5.2
Playing badminton, recreational to competitive	5.2–10.0
Playing basketball, half or full court (more for fast break)	6.0–9.0
Bowling (while active)	7.0
Playing tennis, recreational to competitive	7.0–11.0
Waterskiing	8.0
Playing soccer	9.0
Snowshoeing (2.5 mph, or 4.0 kph)	9.0
Slide board	9.0–13.0
Playing handball or squash	10.0
Mountain climbing	10.0–15.0
Skipping rope	10.0–15.0
Practicing judo or karate	13.0
Playing football (while active)	13.3
Wrestling	14.4
Skiing	
Moderate to steep	8.0–20.0
Downhill racing	16.5
Cross-country (3–10 mph, or 4.8–16.1 kph)	9.0–20.0

Activity	Cal/min*
Swimming	
Leisurely	6.0
Crawl (25–50 yd/min or m/min)	6.0–12.5
Butterfly (50 yd/min or m/min)	14.0
Backstroke (25–50 yd/min or m/min)	6.0–12.5
Breaststroke (25–50 yd/min or m/min)	6.0–12.5
Sidestroke (40 yd/min or m/min)	11.0
Dancing	
Modern, moderate to vigorous	4.2–5.7
Ballroom, waltz to rumba	5.7–7.0
Square	7.7
Walking	
Road or field (3.5 mph, or 5.6 kph)	5.6–7.0
Snow, hard to soft (2.5–3.5 mph, or 4.0–5.6 kph)	10.0–20.0
Uphill, 5–10–15% grade (3.5 mph, or 5.6 kph)	8.0–11.0–15.0
Downhill, 5–10% grade (2.5 mph, or 4.0 kph)	3.5–3.7
Downhill, 15–20% grade (2.5 mph or 4.0 kph)	3.7–4.3
Hiking, 40 lb (18 kg) pack (3.0 mph, or 4.8 kph)	6.8
Running	
12:00 mi, or 7:30 km (5 mph, or 8 kph)	10.0
8:00 mi, or 5:00 km (7.5 mph, or 12.1 kph)	15.0
6:00 mi, or 3:45 km (10 mph, or 16.1 kph)	20.0
5:00 mi, or 3:05 km (12 mph, or 19.3 kph)	25.0

*Depends on efficiency and body size. Add 10% for each 15 lb (6.8 kg) over 150 lb (68 kg); subtract 10% for each 15 lb under 150 lb. Use activity pulse rate to confirm caloric expenditure (see figure 13.1, page 271).

Sources: Ainsworth et al. 1993; Consolazio, Johnson, and Pecora 1963; Passmore and Durnin 1955; Roth 1968; Unpublished data from the Human Performance Laboratory, University of Montana 1964–2005.

Activity, Diet, and Weight Control

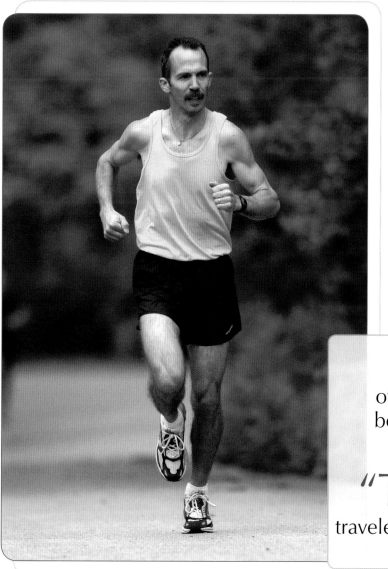

"A journey of a thousand miles must begin with a single step."
Lao-Tzu

"The swiftest traveler is he that goes afoot."
Henry David Thoreau

Weight control is a lifelong journey. The best time to start is when you are young; the next best time is today. Physical activity is the positive approach to weight control. When you decide to do something about your weight, you are committing to a course of action. No other approach is so physiologically sound, so definite, so enjoyable. Action is more psychologically rewarding than avoidance. When you take a walk after dinner you relax, improve your digestion, enhance your vitality, and burn fat and calories. After the walk you feel better both physically and emotionally. Problems loom large when you sit and brood, but how quickly they shrink when you undertake a plan of action!

Dieting carries negative connotations of avoidance, deprivation, and punishment. Dieting creates false hopes, contributes to stress, ruins the disposition, causes fatigue, and often leads to increases in body weight and fat. The ups and downs of frequent dieting (weight cycling, or yo-yo dieting) increase the risk of psychopathology, life dissatisfaction, binge eating, morbidity, and mortality (Brownell and Rodin 1994).

The most exciting part of this chapter deals with the extra benefits that you obtain with improved fitness, benefits that exceed the effects of activity. This material, although not new, is finally coming to the attention of public health and fitness professionals. In our estimation, these extra benefits provide the most convincing case for activity and fitness and their relationship to health.

This chapter will help you

- understand why activity is superior to dieting as a means of weight control,
- determine the effects of activity on the appetite, and
- understand the extra weight-control and fat metabolism benefits associated with improved fitness.

Activity and Weight Control

The only way to remove stored fat is to burn it off. By now you know that exercise increases caloric expenditure and that energy expenditure is related to both the intensity and the duration of activity. As exercise becomes more intense, the duration of participation must necessarily become shorter. Although we may be able to expend as many as 125 calories in one all-out mile (1.6-kilometer) run, we can walk briskly or jog at a comfortable pace for 3 miles (4.8 kilometers) and triple the caloric expenditure without becoming exhausted. This notion explains why we recommend moderate activity instead of high-intensity effort for weight control. The relationship of exercise to caloric expenditure also helps explain why the benefits grow with improved fitness. More fitness allows more activity, and therefore more control over your weight.

The effects of exercise do not stop when the exercise ceases. The excess postexercise oxygen consumption (EPOC), the amount that exceeds the resting level after exercise, indicates a prolonged postexercise elevation in caloric expenditure. Caloric expenditure can remain elevated for 30 minutes or more after vigorous exercise. Long-duration effort such as a distance run will elevate oxygen consumption and body temperature and call forth hormones to mobilize energy and increase metabolism. When the exercise stops, caloric expenditure remains elevated above resting levels during the recovery period. The EPOC is often neglected when the caloric benefits of exercise are tabulated.

Activity Versus Dieting

Some people believe that dieting is better than exercise for controlling weight. They point out, quite correctly, that it is easier to reduce caloric intake by refusing a piece of cake (250 calories) than it is to burn off the cake after eating it, which would require jogging more than 2 miles (3.2 kilometers) at 110 calories per mile. But let's examine the question "Is dieting a better method of weight control?" The answer has been available for over 35 years, and the answer is no.

> "Is dieting a better method of weight control?" The answer has been available for over 35 years, and the answer is no.

Oscai and Holloszy (1969) compared the effects of dieting and exercise on the body composition of laboratory rats. They controlled the experiment so that both groups lost the same amount of weight. Following 18 weeks of either food restriction (dieting) or swimming (exercise), they performed carcass analysis.

The analysis indicated that exercise was a more effective way to lose fat (78 percent of the total weight loss for the exercising group versus 62 percent for the dieting group). Furthermore, the study provided vivid evidence of the protein-conserving effects of exercise, 5 percent protein loss for exercisers versus 11 percent for dieters. The amount of water lost through caloric restriction was 16 percent for exercisers versus 26 percent for dieters. Water loss, a common occurrence among dieters, accounts for the early success of most fad diets and the eventual failure of the overall goal, fat loss. A control group of sedentary, freely eating animals gained weight during the study. Their weight gain consisted of 87 percent fat and 10 percent water. Can we generalize the results of this animal study to human subjects?

A study involving 16 obese patients compared a period of 6 months of dieting with a similar period of dieting and exercise. The exercise group achieved greater fat loss, and the exercise produced other benefits, including a lower resting heart rate and improved heart rate recovery after exercise (Kenrick, Ball, and Canary 1972). And when 25 women created a deficit of 500 calories per day by dieting, exercise, or a combination of the two, all the women lost the same amount of weight but those in the dieting group

The combination of exercise and dieting burns more fat and retains more lean tissue than dieting alone.

lost less fat and more lean tissue. The authors of the study (Zuti and Golding 1976) recommended that those interested in losing weight combine dieting and exercise to ensure greater fat loss and conservation of lean tissue. A more recent study of 24 obese women confirms the superiority of diet and exercise for the reduction of adipose tissue and preservation of lean tissue (skeletal muscle), as compared with diet alone (Ross, Pedwell, and Rissanen 1995).

These studies clearly indicate the need for activity in a program of weight control. Dieting or caloric restriction can lead to loss of weight, but a loss of protein (lean tissue) and water accompanies the weight loss. When the body loses lean tissue, it becomes less able to burn calories and eventually gains more fat weight. Dietary weight loss leads to a disproportionate decline in the metabolic rate and almost certain future weight gain (Leibel, Rosenbaum, and Hirsch 1995). A complication in the loss of lean tissue is a possible resetting of the metabolic thermostat, making weight gain likely with even less caloric intake. Four decades of research show that weight loss with exercise maximizes the removal of fat, minimizes the loss of protein, and helps maintain the metabolic rate. Exercise and dieting combine to provide a positive attack on both causes of overweight: inadequate caloric expenditure and excess caloric intake.

> Exercise and dieting combine to provide a positive attack on both causes of overweight: inadequate caloric expenditure and excess caloric intake.

Metabolic Rate

Exercise has an added benefit in relation to weight control and diet. In one study, several weeks of severe caloric restriction imposed by dieting led to the usual loss of lean tissue and a decrease in metabolic rate. The drop in metabolic rate makes it difficult for dieters to maintain a lower body weight because the more efficient body burns 10 to 15 percent fewer calories daily. On the bright side, however, just 2 weeks of exercise restored the metabolic rate to prediet levels. Moreover, the exercise reduced the loss of protein and increased the use of fat as the source of energy (Móle et al. 1989).

Activity and Appetite

In the past, the use of activity to achieve energy balance and weight control received criticism. Detractors argued that exercise would increase the appetite as the body attempted to keep pace with energy needs. Many assume that the desire for food signifies a real need for nourishment, but it doesn't. Appetite is a psychological desire that is influenced by several factors. The control center for food intake, the appestat, is located in the hypothalamus, an area of the brain that functions like a thermostat to turn on eating behavior and then turn it off when the desire or hunger has been satisfied. Unfortunately, it takes many minutes for the food that you eat to reach the bloodstream, where the appestat can see that you've satisfied the need. You may tuck away several hundred extra calories before the appestat gets the message.

Physiological factors such as low blood sugar, hormones, hours of daylight, cold temperatures, hunger pangs from an empty stomach, and unfilled fat cells can stimulate the appestat. Physical activity also stimulates eating behavior, but the increased caloric intake serves only to maintain body weight. Sedentary individuals take in more calories than they need. More exercise means more food intake, but the appetite doesn't keep pace with energy output. Regular activity seems to help the appestat adjust caloric intake to energy needs. The appestat is rather imprecise at a low level of energy expenditure, but for regularly active people, appetite control is much more related to energy requirements (Mayer and Bullen 1974). An exercise study with obese women cycling at 50 percent of $\dot{V}O_2$max found that 25 of 28 participants ate less during the 12-week program and continued to eat less during a 10-week follow-up (Vailodash 2000). At the high end of the activity scale, where endurance athletes and workers burn 4,000 to 6,000 calories daily in running, cycling, swimming, or work, the appetite usually underestimates energy needs (Ruby, Schoeller, and Sharkey 2001). Conversely, when a sedentary routine is imposed on otherwise active men, no reduction in energy intake occurs, leading to a positive energy balance (Stubbs et al. 2004).

Psychological factors such as the smell, sight, or taste of food can evoke the desire to eat. Habit and emotional factors also condition eating behavior. We eat to celebrate, to prolong feelings of excitement. Appetite is a complex phenomenon, subject to many influences, reflecting more than the need for nourishment. The appestat frequently overestimates energy needs. Weight control becomes possible when you realize that your eyes are bigger than your stomach and that your potential for energy intake is greater than your regular energy expenditure.

Premeal or Postmeal Exercise

Years ago, when the American diet was first implicated as a culprit in the heart disease epidemic, researchers roamed the world studying the relationship between diet and the incidence of heart disease. They found that diet alone did not account for the presence or absence of the problem; other factors such as a lack of tension and stress or physical activity confounded the relationship. Several researchers have focused on the effect of pre- or postmeal exercise on postprandial lipemia, the presence of fat in the blood after a meal. Studies conducted at the University of Florida have shown that exercise before or after a meal is effective in reducing the magnitude and duration of postprandial lipemia (Zauner, Burt, and Mapes 1968). Light exercise proved to be as effective as strenuous effort in this regard. A recent study on females confirms the ability of prior exercise to increase the utilization of dietary fat (Votruba et al. 2002). Recent research also indicates that the effect of exercise on postprandial lipemia is greater than and different from the effect attributable to a comparable caloric deficit. A 90-minute walk reduced postprandial lipemia 20 percent below control levels, whereas caloric restriction reduced it only 7 percent (Gill and Hardman 2000).

Lipemia has long been associated with atherosclerosis, reduced myocardial blood flow, and accelerated blood clotting. Thus anything that reduces the level of fat in the blood seems prudent and advisable. Vigorous premeal exercise may inhibit the appetite and increase the metabolism of fat ingested after the exercise. The metabolic rate remains somewhat elevated after exercise, and the ingested fat is used quickly to restore energy burned during exercise. Mild postmeal effort such as a walk after dinner also serves to reduce lipemia. Both pre- and postmeal exercise increase caloric expenditure and fat metabolism, lead to improved fitness, and contribute to health and weight control.

While we're on the subject of meals and blood lipids, you should know that the number of meals that you eat influences blood fat levels. By spreading the same number of calories over more meals (three to six), you will lower your cholesterol levels. Apparently, we are able to handle fat better in smaller doses. Conversely, if you avoid meals in an effort to lose weight, your metabolic rate will decline and your cholesterol level will climb. Rapid weight gain may follow your temporary weight loss.

Fitness and Fat

The effects of activity on weight control and energy balance are well established. Systematic and progressive exercise leads to improvement in aerobic fitness. This section deals with the extra benefits associated with improved fitness, benefits that provide dramatic evidence of the role that fitness plays in health and prevention of heart disease. These benefits include the following:

- Increased caloric expenditure
- Increased fat mobilization
- Increased fat utilization
- Reduced blood lipids
- Increased lean tissue (muscle)

Caloric Expenditure

Because unfit people tire quickly during exercise, they have limited ability to expend calories. As fitness improves, caloric expenditure rises, with increases in the intensity, duration, and frequency of exercise and because of the inevitable participation in activities that are more vigorous. The fit person does more with less fatigue. Increased fitness undoubtedly contributes to energy expenditure and weight control.

We have studied the effects of training on individuals' perception of effort and fatigue (Docktor and Sharkey 1971), and recent studies confirm the beneficial effects of training on one's perception of effort (Gaskill et al. 2005). As fitness improves, a person can perform more work at the same heart rate and level of perceived exertion. Work levels once perceived as difficult become less so, and once-fatiguing exertion can be managed with ease. After training, a person can accomplish a given task with a lower heart rate as well as a lower level of perceived exertion. Thus the subjects are able to burn more energy without experiencing a greater sense of fatigue.

Further proof of the value of fitness to caloric expenditure is found in the relationship of caloric expenditure to heart rate. Caloric expenditure is related directly to heart rate, but level of fitness also influences the relationship. For people in low fitness categories, a high heart rate does not indicate extremely high caloric expenditure (see figure 13.1). For those in high fitness categories, the same heart rate (HR) indicates much higher energy expenditure:

140 HR for very poor fitness level = 6 to 7 calories per minute expended

140 HR for very good fitness level = 12 calories per minute expended

You can use figure 13.1 to estimate your caloric expenditure in any activity. After several minutes of participation, stop and immediately take your pulse at wrist or throat (use gentle contact) for 15 seconds. Multiply by four to get your rate per minute. Then use the line corresponding to your fitness level to estimate your caloric expenditure per minute. Notice how caloric expenditure will improve (at the same heart rate) as your fitness improves. This finding should convince you that fitness provides extra benefits to those who persevere.

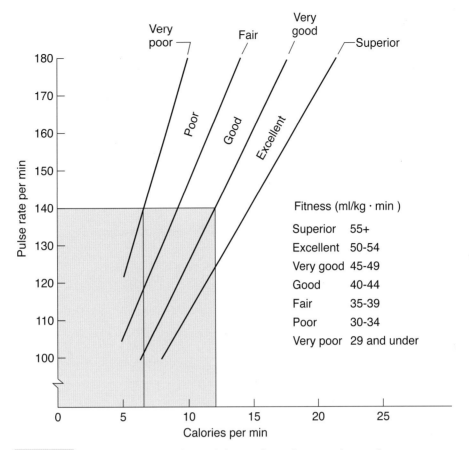

Figure 13.1 Predicting calories burned during physical activity from pulse rate. Reprinted from Sharkey, 1974.

Fat Mobilization

Fat is stored in fat cells in the form of triglycerides (three molecules of fatty acid and one molecule of glycerol). A triglyceride molecule is too large to pass through the wall of the fat cell into the circulation, so when energy is needed, the triglyceride is broken down and the fatty acid molecules pass into the blood for transport to the working muscles. The hormone epinephrine stimulates a receptor in the fat cell membrane and activates the enzyme lipase. Lipase splits the triglyceride molecule, and the fatty acids are free to enter the circulation.

As exercise becomes more intense, we produce lactic acid. The point at which lactic acid begins to accumulate in the blood, the second lactate threshold, indicates when lactate production exceeds removal. At this intensity a significant shift from fat to carbohydrate metabolism has occured. You will recall that the second lactate threshold is related to activity and fitness. It may be below 50 percent of the maximal oxygen uptake for the unfit and above 80 percent for the highly trained. But what does that have to do with fat?

Years ago, researchers discovered that lactic acid seemed to inhibit the mobilization of free fatty acids (FFAs) from adipose tissue (see figure 5.5, page 94). The lactic acid blocked the action of epinephrine, thereby reducing the availability of fat for muscle metabolism (Issekutz and Miller 1962). One of the best-documented effects of training is that more work can be accomplished before lactic acid levels rise. After

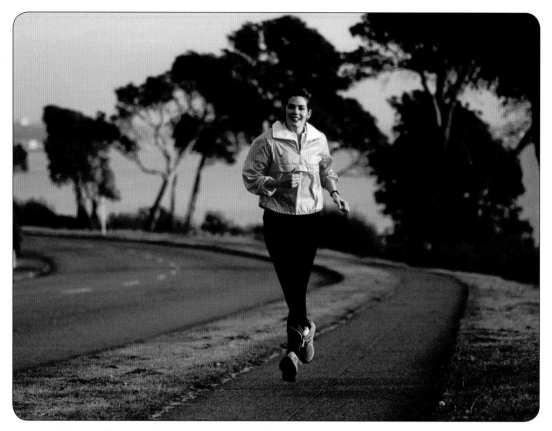

Improved fitness allows people to burn more fat with less perceived exertion.

improving fitness, a person who formerly produced lactic acid at a given workload can accomplish the same workload with little increase in lactic acid. This result may be because of a decrease in lactic acid production or an increase in lactic acid clearance. Whatever the case, improved aerobic fitness allows a person to accomplish more work aerobically. The lactate threshold increases, and more fat is available for use as an energy source.

A study of trained subjects illustrates that moderate levels of lactic acid do not affect FFA mobilization and utilization (Vega deJesus and Siconolfi 1988). The fit subjects were able to mobilize fat at the second lactate threshold (4 millimoles lactic acid), which defines the highest level of exercise intensity that a person can sustain during prolonged exertion. These findings help explain the tremendous increase in endurance associated with training. Fat is the most abundant energy source (50 times more abundant than carbohydrate). Improved fitness allows greater access to that immense storehouse of energy.

Fat Utilization

The mobilization of fat does not ensure its metabolism. How does training influence the utilization of FFA as a source of energy for muscular contractions? Studies have shown that trained animals and humans are capable of extracting a greater percentage of their energy from FFA during submaximal exercise. How, then, does fitness influence fat utilization?

Lactic Acid

Lactic acid is produced when the breakdown of muscle glycogen (to three carbon pyruvic acid molecules) exceeds the ability of the mitochondria to process this metabolite. So the pyruvic acid picks up hydrogen, becomes lactic acid, and begins to accumulate in the muscle and blood. The heart and skeletal muscle can use lactate as a source of energy, and the liver can oxidize it. But when production of lactate exceeds removal, the level in muscle and blood increases. The rising level of acid in the muscle reduces force production by interfering with muscle contractions and decreases endurance by lowering the efficiency of aerobic enzymes.

Lipoprotein Lipase

Earlier we talked about LPL in adipose tissue. In muscle the LPL helps grab circulating fat from the blood and use it for energy. Muscle LPL activity increases with endurance training and enhances the ability of the muscle to use fat as a fuel (Nikkila et al. 1978).

Fat Oxidation

Móle, Oscai, and Holloszy (1971) provided convincing proof of the effect of training on FFA utilization. They found that the ability of rat muscle to oxidize the fatty acid palmitate doubled following 12 weeks of treadmill training. The authors suggested that the shift to fat metabolism was a key factor in the development of endurance fitness and an important mechanism serving to spare carbohydrate stores and prevent low blood sugar during prolonged exertion. Thus the physically fit person is able to derive a greater percentage of energy requirements from fat than the unfit subject can. At a given workload, the fit subject may obtain as much as 90 percent of his or her energy from fat. Free fatty acids are used during all forms of muscular activity, except for all-out bursts of effort such as the 100-yard (100-meter) dash. Training even seems to improve the ability of the heart muscle to oxidize fat (Keul 1971).

When exercise begins, the initial source of energy from fat is from intramuscular fat, a supply that is enhanced with training. When prolonged activity depletes intramuscular fat, the body uses fat that comes from adipose tissue by way of the blood (Coggan and Williams 1995). Improved fitness increases the availability of fat through mobilization of FFAs, as well as an increase in enzyme activity. Both contribute to the rate of FFA utilization.

Maximal Fat Oxidation

To determine when maximal fat oxidation occurred during exercise, moderately trained subjects were exercised on a progressive laboratory bicycle test. Fat oxidation peaked at 55 to 72 percent of $\dot{V}O_2$max, or 68 to 79 percent of maximal heart rate, values higher than those previously noted (Achten, Gleeson, and Jeukendrup 2002). This study, performed after subjects fasted for 10 hours, shows that fat can be a significant source of energy for rather vigorous exercise. Ingesting carbohydrate before exercise lowers the contribution of fat to energy expenditure, so if your goal is oxidation of fat, exercise before breakfast.

Blood Lipids

Blood lipids—cholesterol and triglycerides—have been associated with the incidence and severity of coronary heart disease. They are related to other risk factors, including diet, overweight, and lack of exercise. Recent findings suggest that fitness training also influences the lipids.

Triglycerides

Dietary fat intake shows up in the blood as chylomicrons, large clumps of triglycerides. Most of the triglycerides are removed from the plasma in the capillaries adjacent to muscle and adipose tissue. The liver clears any remains from the circulation. Chylomicrons are responsible for the milky appearance of blood plasma following a meal (postprandial lipemia). Besides containing 80 to 95 percent triglyceride, chylomicrons contain 2 to 7 percent cholesterol, 3 to 6 percent phospholipid, and 1 to 2 percent protein.

Dieting or participation in regular physical activity can reduce fasting serum triglyceride levels. The reduction because of exercise occurs several hours afterward and lasts for about 2 days. With regular exercise, further reductions occur until the person reaches a plateau consistent with his or her exercise, diet, and other factors, including inherited blood lipid patterns.

Earlier in this chapter we established the influence of exercise on postmeal fat in blood. The research supports the hypothesis that regular exercise enhances the removal and utilization of triglyceride by muscle cells, rather than allowing their deposit in adipose tissue or processing by the liver, possibly to synthesize more cholesterol.

A researcher trained sedentary rats for 12 weeks on a treadmill. Following the training, the muscles were analyzed for the activity of lipoprotein lipase (LPL), the enzyme responsible for the uptake of plasma triglyceride fatty acids (TGFA) from plasma chylomicrons and other sources in the blood. The researcher reasoned that an increase in LPL activity would accompany any increase in the uptake of TGFA by skeletal muscle during exercise. The results of the study confirmed the hypothesis. Regular endurance training led to a two- to fourfold increase in LPL activity, indicating that training increases the capacity of muscle fibers to take up and oxidize fatty acids originating in plasma triglycerides (Borensztajn 1975).

Because the fat is used before it can be deposited in adipose tissue, these findings have tremendous significance in the area of weight control. The implications for cardiovascular health are even more exciting, as is the realization that these benefits are associated with an entirely natural, enjoyable, and satisfying experience—aerobic training.

Cholesterol

Cholesterol ingested in the diet is absorbed in the small intestine, finds its way into the lymph system, and then is dumped into the blood. There it joins cholesterol produced by the body in the chylomicrons and in very low density lipoprotein particles (VLDL). Once in the plasma, the same enzymes that act on the chylomicrons attack the VLDL. Much of the triglyceride is removed (within 2 to 6 hours). The VLDL is degraded to low-density lipoprotein (LDL), which the liver removes over a period of 2 to 5 days. Because of the smaller size of the LDL particle and its high concentration of cholesterol, the LDL particle seems to be involved directly in the development of coronary artery disease. The LDL particles find their way into coronary arteries and contribute to the growth of atherosclerotic plaques. Thus LDL is believed to be a major culprit in the development of coronary artery disease.

Until the mid-1970s, diet, weight loss, and drugs were believed to be the major weapons in the fight against cholesterol. Studies on the effect of exercise on cholesterol typically reported a modest reduction but only when the exercise was vigorous and of long duration (3 or more miles, or 5 or more kilometers, of running per day). But remember that the blood transports cholesterol in several ways. A single measure of serum cholesterol does not indicate how the cholesterol is distributed among the several lipoprotein fractions, nor does it indicate the effects of exercise.

Dr. Wood and his associates (1975) of the Stanford Heart Disease Prevention Program compared the lipoprotein patterns of sedentary and active middle-aged men (35 to 59 years old). The active group consisted of joggers who averaged at least 15 miles (24.1 kilometers) per week for the preceding year. As expected, the triglycerides were "strikingly" lower for the active group, while total cholesterol was only "modestly" lower. But when the lipoprotein pattern was analyzed, the joggers exhibited a significantly lower level of dangerous LDL and an elevated level of high-density lipoprotein (HDL). These findings were significant, because there is a direct relationship between LDL and heart disease and an inverse relationship between HDL and heart disease (as HDL goes up, the incidence of heart disease goes down). HDL seems to carry cholesterol away from the tissues for removal by the liver. Dr. Wood noted that the lipoprotein pattern of the active men was similar to that of the typical young woman, who has the lowest risk of heart disease in the adult population.

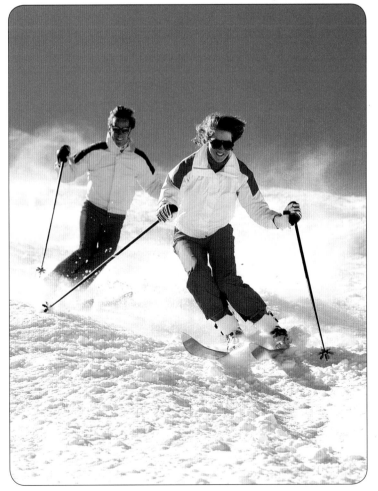

Get active and improve your fitness to help reduce your risk of heart disease.

When researchers studied the effects of 7 weeks of training on the serum lipids and lipoproteins of medical students, triglycerides fell by 27 percent. Furthermore, they found a marked reduction of LDL and VLDL cholesterol, an increase in HDL cholesterol, and no changes in body weight to confuse the results (Lopez et al. 1974). Studies in our lab (Sharkey et al. 1980) agree with those reported by Dr. Wood and many others (Leon et al. 2002). They indicate how training helps shift cholesterol from the dangerous LDL to the favorable HDL, why total cholesterol fails to indicate all the effects of exercise, and how activity and fitness help reduce the risk of coronary artery disease.

How's that for an extra benefit of fitness? Fitness not only allows increased caloric expenditure and enhanced fat utilization but also directly affects the blood lipids and reduces risk of heart disease. In our view, this effect is one of the most important benefits of exercise and fitness. If all this doesn't convince you to become active and improve your aerobic fitness, well, we'll just have to keep trying. For example, evidence indicates that it may be possible to lower serum cholesterol levels enough to reverse the process of atherosclerosis, to remove fatty buildup from the lining of the coronary arteries (Ornish 1993). If it proves to be true that diet and exercise, perhaps with the help of drug therapy, can accomplish this reversal, it will be possible to prevent or cure, not just treat, many cases of the nation's number-one killer.

Leptin

Leptin, a hormone produced by fat cells, helps regulate body weight and metabolism. Named after the Greek word *leptos*, which means "thin," leptin influences hunger, feeding behavior, body temperature, and energy expenditure. Leptin stimulates lipid metabolism and increases energy expenditure, and may limit excess energy storage. Leptin levels are correlated to the amount of fat stored in the body, although not all obese people have increased levels. Studies indicate that exercise lasting 1 or more hours reduces serum leptin concentrations (Hulver and Houmar 2003). Exercise and diet as well as sleep influence leptin levels. High-fat diets reduce the stimulatory effect of leptin on skeletal muscle fatty acid metabolism (Steinberg 2003). Sleep restriction is associated with decreased leptin levels, increased hunger, and greater appetite (Spiegel et al. 2004). Over the past 40 years, self-reported sleep duration in the United States has decreased 2 hours per night. Does lack of sleep contribute to overweight?

Lean Tissue

Finally, let us remind you that muscle is the furnace that burns fat. Whereas dieting leads to loss of muscle, a lower metabolic rate, and reduced ability to exercise and burn fat, fitness training has the capacity to maintain or increase muscle mass and burn more calories and more fat. Aerobic training such as running leads to a small increase in lean body weight. Training with more resistance, such as in cycling, can cause more noticeable changes in muscle. And, of course, muscular fitness (resistance) training leads to impressive changes in muscle mass. Fortunately, activity and training can rapidly reclaim muscle lost in dieting.

Whereas aerobic exercise doesn't have a great effect on the resting metabolic rate, resistance training has been shown to increase strength and metabolic rate and maintain metabolically active tissue in older adults (Campbell et al. 1994). Moreover, resistance training lowers visceral fat, the fat associated with a higher risk of heart disease (Treuth, Hunter, and Kekes-Szabo 1995).

Activity and Diet

Exercise tones muscles, improves your appearance, conserves protein, and increases the utilization of fat. The combination of exercise and sensible caloric intake should be a way of life. Let's see how you can combine diet and exercise in a program of weight loss and weight control.

When you combine exercise and diet, you can eat more and still achieve a weight loss of 2 pounds (.9 kilogram) per week. A program with a caloric deficit of 1,000 calories per day results in a 7,000-calorie deficit per week. Because 1 pound (.45 kilogram) of fat equals 3,500 calories, 7,000 calories equals a 2-pound (.9-kilogram) weight loss. John is 20 pounds (9 kilograms) overweight and in the poor fitness category. He achieves energy balance when his caloric intake equals his typical daily expenditure of 2,500 calories. How should he proceed? John should reduce his caloric intake by 500 calories per day and begin exercising (see table 13.1).

Now that he has achieved his goal, John has several choices:

- Continue to exercise and eat as he pleases
- Continue activity and continue to eat a reduced-fat diet
- Return to sedentary habits and restrict caloric intake—for life
- Return to sedentary habits, eat a high-fat diet, and regain all the weight he has lost and more

If he chooses to remain active (400 calories of activity daily), he will be able to eat the foods that he enjoys and splurge occasionally on extravagant foods. He should still consider a reduction of fat in the diet, but with sufficient activity, such as brisk walking or running 4 to 5 miles (6 to 8 kilometers) daily, he may be able to eat whatever he wishes with no adverse effect on his weight or health. A blood lipid profile (cholesterol, LDL and HDL cholesterol, and triglycerides) will confirm that possibility.

Table 13.1   Sample Weight-Loss Program

20 lb × 3,500 cal/lb = 70,000 cal overweight (20 lb = 9.1 kg)		Cal	Total cal
Weeks 1 and 2	Exercise = 200 cal/day × 7 days	= 1,400	
	Diet = 500 cal/day × 14 days	= 7,000	
		8,400	8,400
Weeks 3 and 4	Exercise = 250 cal/day × 14 days	= 3,500	
	Diet = 500 cal/day × 14 days	= 7,000	
		10,500	18,900
Weeks 5 and 6	Exercise = 300 cal/day × 14 days	= 4,200	
	Diet = 500 cal/day × 14 days	= 7,000	
		11,200	30,100
Weeks 7 and 8	Exercise = 350 cal/day × 14 days	= 4,900	
	Diet = 500 cal/day × 14 days	= 7,000	
		11,900	42,000
Weeks 9 and 10	Exercise = 400 cal/day × 14 days	= 5,600	
	Diet = 500 cal/day × 14 days	= 7,000	
		12,600	54,600
Weeks 11 and 12	Exercise = 450 cal/day × 14 days	= 6,300	
	Diet = 500 cal/day × 14 days	= 7,000	
		13,300	67,900

After 12 weeks = 67,900 cal lost.
Weeks 13 and 14—forget the diet. Exercise just 150 cal/day (14 days × 150 cal = 2,100 cal). 67,900 + 2,100 = 70,000 cal, or 20 lb (9.1 kg).

Summary

In the words of a leading obesity researcher, "Exercise is clearly beneficial as a means of losing weight and keeping it off. Given recent studies showing its association with maintenance, it would be difficult to argue that any factor is more important than exercise" (Brownell 1995, 124).

Activity is the positive way to achieve weight control without losing lean tissue. Dieting is a negative approach that uses deprivation to achieve results. Dieting by itself is seldom successful in the long run. Most weight-loss diets end in failure, with more weight and fat than before the dieting began. Activities such as walking, jogging, or cycling may seem like slow ways to lose weight, but they work. If your activity burns 250 extra calories each day, you'll burn more than 1,500 calories a week. In the course of a year you'll lose more than 20 pounds (9 kilograms). Calories do count, and you should learn how to count them. Turn to chapter 14 for a sensible and effective approach to achieve energy balance and take the first step in your lifelong quest for a trim, healthy body.

Weight-Control Programs

"When the stomach is full, it is easy to talk of fasting."

St. Jerome

This chapter outlines activity, food choices (diet), and behavioral modifications that provide a three-pronged approach to lifelong weight control. If you are slightly overweight, simply increase daily activity to achieve your goal. Twenty minutes of brisk walking each day (at 6 calories per minute) will use enough calories to burn 1 pound (.45 kilogram) of fat each month. If your problem is moderate, use activity and food choices to gain control. Eliminate empty calories, substitute low-fat foods for high-fat foods, and eat moderate portions. This approach alone should help you lose an additional pound each month. Activity and diet can help you lose 4 or more pounds (1.8 kilograms) per month, but you should never attempt to lose more than 2 pounds (.9 kilogram) per week or 8 pounds (3.6 kilograms) per month. Finally, if your problem is significant and long-standing, you should add a behavioral approach to your program. Proper use of any one of the three—activity, food choices, and eating behavior—will help you lose weight, but if you are interested in long-term weight loss, if your weight-control problem is significant, if you want to gain complete and lasting control, consider combining the benefits of all three.

This chapter will help you

- implement the weight-control program best suited to your needs;
- use the essentials of behavior therapy; and
- lose, maintain, or gain weight.

Activity

Your weight-control program should include both aerobic training and muscular fitness training. The aerobic fitness prescription for weight loss or weight control maximizes caloric expenditure (duration) at the expense of exercise intensity. You should extend exercise duration to increase caloric expenditure, and you should increase both duration and frequency of exercise to achieve the maximal benefit of exercise. Thus if your fitness prescription suggests 100 to 200 calories of exercise several days per week, you should try to work at the low edge of your training zone (intensity) and increase the caloric expenditure (duration). Also, increase the frequency to daily or twice daily, if possible, and add supplemental activities. The addition of moderate exercise to a caloric restriction (diet) program provides advantages in fat utilization, fat loss, and caloric expenditure, even in obese individuals (Kempen, Saris, and Westerterp 1995).

The muscular fitness portion of the weight-control program is aimed at maintaining or increasing lean body weight (muscle) and maintaining or increasing the resting metabolic rate (Ryan et al. 1995). Unless you are interested in gaining strength for a particular reason, our recommendation is to engage in muscular endurance training, performing at least one set of 15 to 25 repetitions with moderate resistance. Do this for 8 to 10 exercises, two or three times per week, and you will maintain muscle mass and resting metabolic rate, both of which are important to the long-term success of your weight-control program.

Your daily exercise session is only one of the many ways to increase caloric expenditure. Walk to work, during work, to lunch, during coffee breaks, after dinner. Take an exercise break during the day. Climb stairs, jump rope, do calisthenics. Do anything that increases caloric expenditure. If you expend 200 calories in your training session and another 100 walking or climbing stairs, you have accelerated your exercise weight

Adding an exercise break to your daily routine can increase caloric expenditure.

loss by 50 percent. When you become more fit and are capable of burning 500 calories daily through exercise, you will be able to lose 1 pound (.45 kilogram) per week (500 calories times 7 days equals 3,500 calories) through exercise alone.

The best way to achieve permanent weight loss is to make a change in lifestyle. The change could be to return to old ways of doing things. Avoid using unnecessary

Caloric Cost

You may be encouraged to know that energy expenditure values based on the oxygen cost and caloric expenditure of various activities sometimes underestimate your actual caloric expenditure. For example, when we study the energy cost of running by having highly trained endurance runners run on a treadmill, the values underestimate your cost of running for the following reasons:

- The treadmill is perfectly flat (unlike the road or trail that you may use).
- The air in the lab is still (whereas outside, even on a calm day, the moving body must overcome some wind resistance).
- Trained runners are up to 10 percent more efficient than untrained runners are.
- The lab values don't consider the postexercise period, when your body uses energy to replace stores of energy consumed during the run. The excess postexercise oxygen consumption (EPOC) may be elevated for up to an hour after prolonged, hard exertion. Widely used values for the energy cost of running may be 10 percent too low for many joggers. Over a period of weeks, an error of that size renders a serious disservice to exercise and its role in weight control.

labor-saving devices (remote control, power mower, snow thrower). Seek out and employ energy-using devices such as the snow shovel, the bicycle, or your own two feet. The best advice is never to use a machine when you can do the job yourself. You will be doing yourself a favor, saving energy (electricity, gas, oil, coal), and reducing pollution, all at the same time.

Perhaps the best idea is to find an active hobby or sport and make it an essential part of your life. Try woodworking, racquetball, golf, or dancing. Get a canoe or cross-country skis, or start a garden. Dig out the tennis racket and try it. Go ice-skating in winter or roller-skating any time of year. You'll enrich your life and lower your weight at the same time. Of course, you'll look better too!

The National Weight Control Registry keeps track of people who have successfully lost at least 30 pounds (13.6 kilograms) and managed to keep it off for at least a year. How do they do it? Besides restricting calories, they increase caloric expenditure by engaging in an hour or more of exercise daily. Eat less and get more exercise.

Food Choices (Diet)

If you're searching for one of those fad diets that regularly come and go, don't look here. When we say dieting, we simply mean reduced caloric intake, which people usually accomplish by reducing high-calorie fat in the diet and little else. As we said in chapter 11, each gram of fat contains 9.3 calories, verses only 4.1 and 4.3 for carbohydrate and protein, respectively. Almost 40 percent of the calories in the average diet come from fat. If you've been eating 2,000 calories daily, 800 probably come from fat. We'll tell you how to reduce fat intake later in this chapter. But first let us say what we don't mean by dieting.

When you restrict calories, the daily caloric deficit should not exceed 1,000 calories regularly. Of course, you can restrict caloric intake far below energy needs. If you do that for more than a few days, however, you are on a starvation diet. Your body won't receive essential nutrients, your energy level will sag, your immune system will suffer, and your resistance to infection will decline. Furthermore, the body will interpret the starvation diet as a signal to reduce caloric expenditure. In response, your resting energy expenditure will decline, you'll lose lean tissue, and you'll be on your way to increased weight-loss problems.

Fasting

Fasting, the ultimate form of caloric restriction, is guaranteed to bring about a dramatic weight loss, as much as a pound (.45 kilogram) a day—for a while. An occasional day of fasting will do no harm unless you are under stress or in training for competition. But the risks of fasting are many, especially if you continue it for an extended period. If you are grossly overweight and eager to fast, check into a clinic and proceed. Otherwise, avoid extended periods of fasting.

Diets to Avoid

Almost every popular magazine includes an article on dieting. Many offer a "revolutionary" new diet plan with such promises as "eat all you want," "calories don't count," "quick weight loss," and "super energy." You've heard of the water diet, the drinking man's diet, the high-protein diet, the liquid-protein diet, the low-carbohydrate diet, and others. Unfortunately, these plans reach a far wider audience than do controlled studies, editorials, and warnings in medical journals.

Be suspicious of any diet plan that promises rapid results, more than 2 pounds (.9 kilogram) of weight loss per week. Certainly, you can lose more weight by fasting or by dehydration. Water is heavy, about 2 pounds per quart (about .5 kilogram per liter). We could try to fool you into losing weight by sweating. You could easily lose 2 pounds (.9 kilogram) in an hour; athletes lose 6 pounds (2.7 kilograms) or more in a hard workout. What is so bad about that? Your body needs the water and replaces it as soon as it can. Question any plan that calls for low intake of carbohydrate or protein, encourages high intake of protein or fat, or recommends dehydration as a means of weight loss.

> Be suspicious of any diet plan that promises rapid results, more than 2 pounds (.9 kilogram) of weight loss per week.

Finally, consider the conclusion of a systematic review and evaluation of commercial weight-loss programs. The evidence, in the form of carefully controlled studies, to support the use of commercial and self-help weight-loss programs is suboptimal. Controlled trials are needed to assess the efficacy and cost-effectiveness of these interventions (Tsai and Wadden 2005). Commercial interventions available over the Internet and organized self-help programs produced minimal long-term weight loss.

Low-Carbohydrate Diet

One popular diet advocates near exclusion of carbohydrate. The creator of the diet states that the average overweight man should lose about 7 pounds (3.2 kilograms) in the first week of the diet! (Remember, carbohydrate is stored with water.) The diet allows a liberal intake of fat and all the protein you want—reason enough to question the plan. Low-carbohydrate diets are questionable for another reason: When blood-sugar levels are low, the fatty acid molecules from adipose tissue are shipped to the liver, where they are converted to ketone bodies to provide energy for the manufacture of glucose. Excess ketone bodies spill over into the blood and are carried to the tissues, where they are oxidized. During starvation or a low-carbohydrate diet, the production of ketone bodies can exceed the ability of the body to remove them metabolically. When this happens, the excess appears in the urine and in exhaled air. The condition is called ketosis, and the main danger is lowering of the blood pH (acidosis).

You should avoid simple sugars, but complex carbohydrates (whole-grain products, corn, rice, beans) provide energy and nutrition. They are excellent sources of vitamins and minerals. Many are high in fiber as well. In those areas of the world where the diet consists largely of energy derived from complex carbohydrates, obesity is rare and atherosclerosis and heart disease are virtually nonexistent.

> "To think carbs make you fat is wrong. You're fat because you're not exercising."
>
> *Chris Carmichael*

High-Protein Diet

Advocates of the high-protein (low-carbohydrate) diet argue that carbohydrate stimulates insulin secretion and storage of fat and that a sustained high level of carbohydrate intake may lead to insulin resistance. Although this may be true for some sedentary people who eat excess simple carbohydrate, it is not a problem for the active person. In fact, regular exercise increases insulin sensitivity and reduces the risk of diabetes.

Unless you are engaged in aerobic or muscular fitness training, you don't need more protein than the recommended dietary allowance. Excess protein is stored as fat (NH_3 is excreted in the urine), and because dietary protein often is associated with fat, as in meat or dairy products, you risk taking in more fat. Moreover, higher levels of meat and seafood consumption are associated with increased risk of gout (Choi et al. 2004).

- RDA for protein: 0.8 grams of protein per kilogram of body weight (2 ounces for 155-pound person, or 56 grams for a 70-kilogram person)
- For aerobic training: 1.2 to 1.4 grams per kilogram of body weight (3 ounces for 155-pound person, or 90 grams for 70-kilogram person)
- For strength training: 1.4 to 1.8 grams per kilogram of body weight (4 ounces for 155-pound person, or 110 grams for 70-kilogram person)

Some high-protein diets achieve temporary success because they are also low in calories and because significant water loss is associated with low carbohydrate intake. Unfortunately, they fail to provide the energy and some nutrients that you need to live a vigorous life. These diets appeal to those who intend to remain sedentary.

That idea doesn't mean that you should restrict protein intake. Any diet that restricts protein below the recommended dietary allowance makes no sense. During adolescence, such a plan could stunt normal development. Restricting protein intake is certain to cause muscle loss at any age. Muscle loss reduces resting metabolism and makes future caloric expenditure more difficult, leading to increased fat and body weight. And you cannot achieve the benefits of aerobic or muscular fitness training without adequate protein.

Reduced-Fat Diet

Reducing fat in the diet makes sense, up to a point. Fat is high in calories, and in excess it is related to heart disease, stroke, diabetes, and some cancers, so there are good reasons for reducing the percentage of fat in your diet. Some fat is required for good nutrition, however, especially during early childhood. Essential fatty acids must be part of the diet. Moreover, fat-soluble vitamins are not absorbed unless fat is present. Fats improve the flavor of food and make it more filling. We would never suggest complete removal of fat from the diet, but we do suggest that you begin now to lower your percentage of calories obtained from fat from the 40 percent figure common in this country to 25 or 30 percent, as recommended in the performance diet. We also urge you to reduce your intake of saturated fats to no more than one-third of total fat intake. Do this by substituting a cholesterol-lowering margarine for butter, replacing whole milk with skimmed milk and fatty meat with lean (including fish and fowl), and using more monounsaturated olive and other oils. How far should you go to reduce the fat content of your diet?

Low-Fat Diet

The program recommended by Nathan Pritikin (1979) called for the following daily energy intake (percentage of calories):

- 80 percent from carbohydrate (mostly complex)
- 10 percent from fat
- 10 percent from protein

Researchers at the California-based Longevity Research Institute have reported dramatic results among patients with heart and circulatory disorders and diabetes. The diet is a surefire way to reduce triglycerides and cholesterol. When accompanied by an exercise program, as it is at the institute, the diet may slow or even arrest the progress of atherosclerosis (Leonard, Hofer, and Pritikin 1974). Dr. Dean Ornish supports the low-fat diet (10 percent of calories from fat) for those with elevated risk of heart disease, with claims that the low-fat diet may reverse atherosclerosis (1993).

The low-fat diet has several advantages besides its effect on blood lipids and heart disease. Complex carbohydrate is high in fiber, and low-fiber diets are related to cancer of the colon. The high-carbohydrate diet is an excellent energy diet. When combined with a sensible exercise program, it will not lead to accumulation of fat. In fact, because carbohydrate has only 4 calories per gram, you can eat quite a bit without gaining weight. Finally, because fat seems to inhibit the action of insulin and because this diet reduces the level of fat in the blood, the low-fat diet could reduce the severity of adult-onset diabetes or reliance on insulin.

But the high-carbohydrate diet may not include enough protein for vigorous living. Let's assume that your weight is 70 kilograms (154 pounds) and that your daily caloric intake averages 2,000 calories. If 10 percent of that energy comes from protein, you will take in 200 calories from protein. Protein averages 4.3 calories per gram, so 200 calories divided by 4.3 equals 47 grams of protein. That amount falls below the daily allowance for protein recommended by the National Research Council (.8 gram of protein per kilogram of body weight multiplied by 70 kilograms is 56 grams). For this reason we do not recommend this level of protein intake. Instead we recommend a diet that provides 15 percent of calories from good-quality protein, including lean meat, low-fat dairy, and plant sources.

How much fat does the very-low-fat diet allow? If daily intake is 2,000 calories, 10 percent fat allows 200 calories. Divide 200 by 9.3 calories per gram of fat and you get 22 grams of fat, a very small amount. In our culture, this is a difficult diet. The author of the plan found it necessary to retrain the palates of his subjects because the drastic reductions of fat made food seem bland (Pritikin 1979). When one attempts to apply the diet in a restaurant, every page of the menu produces frustration.

High-Fat Diet

Is there ever a reason to eat a high-fat diet? Perhaps. Athletes tend to select a high-fat diet (50 percent of calories from fat) during periods of prolonged hard training. We've observed cross-country athletes from the U.S. Ski Team eating 50 percent of calories from fat during fall training camps, when they ski 50 or more kilometers (31 miles) daily. Wildland firefighters expend as many as 6,000 calories a day when they are working, and during those periods they eat more fat (Ruby, Schoeller, and Sharkey 2001). Athletes who cross-country skied the entire length of the Iditarod dogsled race in Alaska (1,100 miles, or 1,770 kilometers), pulling a sled with food, tent, and sleeping bag, did so with the aid of high-fat snacks (e.g., balls of butter with bacon bits) to fuel their estimated 10,000-calorie-per-day energy expenditure! During periods of extreme endurance training when energy requirements are high, increasing the percentage of fat in the diet to approximately 50 percent of total energy does not result in adverse changes in blood lipids (Brown and Cox 1998), but a high-fat diet may interfere with the function of the immune system (Pedersen et al. 2000). For health reasons, one should return to a lower fat intake as soon as possible.

Diet Studies

Finally, after years of undocumented claims about various low-carb and other diets, we have some controlled studies to review. One study of obese men and women compared a low-carb diet to a conventional low-fat diet. Subjects on the low-carb diet lost more weight at 6 months (7.0 versus 3.2 percent body weight), but the differences were not significant at 12 months. No differences were found between the groups in total or low-density cholesterol, but increases in HDL cholesterol and decreases in triglycerides were greater on the low-carb diet. Both diets decreased blood pressure and the insulin response to oral glucose. The low-carb diet was associated with more improvements in CAD risk factors. Adherence was poor and attrition was high in both groups (Foster et al. 2003).

In a 6-month study of severely obese subjects, those on a low-carb diet lost more weight than did those on the calorie- and fat-restricted diet, with relative improvement in insulin sensitivity and triglyceride levels. The authors recommended caution in interpretation of findings because of the small magnitude of overall and between-group differences in weight loss and the short duration of the study (Samaha et al. 2003).

In a comparison of several popular diets, including the Atkins (low carb), Ornish (low fat), Weight Watchers (less calories), and Zone (less carb), the authors studied adherence rates and the effectiveness of the diets on weight loss and cardiac risk factor reduction (Dansinger et al. 2005). Each diet group began with 40 overweight or obese participants (22 to 72 years old), and the study lasted 18 months. Although differences among diets were not significant, weight loss ranged from 7.3 pounds (3.3 kilograms) on the Ornish diet to 4.8 pounds (2.1 kilograms) on the Atkins diet. Each diet reduced the LDL to HDL cholesterol ratio about 10 percent. Cardiac risk reduction was somewhat better in the low-carb diets, but all diets reduced C-reactive protein approximately 20 percent. Benefits were limited to those who remained on the diets, but half of the Ornish and Atkins participants dropped out, and 35 percent of the Weight Watchers and Zone participants dropped out after a year. Weight loss predicted improvements in risk reduction. Each diet modestly reduced body weight. Increased adherence was associated with greater weight loss and risk factor reductions for each diet group.

Finally, in a review of low-carb diet studies the authors concluded that evidence is insufficient to make recommendations for or against use of low-carb diets, particularly among participants older than age 50, for use longer than 90 days, or for diets of 20 grams per day or less of carbohydrate. Among the published studies, weight loss on a low-carb diet was associated more with decreased caloric intake and increased diet duration than it was with reduced carbohydrate content (Bravata et al. 2003).

While we await future studies on the effectiveness of diets, consider this 12-week study on subjects with impaired glucose tolerance who had unlimited access to a low-fat, high-carb diet. Those on the low-fat (high-carb) diet lost 7 pounds (3.2 kilograms), whereas the low fat plus exercise group lost 10.6 pounds (4.8 kilograms), without caloric restriction. In addition, thigh fat area decreased in both groups, and no decrease occurred in resting metabolic rate or fat oxidation (Hays et al. 2004).

In our opinion, the low-carbohydrate (high-protein) diet may be a reasonable, short-term approach for people who intend to remain sedentary. But for those who are or intend to be active, we recommend the performance diet (55 to 60 percent of calories from carbohydrate, 15 percent from protein, 25 to 30 percent from fat). The weight-loss results are similar, the carbohydrate provides energy for the active life, and the activity reinforces long-term maintenance of the weight-control plan.

Diet Recommendations

You do not have to change your eating habits overnight, and you don't have to reduce fat intake to 10 percent, unless your risk of coronary artery disease (CAD) is high. Otherwise, a fat intake of 25 percent is both reasonable and attainable. Begin today to reduce the fat content of your diet. Limit saturated fat (avoid hydrogenated or trans-fatty acids) to one-third of total fat calories. Try to make some of the substitutions that we've mentioned. Experiment with complex carbohydrates. Use beans and corn in a Mexican dinner. Try rice and soy for an Asian experience. Become familiar with the glycemic index, use potatoes occasionally (with fat-free sour cream), and use whole-grained products. The proper combination of these low-fat foods provides energy and meets the need for protein, fiber, and other nutrients. Avoid empty calories such as table sugar and soda pop. Substitute a carrot, celery, or fruit for your usual snacks. You can easily reduce fat intake to 25 percent as we await the final word concerning the relationship of dietary fat to health and disease.

The dietary program that we recommend emphasizes maintenance of a moderate diet, including the energy proportions of the performance diet—60 percent carbohydrate, 25 percent fat, and 15 percent protein—and adequate levels of vitamins, minerals, and water. Remember that calories do count. If you cut caloric intake, you will lose weight. If you cut caloric intake substantially, you may live longer.

Assess Food Choices

Take a good look at your caloric intake list. If patterns of behavior are not readily apparent, you should continue to count your calories for several days. Besides recording what you eat, consider when, where, and why you eat (see figure 14.1). Do you have a doughnut on your coffee break just because it's there? Do you have a candy

Figure 14.1 Daily Eating Log

Date _____   Weight _____.

Time	Place (if at home, exactly where were you?)	What did you eat or drink and how much?	What were you doing before you ate?	What did you do while you ate?	Who were you with when you ate?	What did you do after you ate?

From *Fitness and Health, Sixth Edition* by Brian J. Sharkey and Steven E. Gaskill, 2007, Champaign, IL: Human Kinetics.

bar at lunch? Do you have a drink now and then? You may be able to eliminate several hundred calories daily by eliminating or cutting back on unnecessary or ritual eating behaviors. Years ago one of us developed the habit of eating crackers with peanut butter and jelly as a reward for an evening's work. When he realized how quickly the fat calories added up and what could happen to his weight, he vowed to break the ritual. Sure, he still gets the urge, and sometimes he is unable to resist (an addict is never cured). But for the present, he rewards himself with a nutritious but low-calorie treat such as an apple or orange. In this way he has reduced both calories and fat intake.

Sugar-Sweetened Drinks

Soft drinks and fruit punches contain quantities of high fructose corn syrup and other sweeteners that may contribute to overweight and adult-onset (type 2) diabetes. Data from the Nurses Health Study showed that high consumption of sugar-sweetened beverages is associated with greater weight gain and increased risk of type 2 diabetes, probably because of excess calories and rapidly absorbable sugars (Schulze et al. 2004).

Modify Meals

Now that you've eliminated the extras, look at the size and content of your meals. Some think that dieting means avoiding meals, often breakfast. Skipping meals is the worst thing you can do, for several reasons. People work better when they eat breakfast. When you avoid meals, you become weak and hungry and are more likely to grab a doughnut. People who are susceptible to low blood sugar may even notice poor performance in sports skills or work. Eventually, you sit down to a meal and overeat. In addition, when you eat fewer than three meals a day, triglyceride and cholesterol levels are higher than they are when you eat more frequently. By eating meals more frequently, you avoid the feelings of hunger and fatigue often associated with diet and you reduce blood lipid levels.

The easiest way to reduce mealtime calories is to reduce the size and number of helpings that you consume. Use a smaller plate and fill it only once. Refuse second helpings, except for salad or vegetables. And, of course, eliminate high-calorie desserts, toppings, dressings, gravies, and sauces (see table 14.1 for a six-meal plan). Eat all you want of fruits, low-fat cereals, whole-grain breads (try olive oil instead of butter), vegetables, and water. Consider several servings of low-fat dairy products each day. Some think that milk and calcium contribute to fat and weight loss.

Table 14.1   Low-Calorie Six-Meal Plan

Meal	Menu
Breakfast	Egg or cheese
	Fruit
	Slice whole-grain bread
	Coffee or tea
Midmorning	Fresh or dried fruit
	Milk (low fat)
Lunch	Meat, fish, or peanut butter sandwich
	Milk, fruit, or vegetable juice
Midafternoon	Soup, fruit, and salad
Dinner	Meat, fish, poultry, or cheese
	Potato, rice, beans, corn, or whole-grain
	Cereal product
	Fresh fruit
	Vegetables, including leafy greens
	Coffee or tea
Bedtime	Fruit and low-fat yogurt

Avoid eating at establishments that promise all you can eat or offer supersized meals. If you're like us, you'll want to get your money's worth and eat far more calories than you need.

Substitute

The final step in this simple plan is to make substitutions. Substitute low-calorie snacks for high-calorie foods (e.g., pretzels for potato chips or peanuts). Substitute low-fat foods (skim milk, lean meats, nonfat salad dressing, low-fat cheese) for high-fat foods. When you begin to read labels you will be on your way to a low-fat diet. Try to stay below 50 grams of fat daily. (If labels don't tell how much fat is in the food, the list of ingredients will help. Ingredients are listed in order of concentration, from highest to lowest. When fat comes early in the list, you are looking at a high-fat food.) Remember to avoid cottonseed, palm, and coconut oils, which are found in many snack foods, processed products, and coffee creamers. Watch out for hydrogenated oils found in all sorts of packaged foods. Oils that were otherwise safe, when hydrogenated, form a more solid fat (trans-fatty acids), which increases the risk of heart disease.

In food preparation, use olive oil and canola oil; both are high in monounsaturated fat, preferable to oil that is saturated or hydrogenated. Using this approach, you easily can achieve a daily caloric deficit of 500 calories. Because you are eating at least three meals a day, you won't feel weak and hungry. And when you combine the benefits of diet with those of exercise and fitness, you will be delighted with the results.

Finally, don't be tempted by low-fat snacks. Although they contain one-third less fat than the regular versions, they often have just as many calories, using sugar to make up the difference in taste.

Read Labels

To lower the total amount of fat in your diet to 25 percent and to reduce saturated fat to one-third of total fat, begin by reading the labels on everything that you buy (see figure 14.2). Of course, ice cream and potato chips can be loaded with fat, but so are peanuts and many other snacks. If your goal is 25 percent of calories from fat and your daily intake is 2,000 calories, you can eat 500 calories of fat, or about 54 grams (500 divided by 9.3 calories per gram equals 54). If you want to snack, choose pretzels with less than 1 gram of fat per serving instead of chips with 11 grams, or choose low-fat yogurt or ice cream with 0 grams of fat per serving verses 16 for the rich, creamy variety. In time you will grow to prefer the low-fat version.

Behavior Modification

If you follow the instructions and achieve a negative energy balance (caloric deficit), you will lose weight. With a deficit of 1,000 calories daily, you will lose 2 pounds (.9 kilogram) per week. But if you are a

Nutrition Facts	
Serving Size ¹/₂ cup (114g)	
Servings Per Container 4	
Amount Per Serving	
Calories 260 Calories from Fat 120	
	% Daily Value*
Total Fat 13g	20%
Saturated Fat 5g	25%
Cholesterol 30mg	10%
Sodium 660mg	28%
Total Carbohydrate 31g	11%
Dietary Fiber 0g	0%
Sugars 5g	
Protein 5g	
Vitamin A 4%	Vitamin C 2%
Calcium 15%	Iron 4%

*Percent Daily Values are based on a 2000 calorie diet. Your daily values may be higher or lower depending on your calorie needs.

	Calories:	2000	2500
Total Fat	Less than	65g	80g
Sat. Fat	Less than	20g	25g
Cholesterol	Less than	300mg	300mg
Sodium	Less than	2400mg	2400mg
Total Carbohydrate		300g	375g
Dietary Fiber		25g	30g

Calories per gram:
Fat 9 · Carbohydrate 4 · Protein 4

Figure 14.2 To improve your diet, start by reading nutrition labels.

difficult case and need additional help, this section is for you. Even if you have your weight completely under control, you may learn a lot about yourself and your eating behavior by carrying out the exercises in this section. Behavior therapy (once called behavior modification) is the third and last major weapon in the battle of the bulge. The essentials of the behavioral approach include the following:

1. Identify the behavior that you wish to modify, in this case eating behavior. Keep a food diary that indicates the kind and amount of food you eat—when, where, why, and with whom; what you do while eating; your mood; and your degree of hunger (see figures 14.1 and 14.3).

Figure 14.3   Cognitive Supplement to Daily Eating Log

Date _____

Time	What were your thoughts or feelings before you ate?	While you ate?	After you ate?

From *Fitness and Health, Sixth Edition* by Brian J. Sharkey and Steven E. Gaskill, 2007, Champaign, IL: Human Kinetics.

2. Analyze your customary eating behavior and plan new eating behaviors (see the section on diet in this chapter). The new behaviors will include dietary adjustments and activity. To reduce cues or reinforcement for old eating behaviors, try the following:

- Eat in one room only (dining room or kitchen).
- Wrap your utensils in a napkin; wait several minutes before you begin eating.
- Pause and set your utensils down between bites. Don't prepare another bite until you've swallowed the last one.
- Wait 30 minutes before having a nutritious, low-calorie dessert, or have a low-calorie beverage instead of dessert (decaffeinated tea or coffee).
- Concentrate on what you are eating. Take time to enjoy each bite. Save one item to eat later.
- Buy a smaller place setting and eat only from that plate.
- After the meal, remove all dishes to the kitchen and brush your teeth. The meal is over.
- When you feel hungry, try to decide if it is real (stomach hunger) or merely boredom for something to do (mouth hunger).
- Avoid eating in front of the TV or while reading.
- If you must snack, be sure that the snack is nutritious—low in fat, salt, and calories.
- For best results, do not eat after 7 p.m.

3. Plan new reinforcements or rewards to reinforce the new eating behavior. Develop a schedule of reinforcement (see figure 14.4), a plan of frequent rewards for

good behavior. Because your new eating behavior will soon show up on the scale or the tape measure, you can use small units of weight loss and small reductions in girth as indicators of adherence to the new eating behavior. Almost any sort of reward is effective, except food! A tangible, universally accepted reward such as money seems to work for most people. Weigh yourself daily, in the morning after your toilet but before breakfast, and give yourself a monetary reward for each unit of weight lost. A similar plan to reward reduced girth (waist, thigh) provides added incentive. Spend the reward immediately if you wish or save it for something you really want but might otherwise not buy. If the plan seems silly, remember this: You will spend far more than the cost of reinforcement on food and medical bills if you do not lose the weight.

Figure 14.4   Weight-Loss Reinforcement Schedule

Date	Weight	Reward	Girth	Reward	Total

Note: For example, $1 per lb (.5 kg); $1 per 1/2 in. (1 cm) of waist girth. Start new total when you spend the reward.

From *Fitness and Health, Sixth Edition* by Brian J. Sharkey and Steven E. Gaskill, 2007, Champaign, IL: Human Kinetics.

The same general principles apply to those who are having trouble starting or staying with an activity program. Review existing behavior, plan the new behavior, and reward yourself for adherence to the new behavior (e.g., walking, jogging, playing tennis). You may choose a monetary reward or, if you like, a low-calorie favor. See chapter 18 for more suggestions on how to use behavior therapy to reinforce activity.

Gaining Weight

This section is intended to help underweight people achieve sensible nonfat weight gain. The plan is not meant to help you bulk up for sports like football. When normal-weight people bulk up, they assume considerable health risk. Coaches who encourage such procedures should be held responsible for conducting weight-loss programs when the athlete's season or career is over. As with weight loss, the weight-gain program includes exercise, diet, and behavior therapy.

- **Exercise.** Includes a strength-training program to build lean body weight and a reduction in calorie-burning activities (aerobic exercise, sports) to allow a positive caloric balance.

- **Diet.** Includes an overall increase in calories, with 750 extra calories on strength-training days and 250 extra on nontraining days. The extra calories should be largely from low-fat, protein-rich foods (lean meats, eggs, low-fat dairy products, soy protein).

A low-fat protein supplement can be used to provide an extra 20 grams (86 calories) of protein daily.

- **Behavior therapy.** If needed, develop a reinforcement schedule to reward gains in lean body weight. Determine a desirable weight and make steady progress toward that goal.

This program should lead to a gain of about 1 pound (.45 kilogram) of weight each week. If you attempt to gain weight too fast, much of the gain will be fat. So determine current eating behavior and plan needed modifications (e.g., more meals, nutritious snacks). Start strength training and watch the scale go up. Remember to return to aerobic exercise and weight control when you achieve the desired body weight.

Health Clubs and Diet Centers

Do health clubs and diet centers figure in your weight-control program? Although both have experienced considerable growth, you should be a careful consumer of their services. You may be surprised to learn that state or local laws do not govern clubs or centers. No professional competence or qualifications are required. Hairdressers need a state license, but in most states anyone can open and operate a health club or diet center. Here are some suggestions to help you become a discriminating consumer.

- **Health clubs.** To help you differentiate a good club from a bad one—an effective program and qualified staff from a fly-by-night organization—you should do the following. Visit the club for a tour and free introductory session. Is the facility clean and well equipped? Does the equipment meet your needs? Are patrons satisfied? Do they encourage you to join? Ask about the staff's qualifications and credentials. Do they have degrees in the field from reputable institutions? Do they have experience? Are they certified? Are they all trained in emergency response? The American College of Sports Medicine (ACSM) certifies health and fitness instructors and program directors who meet educational and experience standards and successfully complete a rigorous test. ACSM publishes standards for health clubs and has a brochure to help you evaluate a health club. Write to ACSM at P.O. Box 1440, Indianapolis, IN 46206-1440 or visit their Web site (www.acsm.org) to request the brochure or other services.

Talk to club members before you join. When you decide to join a club, avoid long-term contracts. Be wary of discounts and other high-pressure come-ons, which may be signs of a failing business or high member turnover. Sign up for a few months or until you are certain that the club meets your needs. Then become active in a member advisory group that works with management to maintain and upgrade staff qualifications, facilities, and equipment.

- **Diet centers.** Although diet centers provide dieting advice and encouragement, few boast the services of a registered dietitian, and fewer still have an on-site medical director. Most centers sell expensive vitamins, diet foods, and other products to their clients. Some clients lose weight, often at a rapid rate, indicating significant loss of water and lean tissue. Some centers advise against exercise, because clients following their program are often too listless to participate.

If you are considering the services of a diet center, follow the advice that we provided regarding health clubs. Visit, ask questions, and ask about qualifications. Is a registered dietitian on the staff? Is a reputable local physician associated with the center? Most important, ask about the long-term success rate of the program. Then ask to contact some of the diet center's clients. Ask yourself if the center provides any service that you cannot provide for yourself. The existence of so many centers suggests that the simple facts of energy balance and weight control have not reached enough people, that people lack the information, opportunity, or will to take control of their eating and activity behaviors.

Weight-Control Fallacies

Let's review some of the fallacies associated with weight loss. We'll consider false claims (lose girth, not weight), useless devices, drugs, and even smoking. Then we will examine the surgeries that extremely obese individuals sometimes consider.

Lose Girth, Not Weight

The idea that people can lose inches (centimeters), not pounds (kilograms), is the come-on of the figure salon. Such facilities try to appeal to people who don't want to work hard enough to achieve real fat and weight loss. Of course, you may be able to improve your appearance with exercises that merely tone muscles and improve posture. The fallacy is that while you are shaping the body, you are ignoring the engine, worn hoses, and other parts (i.e., the heart and blood vessels) and missing the health benefits associated with exercise and loss of body weight and fat. Typically, people do not lose girth at all; a slightly tighter pull on the measuring tape gives the impression of progress. Fitness and health, like beauty, are more than skin deep.

Spot Reduction

Evidence that fat can be removed from specific areas (spots) by localized exercises is extremely limited. One study showed a mere 1 millimeter of spot reduction after 6 weeks of exercise. Avid tennis players have about the same skinfold on both arms, even though the racket arm is more muscular.

Dunlop's Disease

My friend Ted once tried sit-ups to get rid of what he called Dunlop's disease, in which his belly "done lopped" over his belt. He worked up to 400 sit-ups daily with no success. We showed him a study conducted by Dr. Frank Katch and colleagues at the University of Massachusetts. They collected fat biopsies from several sites before and after a 4-week training program consisting entirely of sit-ups. Posttraining analysis of fat cells revealed that the fat loss came from all the fat storage areas measured, not just abdominal fat (McArdle, Katch, and Katch 1994). What about Ted? He became an ultramarathoner, training for and running 100-mile (161-kilometer) races, and his tummy ceased to be a problem. The moral of this story is that burning off sufficient calories will take care of the spots and inches (centimeters).

The best way to lose weight is through sensible dieting and exercise.

Exercise Devices

You've seen the advertisements for passive exercise—electrical stimulation, vibrating machines, sauna shorts, and body wraps—devices that promise weight or fat loss without effort on your part. Sorry, they just don't work. Passive devices don't burn enough calories, electrical stimulation is not equivalent to voluntary exercise, vibrating devices do not break up fat and wash it away in the circulation, and tight pants or wraps do not remove fat with heat and massage. By spending the same amount of time in moderate exercise, you will get results, including the health benefits that you miss with passive exercise.

The advertising usually claims that with a few minutes of almost effortless activity you will get a firm, healthy, athletic body. The promoters use attractive models, celebrities, or pro athletes to tout the product, and they usually offer a big discount if you act immediately. If you are uncertain, ask your physician or certified health club professional for advice. Our advice is to ask to see the results of research studies and try the product before you buy. Don't sign a long-term contract for any type of exercise program or device. Remember, a brisk walk burns more calories than most passive devices do, and walking is a lot more fun.

Drugs

Laxatives and diuretics remove only water (dehydration). Amphetamines are sometimes prescribed to suppress the appetite, a dangerous approach to lifelong weight control. Reputable physicians prescribe anorectic agents (appetite suppressants) as part of a total program with diet, exercise, and behavior therapy. But they need to avoid increasing doses and the risk of dependency. Recently a weight-control drug combination was associated with development of heart valve problems. Weight-control drugs, when they work, have to be taken forever to achieve lifelong weight control. Research on the genetic component of obesity may lead to future therapies, but such treatment will never remove the need to balance caloric intake and expenditure.

Eating Disorders

The most tragic fallacy is the adoption of dangerous eating behaviors in an effort to achieve an unattainable ideal—a slim, trim figure. When being thin becomes an obsession, when self-worth becomes associated with slimness, the stage is set for eating disorders. Bulimia is a disorder characterized by a binge–purge cycle. Those with mild cases purge (vomit) occasionally to avoid weight gain, and those with more serious cases combine binge–purge with laxatives or diuretics, risking serious metabolic and psychological problems.

Anorexia nervosa is a serious psychological problem characterized by a distorted body image and a refusal to eat. Sometimes the behavior is associated with drugs or with obsessive exercise. If not treated, the person may experience serious medical complications, including death, as starvation compromises the heart and other organs. Eating disorders are more common among young women who seek to please others, who try to be perfect. Fortunately, psychological therapy and medical treatments are available to victims who seek help.

Smoking?

Seeing people smoking cigarettes is sad, but it is tragic to hear that they continue the habit to avoid weight gain. Although it is true that smokers gain some weight when they quit, the amount is not so excessive that they can't eliminate it with diet and exercise. Moreover, the health consequences of smoking far outweigh the effect of any weight gain. Those who smoke should develop an addiction to exercise to replace the addiction to nicotine.

To avoid contributing to the development of eating disorders, don't nag teenagers about weight problems. Minimize the emphasis on body weight, girth, body fat, and BMI values and focus on how they feel and function. Schedule family activities followed by sensible family meals. Use desserts sparingly and stock fruits instead of high-fat or high-sugar snacks. Be aware of eating behaviors and seek help early if eating disorders arise.

Surgery

Lipectomy and liposuction are surgical techniques used to remove unwanted fat. Although lipectomy certainly removes fat and reduces weight, some studies suggest the fat may be regenerated, especially if caloric intake continues to exceed expenditure. Liposuction, which involves vacuuming of fat cells from abdominal, thigh, and other deposits, is generally safe, but no surgery is without risk. A recent study of liposuction on obese women concluded that the procedure, which led to a 19 percent decrease in total fat (22 pounds, or 10 kilograms), did not improve obesity-associated CAD risk factors, blood lipids, blood pressure, blood glucose, and insulin sensitivity (Klein et al. 2004). Surgical removal of superficial fat will not change heart disease or other risk factors, unless diet and exercise accompany it.

Other forms of surgery are reserved for cases of morbid obesity, defined as more than 100 pounds (45 kilograms) overweight, or a BMI over 40. One popular operation employs staples to fashion a smaller stomach. The procedure seems to work, for a while, but over time food intake increases. Obviously, this type of surgery is an expensive and potentially dangerous approach to weight control.

Summary

This chapter has presented ways to use activity, dieting, and behavioral therapy in your lifelong effort to achieve energy balance and weight control. In years past, young folks were more active and had more metabolically active tissue, so weight control wasn't a big problem. With inactivity and poor food choices, overweight and obesity are epidemic. As adults we face new responsibilities, less time for activity, and a further decline in metabolically active tissue, including muscle. Eventually, winter weight gains fail to melt off in spring, and energy balance becomes a major issue. We've reached the stage of life where we must exercise more or eat less if we want to maintain body weight, waist size, blood lipids, and self-respect. Because some of us already engage in a considerable amount of exercise and have reduced the fat in our diets, we are faced with the unhappy prospect of life with fewer calories. But don't feel sorry for us. We've come this far enjoying an enormous appetite and a great love of food. It is time that we learn some self-control. Guess we'll have to review the section on behavior therapy.

Part V

Performance

In a typical day, most of us spend about 8 hours in sleep and 8 hours at work. The rest is largely dedicated to preparation for one or the other, or to so-called leisure-time pursuits, including activity and sport. If you improve fitness to enhance performance in sport or work, sleep will take care of itself.

You may want to go beyond health, even beyond fitness, to perform at a high level and achieve your potential. To do this, you must set goals and then design and carry out a systematic plan to achieve them. The final step is to achieve what you trained for, sometimes in a public performance or event. We usually think of performing in sports, races, or other competitions, but some people train for cross-country bicycle trips, mountain climbs, or other private personal goals. Far too few train to improve their work capacity, to be industrial athletes capable of impressive performance in the workplace.

This section will help you improve your performance. We'll show you how to use simple psychological skills so that you can play your best game more often. And we'll discuss how to prepare for and perform in a variety of terrestrial environments, including heat, cold, and altitude.

Performance in Sport and Work

> ## "Don't play
> sports to get in shape; get in shape to play sports!"
> *Anonymous*
>
> ## "The reason
> why worry kills more people than work is that more people worry than work."
> *Robert Frost*

In this chapter we tell you how to prepare for athletic competition safely and effectively so that you can enjoy the intense pleasure and excitement of sport and competition, without the risk of fatigue, overtraining, injury, or illness. In athletic competitions, adults participate according to age group, and we often find active athletes of 60, 70, and even 80 years of age. A few continue to participate in races beyond their 100th birthdays, as did the late Larry Lewis, an indefatigable runner and a waiter at a posh San Francisco hotel. If you like to train and enjoy the thrill of competition, of getting high on your own hormones, this section is for you. But remember, you must train before you compete.

In this chapter, we also tell you how to train and compete in the workplace. Today, when men and women go to work, few engage in arduous muscular effort. Occupational physiologists, psychologists, and engineers combine to study men and women in their working environment, with the goal of adapting the job to the ability of the average worker. At the same time, laborsaving devices have eliminated the need for muscular work at home, and the automobile makes the task of getting to and from work physically effortless. The consequences of these trends are obvious: The average worker is incapable of delivering a full day of effort in a physically demanding job. Perhaps it is time for a change; perhaps we could benefit by working up to job requirements, not down. Perhaps it is time to adapt the worker to the job rather than adapt the job to the worker. Indeed, some companies have begun to view their workers as highly trained industrial athletes. They recruit, train, maintain, and cross-train those with the physical capacity to do the work. If your work is physically demanding, fitness can help you and your employees improve performance.

This chapter will help you

- use the principles of training,
- improve performance in your favorite sport,
- use diet to enhance performance,
- develop psychological skills to help you play your best game more often, and
- understand the relationship between fitness and work capacity.

Training Principles

This section introduces 13 important physiological principles that you should follow to make steady progress in your training and to avoid illness and injury. The principles are based on research studies and the insights of successful coaches. By the end of this section you should be ready to improve your performance or help others do the same. We focus on the adaptations and individual response to training.

PRINCIPLE 1: READINESS The value of training depends on the physiological and psychological readiness of the individual. Because readiness comes with maturation, physically immature (prepubertal) people lack the physiological preparedness to respond completely to training. Readiness also implies the need for adequate nutrition and rest to benefit from training.

PRINCIPLE 2: ADAPTATION Training induces subtle changes as the body adapts to the added demands. Dr. Ned Fredrick, a friend and a noted sport scientist, calls training for sport a gentle pastime in which we coax subtle changes from the body.

The day-to-day changes are so small as to be immeasurable; weeks and even months of patient progress are required to achieve measurable adaptations. If you try to rush the process, you risk illness, injury, or both. See chapters 5 and 9 to review adaptations to training. The principle of adaptation tells us that we can't rush training. We must follow a sensible program and be satisfied with the results. Trying to do it all in one season is likely to do more harm than good.

PRINCIPLE 3: INDIVIDUAL RESPONSE   People respond differently to the same training for some of the following reasons: heredity, maturity, nutrition, rest, sleep, level of fitness, environmental factors, illness or injury, and motivation. See our new book *Sport Physiology for Coaches* (2006) for more on this and other principles.

PRINCIPLE 4: OVERLOAD   Training must place a demand on the body system if desired adaptations are to take place. To begin, training must exceed the typical daily demand. As you adapt to increased loading, you should add more load. Three factors affect the rate of improvement: frequency, intensity, and time, or FIT. Remember, "If you always do what you always did, you will always get what you always got." To improve, you will have to train more frequently, more intensely, or for more time.

PRINCIPLE 5: PROGRESSION   To achieve adaptations using the overload principle, training must follow the principle of progression. When you increase the training load too quickly, the body cannot adapt and instead breaks down. You must observe progression in terms of FIT, or increases in frequency (sessions per day, week, month, or year), intensity (training load per day, week, month, or year), and time (duration of training in hours per day, week, month, or year).

PRINCIPLE 6: SPECIFICITY   Exercise is specific. When you train, adaptations will take place in the muscle fibers used during the exercise. The adaptations to endurance training are different from adaptations to strength training. This concept means that the type of training you undertake must relate to the desired results. Specific training brings specific results. Of course, you can take any rule or principle to the extreme. Specificity does not mean that you should avoid training opposite or adjacent muscles. In fact, you should train other muscles to avoid muscle imbalances that could predispose the body to injury. You can train adjacent muscles to help you adapt to changes in conditions and provide a backup when the primary muscle fibers become fatigued.

PRINCIPLE 7: VARIATION   You should vary your training program to avoid boredom and to maintain your interest. The principle of variation embraces two basic concepts: work and rest, and hard and easy. Adaptation comes when rest follows work, when easy follows hard. Failure to include variation leads to boredom, staleness, and poor performance. Successive sessions of hard work, if not followed by adequate time for rest and recovery, are certain to hinder progress in training. When workouts become dull, do something different. Use variety (cross-training) to diminish monotony and lighten the physical and psychological burdens of heavy training.

PRINCIPLE 8: PERIODIZATION   To achieve optimal performance, you should vary training systematically. Periodization describes the process of planning systematic variation into training. You program this variation at several levels: daily, weekly, seasonal, and career. Daily periodization varies the stress so that easier days for recovery follow days of hard training. Weekly periodization involves planned variation of the weeks. Most athletes use a 3-week cycle with week 1 being a moderate (average) training load, week 2 involving a greater load, and week 3 being a recovery week. Seasonal variation is the planning of your training season into periods with specific goals.

The general plan starts with a postcompetition (off-season) period of easy, non-specific training followed by a period of basic training (often called the preseason) to develop the aerobic base and foundation for strength. After laying the foundation, athletes increase anaerobic capacity, power, and speed during the period leading into and including the early competitions (early competition period). Finally, the peak performance period is a time of reduced total training volume, increased speed and power work, and, most important, increased rest and recovery to allow optimal performance (figure 15.1).

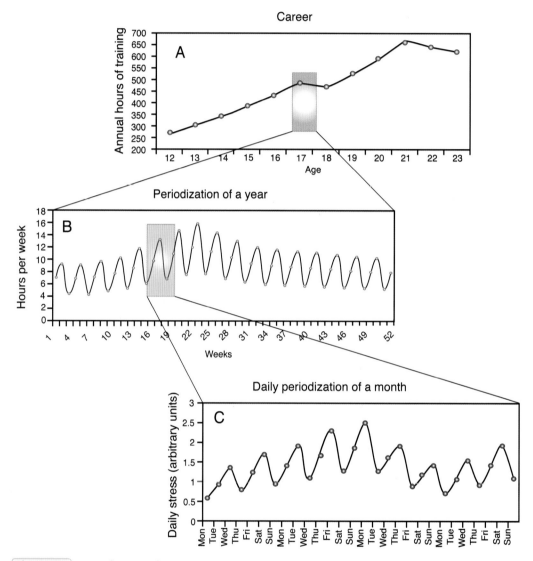

Figure 15.1 Periodization of training. Periodization includes annual, seasonal, weekly, and daily cycles. Graph A shows a hypothetical increase in training hours per year for a developing athlete. The dips in the progression indicate years during which training volume was decreased to reduce stress and increase performance. Typical years for reducing volume might include senior years in high school and college and Olympic years.

Graph B show weekly hours for a single training year. Note the overall progression, with total volume peaking around week 25, and then a gradual reduction of volume as more high-intensity training is done to prepare for competitions. Note also the 3-week cycle of medium-, high-, and low-volume weeks to allow for stress and recovery.

Graph C shows the daily periodization of a month of training. Note the 3-day cycle of medium, hard, and easy days within the larger weekly cycles.

PRINCIPLE 9: WARM-UP AND COOL-DOWN   A warm-up should always precede strenuous activity to increase body temperature; increase respiration and heart rate; and guard against muscle, tendon, and ligament strains. The warm-up should consist of calisthenics, gradually increasing exercise intensity, and stretching. Stretching is more effective after the warm-up.

The cool-down is just as important as the warm-up. Abrupt cessation of vigorous activity leads to pooling of the blood, sluggish circulation, and slow removal of waste products. It may also contribute to cramping, soreness, or more serious problems. High levels of the hormone norepinephrine are present immediately after vigorous exercise, making the heart more subject to irregular beats. The cool-down helps remove excess norepinephrine and reduce body temperature. Light activity and stretching continue the pumping action of muscles on veins, helping the circulation in the removal of metabolic wastes.

PRINCIPLE 10: LONG-TERM TRAINING   Changes resulting from the gradual overload of body systems lead to impressive improvements in performance. But it takes years of effort to approach high-level performance capability. Long-term training allows for growth and development, gradual progress, acquisition of skills, learning of strategies, and fuller understanding of the sport. So don't rush the process; too much training too soon may lead to mental and physical burnout and early retirement from the sport. Excellence comes to those who persist with an enjoyable, well-planned, long-term training program.

PRINCIPLE 11: REVERSIBILITY   Most of the adaptations achieved from months of hard training are reversible. In general, it takes longer to gain endurance than it does to lose it. With complete bed rest, fitness can decline at a rate of almost 10 percent per week! Strength declines more slowly, but lack of use will eventually cause atrophy of even the best-trained muscles. To avoid this problem, maintain a year-round program, with periods of hard work followed by periods of relative rest and variety.

PRINCIPLE 12: MODERATION   The principle of moderation applies to all aspects of life. Too much of anything can be bad for your health. Temper dedication with judgment and moderation. If you train too hard, too long, or too fast, the body will begin to deteriorate. Practice moderation in all things. Remember, even elite athletes vary their training, taking easy days between hard training sessions.

PRINCIPLE 13: POTENTIAL   Every person has a potential maximal level of performance. Most of us never come close to that potential performance. Regular participation in physical activity will help you achieve your potential and improve the quality of daily living.

Training Fallacies

You may hear about other so-called principles of training, but you should be aware that some of them are fallacies or misconceptions. These often-quoted statements are not true and have no basis in medical or scientific research.

FALLACY 1: NO PAIN, NO GAIN   Although often difficult and sometimes unpleasant, serious training shouldn't hurt. Well-prepared athletes can perform difficult events in a state of euphoria, free of pain and oblivious to discomfort. Marathon winners sometimes seem to finish full of vitality, whereas others appear near collapse. Pain is not a

Senior Success

Dr. Thomas K. Cureton was a pioneer in exercise physiology and the study of fitness, spending his illustrious career at the University of Illinois during the 1950s and 1960s. During the week this vigorous teacher and researcher taught classes, conducted research studies, and wrote books and articles about exercise and fitness. On weekends he took to the road to preach the gospel of fitness and health to the lay public. His YMCA workshops were legendary for the enormous energy exhibited by this traveling prophet of fitness. He was so busy that he had little time for himself.

Sometime after his retirement he returned to the pool, site of youthful success in competitive swimming. Before long he was setting national and then world records in his age group. We'll never forget his contributions or his delight at finding athletic success in his eighth decade. It's never too late to start, or to start over.

natural consequence of exercise or training; it is a sign of a problem that you shouldn't ignore. During exercise the body produces natural opiates, called endorphins, that can mask discomfort of the effort. If you experience real pain during training, you should back off. If the pain persists, have the problem evaluated.

Discomfort, on the other hand, can accompany difficult aspects of training such as heavy lifting, intense interval training, or long-distance effort. Discomfort is a natural consequence of the lactic acid that accompanies the anaerobic effort of lifting or intervals, or of the muscle fatigue, microscopic muscle damage (microtrauma), and soreness that come with long-distance training. We would accept this statement: No discomfort, no excellence. Overload sometimes requires working at the upper limit of strength, intensity, or endurance, and that state can be temporarily uncomfortable. If exercise results in pain, it is probably excessive. The next two fallacies are also associated with the "no pain, no gain" misconception.

FALLACY 2: YOU MUST BREAK DOWN MUSCLE TO IMPROVE Microtrauma sometimes occurs in muscle during vigorous training and competition, but it isn't a necessary or even a desirable outcome of training. Runners have shown significant microtrauma at the end of a marathon with long downhill stretches that require eccentric muscular contractions (contractions of a lengthening muscle). Eccentric contractions are a major cause of muscle soreness, which is associated with muscle trauma, reduced force output, and a prolonged (4- to 6-week) period of recovery. Excessive trauma doesn't help training; it stops it.

Weight lifters can traumatize muscle with excess weight or repetitions, but that result is not a necessary stage in the development of strength. Neither pain nor injury is a normal consequence of training, and you should avoid both.

FALLACY 3: GO FOR THE BURN The popular maxim to "go for the burn" is often heard among bodybuilders who do numerous repetitions and sets to build, shape, and define muscles. The burn they describe is probably due to the increased acidity associated with elevated levels of lactic acid in the muscle. Although this sensation isn't dangerous, it isn't a necessary part of a strength program designed to improve performance.

FALLACY 4: LACTIC ACID CAUSES MUSCLE SORENESS This fallacy has been around for years, without any basis in fact. Although contractions that lead to soreness may produce lactic acid, the lactic acid isn't the cause of the soreness. Lactic acid is cleared from muscle and blood within an hour of the exercise. Soreness comes 24 hours or more after the effort, long after the lactic acid has been removed or metabolized. Soreness follows unfamiliar exertion or a long layoff and is probably associated with microtrauma to muscle and connective tissue and the swelling that results. After recovery, additional exposure to the activity will yield less soreness.

FALLACY 5: MUSCLE TURNS TO FAT (OR VICE VERSA) Another common misconception is that when an athlete stops training, muscle can turn to fat. Muscle will no more turn to fat than fat will turn to muscle. Both are highly specialized tissues

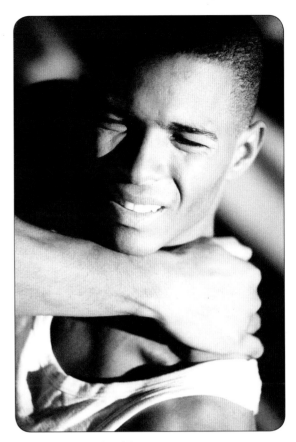

Normal training should not cause pain or injury.

with specific functions. Muscles are composed of long, spaghetti-like fibers with contractile proteins designed to exert force. Fat cells are round receptacles designed to store fat. Training increases the size of muscle fibers (hypertrophy), and detraining reduces their size (atrophy). Excess caloric consumption causes fat cells to grow in size as they store more fat. The cells shrink when you burn more calories than you eat. But long, thin muscle fibers do not change into spherical blobs of fat, or vice versa.

FALLACY 6: I RAN OUT OF WIND Athletes often have the sensation of running out of wind when they run too fast for their level of training. The sensation comes from the lungs and reflects another discomfort of exertion. But this circumstance is more likely to be due to an excess of carbon dioxide than it is to lack of oxygen or air. Carbon dioxide is produced during the oxidative metabolism of carbohydrate, and it is the primary stimulus for respiration. So when carbon dioxide levels are high, as they are during vigorous effort, they cause distress signals in the lungs. The respiratory system thinks that ridding the body of excess carbon dioxide is more important than bringing in more oxygen. Excess carbon dioxide is a sign that you have exceeded your lactate threshold, that you are working above your level of training. Become familiar with the sensation and what it is telling you; ignore it, and you will soon become exhausted.

Physiology of Training

The physiology of training is the study of the response of the body to training. Working together, coaches, athletes, and sports scientists have contributed to a growing body of knowledge about how the body responds to the demands of systematic training. This section provides an overview of training to guide the development and conduct of your program.

Energy Training

To tailor a training program suited to your needs, you first must know the energy sources required in the activity. Figure 15.2 illustrates the relative contribution of anaerobic and aerobic energy sources in relation to the distance or duration of running events (use the time scale to estimate energy sources for other activities). Next, it helps to know something about your individual capabilities, both anaerobic and aerobic. If you are eager to prepare for a marathon, for which the energy source is primarily aerobic, you should be as strong as possible in aerobic fitness. If your event is primarily anaerobic, like a 100-meter swim, you will need anaerobic capability, along with the aerobic capacity to support training and enhance recovery. When you know the energy sources used in the activity and your own capabilities, you can begin to design your training program.

Figure 15.2 Anaerobic and aerobic energy sources in relation to distance and duration of events. Shorter events are primarily anaerobic. For distances greater than 1,500 meters (longer than 4 minutes), training should concentrate on aerobic fitness.

Year-Round Training

Although you can make significant improvements in aerobic energy sources in as little as 2 to 3 months, a year-round program is bound to be safer and more effective (see figure 15.3). All training begins with an aerobic buildup, a period of slow distance work that builds stamina and neuromuscular efficiency. Figure 15.3 shows relative volumes for each training type during each season of training.

After you establish a sound aerobic foundation, you are ready to train the upper end of your aerobic capability, the second lactate threshold. You do this by interval training, using long intervals (2 to 10 minutes). You should do the long lactate threshold intervals at a pace that is only slightly above (2 to 5 percent) your current time-trial pace. Anaerobic training then follows with shorter and faster efforts (30 to 90 seconds). Finally, and only if you'll need speed in the event, you can add sprints to the program (table 15.1).

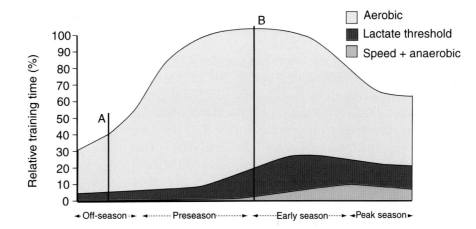

Figure 15.3 Seasonal energy training. The volume of aerobic, second lactate threshold, and speed/(anaerobic) training for each period is relative to the largest volume that you might do during the year. Thus, if your maximum weekly load was 10 hours (line B) you would be doing about 8 hours of aerobic training, 1.6 hours of threshold training, and 25 minutes of speed/(anaerobic) work during a week. During the off-season (line A) you would be training for about 4 hours, with 3.5 hours of aerobic training, 27 minutes of threshold training, and a few minutes of speed training each week. This graph is a general plan that you would adjust based on your goals, sport, and individual capabilities.

Table 15.1   Seasonal Training for Energy Fitness

Season	Training goals	Training methods
Off-season	Aerobic fitness of slow-twitch fibers	Long, slow distance; medium distance; fartlek*; hills
Preseason	Raise anaerobic threshold and aerobic fitness of fast oxidative glycolytic (FOG) fibers	Long intervals (2–10 min), fartlek, pace work, fast distance
Early season	Anaerobic capability and short-term energy and speed	Medium intervals (60–90 sec), short intervals (30–60 sec), sprints
Peak season	Maintain training gains and achieve peak performances	Reduce training volume; emphasize quality not quantity

*Fartlek—a medium-distance effort that consists of faster sections followed by slower ones for recovery.

The year-round approach to training provides the strong foundation needed to compete successfully. Persistent effort minimizes the risk of injury that accompanies anaerobic and speed training. The year-round approach leads to a competitive peak that you can sustain for a month or more and allows a postseason recovery period before a renewed training effort. If you are involved in several activities and cannot devote 12 months to any one, use the same approach but shorten each phase. Always allow at least 1 month each for aerobic and lactate threshold build-ups. If necessary, use the first few weeks of the competitive season for anaerobic and speed training, but don't expect your best performances until later in the season (Sharkey 1986).

Heart Rate Monitors

Athletes often use heart rate monitors (see figure 15.4) to make sure that they are training at the correct intensity. The best monitors are those that use the electrical signal from the heart (ECG). One popular version transmits the signal from the chest to a wrist monitor that displays the rate and stores heart rates for later analysis. If you decide to use a monitor, you will still need to listen to your body, to become familiar with respiratory and other signs of distress. Use the monitor to estimate your lactate threshold and then become aware of your breathing at that level of exertion. You'll need to be able to sense your effort when you race.

Figure 15.4   Athletes use heart rate monitors to gauge the intensity of training.

"No race was ever won or judged by heart rate: speed is the only criteria. Heart rate monitors are good to help athletes go slow, but to go fast you need to monitor speed."

A. Lepavouri, Finnish National Ski Coach

Race-Pace Training

To ensure the specificity of training and the development of needed energy sources, be sure to spend part of your time on race-pace training. If your goal is to ski or run 10 kilometers (6.2 miles) in 35 minutes, you'll have to average 3 minutes and 30 seconds per kilometer during race-pace training. To provide the physiological and psychological base for the effort, do a number of kilometers at that pace or slightly faster. If the pace sometimes feels difficult, remember that the excitement of the race and the competition provided by others will elicit hormonal support to help ease the burden.

Lactate Threshold Training

To run, ski, swim, or cycle fast, you'll need well-trained fast-twitch muscle fibers. Faster training (long intervals, pace training) will train fast oxidative glycolytic (FOG) fibers and raise the second lactate threshold, which defines the upper end of sustainable aerobic effort (see table 15.2).

Because each sport and distance has specific requirements, we recommend that you do threshold training slightly faster than your current performance threshold, your current time-trial or race pace. Do a time trial every 3 to 4 weeks. Determine your pace and then do intervals of 2 to 10 minutes at a pace 3 to 5 percent above your performance pace. Be sure to recover fully between intervals.

Anaerobic Training

Whereas you develop aerobic energy sources in long runs, in runs in which you alternate fast and slow running, and in long-interval training, you perform anaerobic training at higher intensities, when you exceed the second lactate threshold. Because high-intensity effort is fatiguing, you should alternate short periods of intense exer-

Table 15.2 Interval Training Guidelines

Intervals	Train	Repetitions	Duration	Work to rest ratio[*]	Max speed (%)	Max heart rate (%)
Long	Performance threshold	4–6	2–10 min	1:1–2	>race pace[**]	85–90
Medium	Glycogen pathway	8–12	60–90 sec	1:2	80–90	95
Short	High energy	15–20	30–60 sec	1:3	95	100
Sprint	Speed	25 or more	10–30 sec	1:3	100	100

[*]A ratio of 1:1 means that the rest lasts as long as the work interval. A ratio of 1:3 means that the rest is three times as long as the work interval.

[**]Race pace is 3 to 5% faster than current aerobic race pace.

tion with periods of active rest. Allow a gradual anaerobic buildup, beginning with longer intervals and rest periods. Increase the pace and shorten the distances as training progresses. Always use active rest (walk or slow jog) to hasten removal of lactic acid.

The interval training prescription includes the rate and distance of the work interval, the length of the rest period, and the total number of repetitions (e.g., run 400 meters six times, each in 75 seconds, with 2 minutes active rest after each). Because you do interval runs at a faster pace, they require a period of psychological adjustment. Some people never learn to enjoy this form of training. We find it tolerable when we do the workouts with others of similar ability. Incidentally, swimmers often do their intervals in set periods, such as four sets of 100 meters, each in 80 seconds. If they swim fast, the rest is longer; if they swim slowly, they have little time for rest.

The interval-training concept allows a great deal of adaptability to meet individual needs and abilities. Training can be relatively mild (e.g., run 400 meters in 90 seconds four times) for the neophyte, and it can be made more interesting with a variety of distances (e.g., 200s, 300s, 400s, 600s) and paces. Interval training can also be mind numbing, like the program that Buddy Edelen used to prepare for the Tokyo Olympic marathon. Buddy would run 400 meters 25 times to "break the monotony" of long-distance training. Roger Bannister trained until he could run 440 yards 10 times at 60 seconds to prepare for the first 4-minute mile. You, too, can use interval training to prepare for athletic competition. But approach this intense training with moderation, never doing more than two or three intense workouts per week.

Training Plateau?

If your training has reached a plateau and you aren't making satisfactory progress, try adding additional high-intensity training. Cross-country skiers who had not responded well to high-volume, low-intensity training switched to a program with twice the volume of high-intensity training. They demonstrated improvement in $\dot{V}O_2$max, anaerobic threshold, and competitive results (Gaskill et al. 1999). Add intensity with long intervals, pace work, fartlek (speed play), time trials, and races, but be sure to cut back on overall volume to avoid fatigue and overtraining.

Diet and Performance

This section presents a few basic facts concerning diet and performance. One fact is that athletes use the same sources of energy and nutrients as everyone else does. They need more calories to fuel hard training and may need additional nutrients, but those usually come with an increase in nutritious foods (see chapter 11). Here are some ways to ensure adequate energy for performance.

Carbohydrate Loading

Years before it became popular, researchers observed that the best endurance performances occurred when athletes were on a high-carbohydrate diet, such as the performance diet discussed in chapter 11. That diet provides sufficient energy for continuous events lasting up to 1 hour. Carbo loading goes a step further to raise muscle glycogen levels for high-intensity performances lasting more than 1 hour. Using a needle to get a sample of muscle tissue (see muscle biopsy photo in chapter 5, page 88), researchers studied how performance depends on muscle glycogen levels and how glycogen levels depend on carbohydrate intake.

Here is what you can do to ensure proper glycogen levels for competition. For events lasting 1 to 2 hours, do a long, hard workout several days before the event to deplete muscle glycogen stores. This activates an enzyme responsible for packing glycogen into muscle fibers. Next, begin immediately to raise your carbohydrate intake for the next few days by adding extra carbohydrate to the diet. Be sure to drink lots of water, because carbohydrate is stored with water (hydrated). This scheme will double muscle glycogen stores as long as you reduce (taper) training before the event.

For events longer than 2 hours, start your depletion effort 6 days before the event. Do another hard workout the next day to deplete muscle glycogen stores further. Keep carbohydrate intake down for those 2 days. Then after the second depletion effort, return to a high-carbohydrate intake, with water, and taper your training to allow maximum carbohydrate loading. This scheme has raised muscle glycogen levels three to four times, enough to fuel an entire marathon.

Be aware that carbo loading takes place only in the muscles that you deplete with exercise. Other muscles can't easily use the glycogen, so the effect is specific. If you plan to carbo load for an important race, be certain to try it first in a less important event. Some people feel bloated and heavy when they carbo load, but the best performances take place when muscle glycogen levels are highest. One study has shown that inactivity combined with high intake of carbohydrate (up to 10 grams of carbohydrate per kilogram of body weight, with emphasis on foods with a high glycemic index) enables trained athletes to attain maximal muscle glycogen levels within 1 day (Bussau et al. 2002).

Women tend to use more fat and less carbohydrate during submaximal endurance events. The female's preference for fat utilization appears to be hormonally controlled and diminishes as training progresses (Ruby and Robergs 1994). A recent study shows that aerobically trained women increase muscle glycogen in response to high carbohydrate intake (78 percent carbohydrate), but the magnitude was smaller than that previously observed in men. The increase in muscle glycogen from the high-carbohydrate diet was associated with increased cycling performance to exhaustion (8.4 percent) when compared with the moderate-carbohydrate intake (48 percent carbohydrate diet) (Walker et al. 2000).

Pre-, During, and Postevent Feeding

Generally speaking, you should eat the precompetition meal that works for you. Eat at least 3 hours before the event to ensure an empty stomach at race time. Emphasize carbohydrate and avoid difficult-to-digest fats and excess protein. Especially nervous people may want to use a liquid meal before competition. A peanut butter and honey sandwich works for shorter events, and pancakes plus an egg (to slow entry of glucose) works for long events, such as a 50-kilometer (31-mile) ski race.

- **Preevent.** Drink 1 to 2 cups (240 to 480 milliliters) of water before an event, but avoid high carbohydrate intake that might raise insulin levels, lower blood glucose, cause hypoglycemia, reduce free fatty acid availability, and increase reliance on muscle glycogen.

- **During the event.** Drink a cup (240 milliliters) or more of water every 15 to 20 minutes. In longer events drink a sport drink with 6 to 8 percent (60 to 80 grams per liter) carbohydrate every 15 to 20 minutes to maintain blood glucose levels. Cyclists and skiers are able to tolerate more carbohydrate in drinks or solid food (bananas, energy bars, gels) during competition. The carbohydrate provides energy for muscles and the nervous system and helps to enhance the immune system and cognitive function. Recent studies suggest that some protein intake during the event may improve endurance performance.

- **Postevent.** Immediately after the event, begin to consume carbohydrate and some protein (a ratio of four grams carbs to one gram protein) to maximize replacement of muscle glycogen and speed muscle recovery (Ivy et al. 2002). The maximal rate of replacement occurs in the first 2 hours after the event. Select foods with a high glycemic index to maximize replacement of muscle glycogen. Drink lots of juices and water to ensure fluid replacement, but avoid alcoholic beverages, which function as a diuretic.

Muscular Fitness Training

As sport becomes more competitive at every level, participants must invest more time in muscular fitness training. You should evaluate the muscular demands of your sport as well as your strengths and weak points. Then you can proceed to develop a program to improve the strength, muscular endurance, power, or speed that you need to reach your goals. Figure 15.5 on page 313 illustrates such a plan for the seasons of training.

- **Off-season.** The period when you are not competing is the time for strength training. Select important muscle groups in the upper body, core (abdomen and trunk), and legs and engage in a program following the prescriptions presented in chapter 10. When your strength is adequate for the sport, move on to the next phase of training.

Blood Sugar

We have noted how endurance training improves the ability to mobilize and metabolize fat, thereby conserving blood sugar. Nerve tissue depends on the blood sugar (glucose) as its source of energy. This means that the brain and nervous system require a constant supply of glucose. Blood glucose rises after a meal and then drops until it reaches a normal resting level (about 80 milligrams). Thereafter the liver strives to maintain that level, at least until its supply is depleted. The symptoms of hypoglycemia (see table 15.3) indicate the influence of low blood sugar on behavior and performance.

Table 15.3   Hypoglycemia: Common Symptoms

Nervousness	Anxiety
Irritability	Confusion
Exhaustion	Rapid pulse
Faintness, dizziness	Muscle pains
Tremor, cold sweat	Indecisiveness
Depression	Lack of coordination
Vertigo	Lack of concentration
Drowsiness	Blurred vision
Headaches	

Muscles can use blood sugar as an energy source, so long runs, bike rides, or hikes certainly can lead to hypoglycemia. High-energy snacks such as energy bars lead to a big boost of blood sugar, but they also call forth a large secretion of insulin. The insulin speeds the sugar into the muscle, and within a couple of hours one begins to sag again (reactive hypoglycemia). To avoid the problem, simply eat at regular intervals and use energy snacks and carbohydrate drinks to maintain blood sugar levels.

■ **Preseason.** By now you should be moving into power or muscular endurance training. As the season approaches, make the exercises more sport specific, more like the movements of the sport. You develop power with 15 to 25 repetitions maximum (RM) sets done as fast as possible. You improve short-term (anaerobic) endurance in sets of 8 to 15RM.

■ **Early season.** From now on the emphasis is on speed and maintenance of gains in strength, endurance, and power. Practice sport skills at high speed to become more comfortable with speed and to improve neuromuscular coordination. Once-a-week maintenance sessions will retain strength and power gains.

In a study of junior cross-country skiers, sport-specific muscular fitness training (arm work on an inclined ramp) was found superior to lifting weights or even roller skiing to improve arm power and performance. The athletes first developed strength on a steeply inclined ramp and then focused on power with explosive contractions on

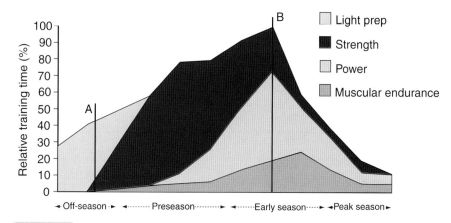

Figure 15.5 Seasonal muscular fitness training plan. The volume of light preparatory, strength, power, and muscular endurance training for each period is relative to the largest volume that you might do during the year. Thus, if your maximum weekly load was 5 hours of muscular fitness training (line B), you would be doing about 1.5 hours of strength training (2 to 6RM), 2.5 hours of power training (8 to 15RM), and 1 hour of muscular endurance training (15 to 25RM) during a week. During the off-season (line A) you would gradually increase lifting of light weights to about 2 hours a week, slowly increasing the weights to a point where you are ready to begin strength training. This graph is a general plan that you would adjust based on goals, sport, and individual needs.

a lesser incline. They finished the final weeks with muscular endurance sets. Specific training and a periodized program improved performance 15 percent (Nesser et al. 2004).

Evaluate the muscular demands of your sport and get started on a program. As you proceed to develop particular muscle groups, don't ignore flexibility and core strength. Don't forget to maintain muscular balance by training muscle groups on opposite sides of the joint. Excessive attention to one muscle group, such as the quadriceps on the front of the thigh, could lead to muscle imbalance and greater risk of injury. In table 15.4 you'll find a format that you can use to develop a program for your sport. Figure 15.6 provides a worksheet for program development, and figure 15.7 illustrates a sample program.

Table 15.4   Developing Your Muscular Fitness Program

1. Determine the muscular fitness requirements of the sport or activity.
2. Identify the major muscle groups and movements involved.
3. Select exercises to develop muscular fitness in upper body, trunk, and legs.
4. Make adjustments for strengths and weaknesses.*
5. Establish training goals, set up a schedule, and get started. Remember to keep good records and to test progress every few weeks.

For more on training for sports, see Sharkey and Gaskill 2006.

*Use fewer sets for strong areas, more for those in need of extra help.

Figure 15.6   Muscular Fitness Program Planner

Sport _____   Position _____

Season _____   Goals _____

Individual strengths _____

Weak points _____

Body part	Exercises	Muscle group	Purpose
Arm and shoulder	_____	_____	_____
	_____	_____	_____
	_____	_____	_____
	_____	_____	_____
Trunk	_____	_____	_____
	_____	_____	_____
	_____	_____	_____
Legs	_____	_____	_____
	_____	_____	_____
	_____	_____	_____
Other	_____	_____	_____

From *Fitness and Health, Sixth Edition* by Brian J. Sharkey and Steven E. Gaskill, 2007, Champaign, IL: Human Kinetics.

Concurrent Strength and Endurance Training

Many athletes conduct concurrent strength and aerobic endurance training in the same muscle group. Early research suggested that endurance training interfered with full development of strength (Hickson 1980). A recent study of 45 male and female subjects supports the contention that combined strength and endurance training can suppress some of the adaptations to strength training. Gains in strength were greater with strength-only training. With female subjects the combined training raised the level of the stress hormone cortisol. Surprisingly, the combined training augmented the number of capillaries per muscle fiber, a measure important to endurance (Bell et al. 2000). If you need high levels of strength, focus on strength training. Experienced athletes seem to be able to thrive in concurrent strength and endurance training. Because concurrent training requires synthesis of strength and endurance proteins, consuming up to 1.8 grams of good-quality protein per kilogram of body weight daily is important.

Figure 15.7   Muscular Fitness Program Planner

Sport _____ *Basketball* _____   Position _____ *Forward* _____

Season _____ *Off-season* _____   Goals _____ *Strength and power* _____

Individual strengths _____ *Shooting* _____

Weak points _____ *Rebounding* _____

Body part	Exercises	Muscle group	Purpose
Arm and shoulder	Lat pull-downs (with basketball)	Hands, arms, chest, and lats	Pull down rebounds
	Biceps curl	Arm flexors	Rebounding
Trunk	Abdominal curl (machine)	Abdominals	Pull down rebounds
	Backups	Lower back	Back strength
Legs	Leaper or power squats	Leg extension and jumping muscles	Sustained power for jumping
	Plyometrics (down jumping)	Leg extension and jumping muscles	Preload and jumping
	Hill (or stair) running	Leg extension and jumping muscles	Sustained power
Other	Rebounding and fast-break drills		Sustained power and endurance in game situations

Note: When you acquire sufficient strength, shift to an endurance, power, or power–endurance program in the preseason (achieve power–endurance by performing 15 to 25 reps as fast as possible).

Psychology of Performance

Psychologist Nathaniel Ehrlich (1971) draws a distinction between competitors and performers in athletic competition. Competitors evaluate their performances strictly on a relativistic, win-loss basis, with little regard given to the absolute level of performance. Performers attach secondary importance to winning. They evaluate their performances against an absolute scale, an ideal.

The competitor subscribes to the Vince Lombardi dictum "Winning isn't everything; it's the only thing." The performer, on the other hand, would give the nod to "It isn't whether you win or lose; it's how (and how well) you play the game." Ehrlich draws an analogy between Maslow's self-esteem and self-actualization levels of motivation (see chapter 18). The competitor seeks esteem, whereas the performer seeks to realize his or her potential. We would hope to find a mature, self-actualizing approach to competition among adult athletes. Each would be seeking his or her potential, and competition would serve as a means to that end. Performers seek good competition because it helps them achieve their potential. Competitors fear good competition because it threatens their self-esteem.

If you value your mental health and don't want to be frustrated by defeat and lose your self-esteem, become a performer. Performers never fail. If their performance is flawed, they know that time and practice will bring them closer to their goal. Become a performer by focusing on the quality of the experience, not the outcome. Don't get angry when you lose; you need good competition to improve. Analyze but don't judge your performance. Approach weaknesses positively (I need to get my racket back earlier), not negatively (my forehand stinks). Set goals in terms of performance instead of wins, medals, or trophies. You may find that the wins and trophies come as performance improves. If not, you can still find satisfaction in the game, and you won't feel regret when it's over.

Play Your Best Game

Have you noticed that you do well on some days and poorly on others? Have you ever wished that you could play your best game more often? Sport psychologists Tutko and Tosi (1976) offered suggestions to help you do just that and improve your ability to deal with the emotional side of your game.

- **Relax.** Contract and then relax your muscles and say, "Let go" as you learn muscle relaxation (Jacobson's progressive relaxation, 1938). Concentrate on your breathing and say, "Easy" with each exhale (Benson's relaxation response, 1975). Eventually, you can use the relaxation techniques in competition to help relieve tension.

- **Concentrate.** Focus your attention on an object in the game (e.g., tennis ball) to free the mind of fears and negative judgments and to allow your best performance. When your opponent tosses the ball for the serve, say (to yourself), "Ball," concentrate on the ball, and let your body do what it has learned to do.

- **Mentally rehearse.** Rehearse mentally before and during practice and before competition to help focus on key elements of the game. Imagine yourself performing well.

- **Physically rehearse.** Use physical rehearsal to hone skills in days preceding competition and as skill rehearsal in the warm-up just before the event.

You will notice that these sport psychologists neglected to include advice on how to psych yourself up for the game or how to psych out your opponent. Did they forget? Probably not. Most of us fail because we are overaroused. We are so psyched up and concerned that we are literally tied in knots, unable to execute the skills that we worked so hard to perfect. If we think too much and try too hard, we are bound to fail. So Tutko and Tosi provide advice aimed at helping you to free your mind, to relax, and to reach the state called flow. Then and only then can you produce your best performance. You'll find yourself saying, "I played over my head," "I was out of my mind," "I couldn't miss; everything I hit went in." Don't get us wrong; we're not suggesting that you enter an event and then forget why you're there. On the contrary, you're there to play well and have fun. You should savor every moment.

The theory behind this approach is based on the different roles played by the right and left brains. The left brain is absorbed with details. It is analytical and judgmental, whereas the right brain is concerned with movements, patterns, and the overall picture. After we learn skills, we should perform them without the critical review of the left brain. Relaxation and concentration allow us to play our best game more often.

Successful distance runners tend to "associate" during a race. They tune in to their bodies so that they will know how fast they dare run. They are consciously aware of pace, position, key opponents, and features along the course. Less-successful runners tend to "disassociate," to lose track of time and place. Form becomes less efficient, and their pace slows.

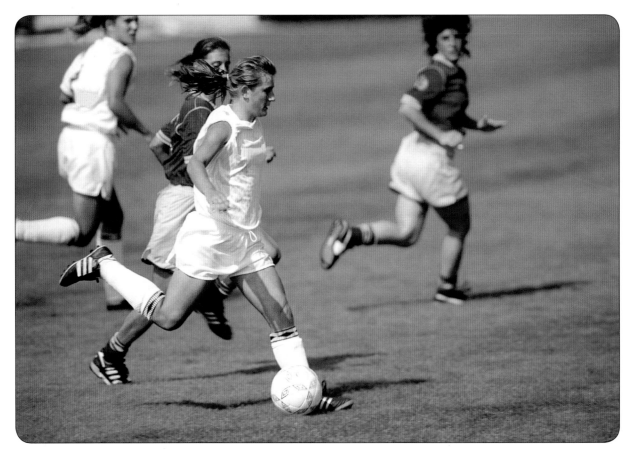

Focusing on the ball during a game can help you eliminate fears and reach your potential.

By learning to handle your emotions, you'll enjoy the game more. Eliminate the tensions, fears, and frustrations, and you may win more often. If you can do all these things and devote sufficient time to practice and training, you will be well on your way to achieving your potential. More important, the enjoyment and success that you experience will keep you involved in a lifelong pursuit of excellence.

Performance Potential

Researchers published a fascinating account of the restraints on performance in running (Ryder, Carr, and Herget 1976). Using running records from the previous 50 years, they plotted the rate of improvement and made some surprising conclusions. On average, the rate of improvement in distances ranging from 100 meters to 30 kilometers has been a steady but slow .75 meter per minute per year. Because record breakers seldom participate in further assaults on the record, the investigators concluded that good runners just don't work as hard after they have set a record. The researchers contend that running records are still well below human physiological limits, that the restraints on performance are largely physiological and pathological. The major obstacle is not the race but the amount of time devoted to daily training. In recent years, athletes have had to train many hours a day to achieve record-breaking status. After achieving the record, the athlete is likely to turn attention to other, more mundane matters, such as starting a career, earning a living, getting married, and having a family.

Thus, time is the obstacle, time and the injuries associated with overuse and overtraining. If you feel stymied in your training, if you are stuck on a plateau, invest more time to resume your progress. Barring injury, you should be able to improve. Following this line of reasoning, progress in world records will begin to slow when men and women have invested as much training time as is humanly possible. Thereafter, progress will depend on improved equipment and new techniques. Today, some 30 years after this analysis, training has become a full-time job for world-class athletes, and world records continue to decline. Of course, specialists in sports medicine are actively engaged in repairing the bodies battered by relentless training.

Most of us are unable to invest excessive time in training, so we must define our potential as the level that we attain following the maximum possible time and effort. Given the limitations imposed by job and family as well as by heredity, physique, gender, and age, you can still make dramatic progress toward your potential. Consider the case of petite Michiko Suwa from Japan. She came to the United States at the age of 28, met and married Mike Gorman, and changed her first name to Miki. Five years later she began jogging, and in 1973 at age 38 she ran her first marathon. Later that year she astounded the running world with a woman's world record. Neither physique nor age predicted her potential. Look at Priscilla Welch, a two-pack-a-day smoker who quit smoking, started running, and went on to become a world-class competitor in the marathon. Or consider Sister Marion, a nun who started running in 1979. Within 5 years she qualified for the 1984 Olympic marathon trials, at the age of 54!

Overtraining

Training, when overdone, can be a stressor that reduces the ability of the immune system to resist infection. Yet athletes at all levels seem prone to overtrain. We grew up believing the old fallacy "No pain, no gain." Yet the risks of overtraining are many, including illness, injury, and lost time.

Symptoms of overtraining include lethargy, fatigue, poor performance, sleep loss, loss of appetite, and illness. Because the symptoms arise slowly, overtraining is difficult to diagnose. Causes of overtraining include boredom, overwork relative to rest, immune suppression because of exhaustion and stress, hormonal imbalance, poor nutrition, rapid weight loss, and inadequate hydration. Scientists have used measures such as the wake-up heart rate and temperature, cortisol to testosterone ratio, and mood scales to try to help people avoid overtraining.

Increases in the cortisol to testosterone ratio has been correlated with overtraining. Blood levels of cortisol, a hormone from the adrenal gland, increase when the body is under physical or psychological stress (Neary et al. 1994). Testosterone is an anabolic (growth-stimulating) hormone that decreases with overtraining. The ratio is a sensitive but expensive indicator of overtraining. If you undertake serious training, you should become familiar with some simple ways to detect overtraining and use them regularly (see table 15.5).

The treatment for overtraining is relative rest. Serious cases demand time off or bed rest, but most people respond to reduced training, more time for recovery, attention to nutrition, and a change of pace. Remember that you should approach training as a gentle pastime. Make haste slowly, and you will eventually reach your goals. Overtrain, and you'll lower your resistance to infection. For more about training and overtraining, see our new book, *Sport Physiology for Coaches* (2006).

Mood States

The profile of mood states (POMS) has been used to study the effects of overtraining. The POMS test uses the responses to 65 words, such as *tense, hopeless, bitter, lively, worn out*, and *bewildered*, to yield mood scores. Subjects are asked to indicate the answer that best describes to what degree they have experienced those particular moods during the past week, including the day of the test. Response options are 0—not at all, 1—a little, 2—moderately, 3—quite a bit, and 4—extremely. Responses are categorized into six mood scores: tension–anxiety, depression–dejection, anger–hostility, vigor–activity, fatigue–inertia, and confusion–bewilderment. The classic iceberg profile depicts an athlete low in all scores except vigor. Overtraining lowers vigor while it raises all the other scales (Morgan et al. 1988).

Table 15.5   Overtraining Indexes

Index	How to use
Pulse index	Take your pulse rate daily (for 60 sec), in the morning before rising. Average the daily rates. When the morning pulse is five or more beats above normal, you should suspect illness or overtraining. Take an easy day to get back to normal.
Weight index	Check your weight daily, in the morning (after toilet but before breakfast). Average daily weights. A rapid or persistent weight loss could indicate impending problems because of poor eating habits, failure to replace fluids, nervousness, or excessive fatigue.
Temperature	Take your morning temperature daily for a week to establish your normal reading. Then use it to determine whether the morning temperature is elevated. A fever usually indicates infection. Take a day off.
Fatigue index	Rate your tiredness after you arise. Ready to drop — 9 Extremely tired — 8 Very tired — 7 Slightly tired — 6 About average — 5 Somewhat fresh — 4 Very fresh — 3 Extremely fresh — 2 Full of life — 1
Step test	After rising in the morning, but before breakfast and coffee, do this step test. Step up and down on the bottom step of stairs (8 in., or 20 cm). Use one step per second, with both feet up on the 2nd second and both down on 4th second. Continue for 1 min and then immediately take your pulse (for 15 sec and then multiply by four to obtain the rate per min). Average the daily rates for a week to get a baseline. When the posttest pulse is 10 or more beats above the normal baseline, you should suspect illness or overtraining. Take a day or two of easy training until your step test pulse is back to normal.

Other useful signs include boredom, weakness, pain in joints, color of urine (dark, concentrated, or cloudy), and skin color (pasty, pale).

Neck Check

What should you do with an upper respiratory tract infection? Dr. Randy Eichner recommends the neck check. If symptoms are above the neck, such as a stuffy nose, sneezing, or a scratchy throat, try a "test drive" at half speed. If you feel better after 10 minutes, you can increase the pace and finish the workout. If symptoms are below the neck, with aching muscles or coughing, or if you have a fever, nausea, or diarrhea, take the day off (Eichner 1995). You can return to training when the fever is gone for at least 24 hours without the aid of aspirin or other antifever medications.

Cross-Training

As the triathlon attracted multisport athletes, the concept of cross-training gained attention. Cross-training can be viewed as systematic variety designed to avoid overuse injuries. It allows addicted athletes to train hard every day with little risk of overuse or repetitive trauma injuries. Some people extol the virtue of training a variety of muscle groups, as in swimming, cycling, and running. Triathletes train for all three disciplines, and they do sport-specific weight training to enhance performance. Cross-training allows athletes and fitness enthusiasts the option to train more than they could in a single sport and to achieve balance in their training.

Does cross-training provide special performance benefits? Probably not. Specificity is still the best rule to follow if you want to improve in a sport. Swimming will not improve performance in running or cycling, and vice versa. Activities that use similar muscles may contribute some to performance, but not to the same degree as increases in specific training (Foster et al. 1995). Of course, cross-training is a necessity if you are preparing for a multiple-discipline event, and it is a great way to remain active and fit as you grow older.

Fitness and Work

Workers in construction, agriculture, forestry, firefighting, law enforcement, and the military are often required to engage in strenuous effort. Without proper conditioning, the stress of arduous work can be unpleasant or worse, so concern for employee health and safety has prompted screening procedures to make sure that the worker is capable of meeting job demands. Some companies have instituted employee fitness programs to help workers meet and maintain required levels of work capacity.

Work Capacity

Work capacity is defined as the ability to accomplish production goals without undue fatigue and without becoming a hazard to oneself or coworkers. Work capacity can also be viewed as sustainable capacity, the level of effort that one can sustain throughout the work shift. Work capacity is the product of a number of factors, including natural endowment, skill, nutrition, aerobic and muscular fitness, intelligence, experience, acclimatization, and lean body weight (Sharkey 1997b). However, a worker may rate high in aerobic or muscular fitness, acclimatization to heat or altitude, even skill and experience but may fail to produce adequately because of lack of motivation. On the other hand, even the most highly motivated workers will fail if they lack strength or endurance, ignore the need to acclimatize to a hot working environment, or lack the physical skills required for the job.

Aerobic Fitness and Work Capacity

When heavy work is required, people with a low level of aerobic fitness are able to sustain only 25 percent of capacity for 8 hours. Those of average fitness can work at about 33 percent, and those with above-average fitness can maintain 40 percent of their capacity for 8 hours. Only highly conditioned and motivated individuals can sustain levels as high as 50 percent of their aerobic fitness level for 8 hours (table 15.6). Those with higher fitness levels have the capacity to do more work and to assist others in emergencies. In some jobs the fit worker is able to produce four to six times more than the unfit worker (Sharkey et al. 1980). Which one would you hire?

Table 15.6   Aerobic Fitness and Sustainable Work Capacity

Aerobic fitness ($\dot{V}O_2$max-ml · kg^{-1} · min^{-1})	Sustainable %	Work output (ml · kg^{-1} · min^{-1})	Calories/min
Low (<35)	25%	<8.7	3
Average (45)	33%	15	5
Above average (50)	40%	20	7.5
Highly fit (>55)	50%	>27.5	10

Muscular Fitness and Work Capacity

Dynamic muscular strength is clearly related to work capacity when the worker must lift very heavy loads or use heavy tools. For repeated lifting, however—as in work with hand tools—strength, muscular endurance, and aerobic fitness combine to set the limits of work capacity (figure 15.8). Combinations of work rate and percentage of maximum strength that fall to the right of the line that represents a person's fitness level cannot be sustained for a full working day. Highly fit workers (55 milliliters per kilogram per minute) can produce more by working at a

Figure 15.8 Interrelationships of strength, aerobic fitness, and work rate.

higher rate. Stronger individuals can lift more with each contraction. The ideal combination includes a balance of aerobic fitness and strength adequate to the task.

Lean Body Weight and Work Capacity

Excess fat certainly limits work capacity. When considerable muscular strength is needed the person with high lean body weight (LBW) is more likely to excel (LBW equals body weight minus fat weight). LBW indicates how much muscle a person brings to the job. Body weight or percent body fat can be misleading. Twenty percent fat sounds high, unless it's on top of 200 pounds (90.7 kilograms) of lean weight (muscle). In a study of wildland firefighters, we found that work capacity was highly related to LBW (Sharkey 1981).

> ## First Lactate Threshold and Work Capacity
>
> Although aerobic fitness ($\dot{V}O_2$max) tells a lot about work capacity, the first lactate threshold is a better predictor of long-term performance. The first lactate threshold indicates the early rise in blood lactate during a progressive exercise test (see figure 4.1 on page 73). Those who can do more work before the lactic acid level rises will be able to sustain a higher level of production in prolonged arduous work. Conducting a laboratory test to determine long-term work capacity isn't necessary. An employer could simply select a job-related work sample and measure performance, the amount of work that the candidate accomplished in 30 to 45 minutes.

Fitness Is Good Business

Experience shows that unfit workers can be a safety hazard to themselves as well as to coworkers. In physically demanding jobs, as well as in office jobs, fit workers are more productive than their sedentary colleagues, are absent less often, and are far less likely to incur job-related disabilities or retire early because of heart or other degenerative diseases. Moreover, physically fit workers have a more positive attitude about work and life in general.

Fit employees are a good investment. Thousands of companies spend billions on employee health and fitness (wellness) programs. The expenditure is justified on several grounds. Each dollar spent on employee health and fitness in the workplace saves several dollars. A return of $5.97 resulted from every dollar invested in multiple category programs (Pronk 2003). Fit workers are less likely to smoke, and smoking costs business and industry billions for health and other costs. Workers who maintain or become fit are less likely to have physician visits or overnight hospital stays, compared with those who are unfit (Mitchell et al. 2004), and fit employees are more productive in any line of work. Our studies with wildland firefighters show that fit workers are able to accomplish more than average workers, and several times more than marginal workers.

Fit employees are also a good investment for safety, health, and morale reasons. Fit workers are less likely to experience debilitating low-back and other injuries. When injured they rehabilitate quickly and miss fewer days of work. Fit wildland firefighters are better able to reach a safety zone and help others to safety (Ruby et al. 2003). Fit workers miss fewer days of work and are far less likely to suffer from musculoskeletal problems or degenerative problems such as heart disease. They also spend a smaller share of the company's health care costs. In one study, active workers spent $250 less than sedentary employees did and $450 less than obese workers did (Wang et al. 2004). Morale is higher among fit employees and those engaged in fitness programs. Fitness and health programs increase loyalty and reduce turnover. If your company doesn't already have an employee health and fitness or wellness program, talk with management, assemble a group of interested coworkers, and get started.

> Fit employees are a good investment for safety, health, and morale reasons.

Occupational Physiology

Physiology, the study of the human body, is becoming increasingly important in the workplace to determine job demands and aid in the selection of workers; to work harden, train, and cross-train workers to improve performance and reduce injuries; to rehabilitate injured workers; and to confront job discrimination according to age, gender, race, or disability. This section considers some of the current issues and provides a fair approach to hiring by examining how to use valid work capacity tests to help prevent discrimination.

A major feature of the workplace during the past 30 years has been the effort to provide equal employment opportunities and prevent discrimination based on age, gender, race, or disability in compliance with federal laws. The Age Discrimination in Employment Act (ADEA) of 1967 outlawed job discrimination based on age, except when age was a bona fide occupational qualification (BFOQ). Yet a large study commissioned by the Equal Employment Opportunity Commission (EEOC) found that age was poorly correlated with performance and that job-related tests accurately reflected work capacity (Landy 1992).

In the 1970s, with the help of the Civil Rights Act of 1964, women began to seek employment in previously male-dominated jobs such as firefighting, law enforcement, construction, and the military. Just as female athletes train to build muscle strength and endurance, female workers can train to compete in formerly male-only jobs. Employers should establish valid job-related tests, advertise the standards, and provide preemployment training programs. If few women qualify, the employer should not lower the standards, but hold firm and watch as women come forth to accept the challenge.

In strenuous jobs, such as firefighting, fit workers create a safer work environment. Fit workers in any environment are more productive than their unfit colleagues.

Studies in work physiology do not suggest racial or ethnic differences in work capacity. Clearly, job-related work-capacity tests do not unfairly affect racial or ethnic groups. Indeed, valid work-capacity tests are color blind. The Americans With Disabilities Act (ADA) of 1991 was enacted to ensure employment opportunities and reasonable accommodations for persons with disabilities. The ADA endorses the use of valid preemployment tests as an objective way to determine a person's ability to do a job.

Finding the right person for the job can often be difficult. When the job demands physical performance, many employers turn to job-related tests to aid the selection process. Development of a valid test of work capacity begins with a job task analysis to select important work tasks. The candidate test is then administered to successful employees to ensure its usefulness and to select a cutoff score. Thereafter, the test can be used to select new employees, to ensure that current employees maintain work capacity, and to evaluate employees returning to work following injury or illness.

Job Demands

Dr. Paul Davis has developed a job-related test for structural firefighters. The test incorporates actual elements of the job, including carrying hoses up several flights of stairs, a chopping task, pulling a heavy hose, and a victim carry. Many departments use this or a similar test to select among the many candidates for the job. Unfortunately, only a few departments demand that their firefighters pass the test annually (Dotson, Santa Maria, and Davis 1976). Dr. Davis' studies show that the fitness and health of public service personnel (police, fire) decline at about the same rate as they do in the sedentary, overweight population (Davis and Starck 1980).

The only way to maintain physical work capacity throughout a worker's career is to require annual testing and participation in a job-related fitness program. Fire departments are known for the care that they give their equipment. Yet they will hire employees who barely pass a selection test and then ignore the need for ongoing physical maintenance. A recent U.S. Fire Administration study found that cardiac arrest or heart attacks accounted for 47 percent of deaths among structural firefighters but only 7 percent of deaths among wildland firefighters (USFA 2002). The report cited the extremely high standards of physical fitness in wildland firefighting agencies as a factor in the lower death rate. A well-designed program maintains or builds the aerobic and muscular capability needed on the job while meeting the employees' health and wellness needs.

Summary

In this chapter we've presented a simple approach to the development of a year-round training program that provides for the systematic development of aerobic and anaerobic energy sources and for muscular strength, endurance, and power. If you are ready for some SERIOUS training, consider the program recommended by Rob Sleamaker (1989). The SERIOUS training program includes the following:

Speed

Endurance

Race or pace

Intervals

Overdistance

Up or vertical (e.g., hills) if applicable

Strength

For more detailed information on training and programming consult our new book, *Sport Physiology for Coaches* (Sharkey and Gaskill 2006).

If you are not that serious, forget speed and pace, but don't ignore variety in your training. Alternate hard with easy, short with long, speed with distance—and don't forget to include rest days for recovery. Outline a program and get started. Keep simple records, and change the program as your goals change. As your interest grows, look for books or magazines that focus on your activity. In time you will become an expert on training and your body's response. Knowledge, coupled with adequate training, will improve your performance.

In the final section of this chapter we showed you that performance in physically demanding work is related to fitness. The harder the work, the higher the relationship to measures of aerobic and muscular fitness. Therefore, when selecting employees for hard work it makes good sense to use a job-related work-capacity test to hire those most suited for the work. But selection isn't enough. An ongoing job-related fitness or physical maintenance program is necessary to make certain that employees maintain the capacity to do the job.

Environment and Performance

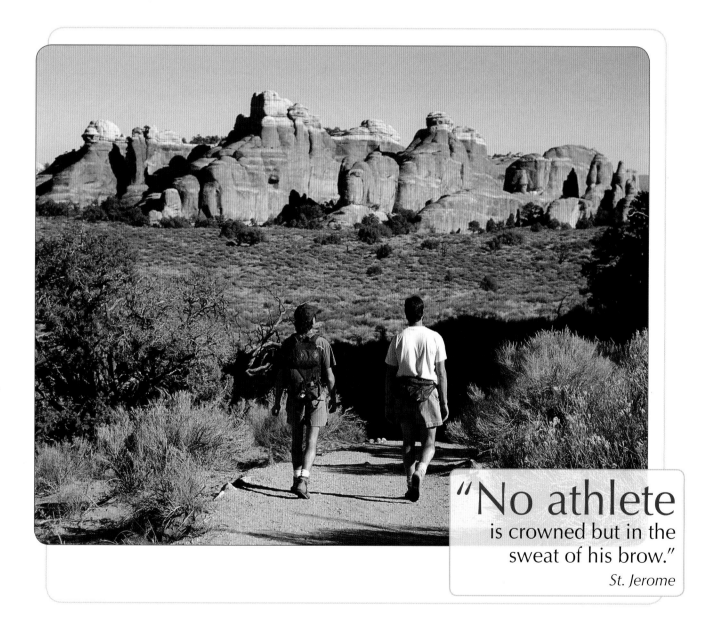

"No athlete is crowned but in the sweat of his brow."

St. Jerome

When you move to Montana you expect to face a cold and sometimes hostile environment, and you know that you will have the opportunity to spend time at higher elevations. But would you expect high temperatures in the summer or air pollution in a state with only 900,000 residents spread out over 150,000 square miles (388,500 square kilometers) of open space? Over the years we've learned some tricks for coping with and even enjoying environmental extremes.

Environmental factors such as heat and cold, humidity, altitude, and air pollution can profoundly affect health and performance. Failure to consider these effects can lead to serious problems, even death. On the other hand, you can adjust or acclimate to the environment, enabling you to perform well and comfortably under a wide range of conditions. Let's consider the problems caused by extremes of temperature, humidity, altitude, and air pollution to see how fitness and proper planning can minimize their effects.

This chapter will help you

- anticipate the effects of the environment on performance,
- take appropriate steps to minimize environmental effects, and
- understand how fitness enhances your ability to acclimatize and perform in difficult environments.

Regulating Temperature

The body's temperature-regulating mechanism consists of four parts:

- A regulating center located in the hypothalamus, an area at the base of the brain that serves as a thermostat to maintain body temperature at or near 37 degrees Celsius (98.6 degrees Fahrenheit)
- Heat and cold receptors located in the skin to sense changes in environmental temperature conditions
- Regulators such as muscles that increase body heat with shivering or exercise
- Vasomotor (nervous system) controls that constrict or dilate arterioles to conserve or lose body heat

The temperature-regulating center responds to the temperature of the blood flowing by the hypothalamus. If the blood cools, the thermostat sends information for the body to conserve heat by constricting blood vessels in the skin and the extremities. Shivering also can generate some heat.

If the blood temperature rises above the desired level (sometimes called a set point), the regulating center can cause dilation of cutaneous (skin) blood vessels and stimulate the production of sweat. Consequently, blood moves from the warmer core of the body to the surface, allowing heat loss by conduction, convection, and radiation as well as by evaporation of sweat from the surface of the skin. Complete evaporation of 1 liter of sweat leads to a heat loss of 580 calories. When the sweat does not evaporate and drips off the body little heat is lost.

Heat and cold receptors in the skin also help maintain body temperature. The cold of the ski slopes will cause constriction of blood vessels, especially in the hands and feet.

The extremities will stay cold until you raise body temperature, warm the blood, and reopen the blood vessels. The best way to do this is by vigorous exercise. Of course, you can put on more clothing or seek relief in the lodge.

The stifling heat of the tennis court will cause dilation of blood vessels, which diverts a significant amount of blood from the muscles to the skin. The heart rate increases in an effort to maintain blood flow to the working muscles and the skin. Sweating will eventually reduce blood volume, and unless you replace the water, your performance will suffer. If you persist in the activity and fail to replace the water loss, you may end up with heat exhaustion or heatstroke. So you are wise to listen to your body's call for rest, shade, and fluid replacement.

Individual differences in body fat, number of sweat glands, fitness level, and possibly gender may influence your response to heat.

- **Body fat.** Body fat serves as a layer of insulation beneath the surface of the skin. People with more subcutaneous fat may have better insulation from the cold, but they are not significantly less prone to lose excess heat to the environment because the body learns to route blood around the fat for cooling purposes. Excess fat is a handicap because the body needs extra energy just to carry it around.

- **Sweat glands.** Each of us inherits a certain number and pattern of sweat glands. Because evaporative heat loss is the most important protection against heat stress, a good supply of active sweat glands is important. Like almost everything else, sweat glands respond to use. If you use them a lot, they become more efficient.

- **Physical fitness.** Fitness seems to enhance the ability to regulate body temperature during work in the heat. It does so by lowering the temperature (set point) at which sweating begins. Thus fit people can work or play with lower heart rates and core temperatures than those of their unfit counterparts. In our lab a highly fit subject had a heart rate of 118, whereas less fit people had rates of 170 beats per minute while doing the same work on the treadmill (Cordes and Sharkey 1995). Acclimatization further lowers the point at which sweating begins. Therefore, the physically fit and heat-acclimated person is even better prepared for work in the heat (Nadel 1977). Recent evidence indicates that fitness hastens the process of acclimatization.

> Fitness seems to enhance the ability to regulate body temperature during work in the heat.

- **Gender.** Men produce more sweat than women do for a given increase in body temperature, perhaps too much. Women are efficient sweaters. Their sweat production is more suited to the heat load, so they don't waste water. When men and women are compared on the same task, men seem better able to work in the heat, but the difference may be due to fitness, not gender. When the fitness level is the same or when the workload is equal in terms of a given percentage of maximal oxygen intake, women are quite able to work in the heat. In several recent marathons, women seemed to tolerate the heat as well as or better than many men did, probably because they sweat more efficiently.

Other factors that can influence your response to heat are illness, medications, drugs, and alcohol. If you have been ill, your thermoregulatory system will take several days to recover. Many prescription and over-the-counter medications, as well as all recreational drugs and alcohol, can influence the body's response in a hot environment. If you are in doubt about medications or drugs, check with a physician or pharmacist before you risk exposure in a hot environment.

Exercising in the Heat

When exercise begins, the temperature-regulating center increases the usual set point of the body, allowing body temperature to increase. The rise in temperature depends on the intensity of exercise. In a moderate environment, the temperature will increase about 1 degree Celsius (1.8 degrees Fahrenheit) at 50 percent of maximal oxygen intake and will rise to about 39 degrees (102 degrees Fahrenheit), a rise of 2 degrees Celsius (3.6 degrees Fahrenheit), at the maximal level. This resetting of the core temperature during exercise can be viewed as an adjustment favorable to the enzyme activity within the muscles. The higher set point also serves to reduce the problem of heat dissipation. Under moderate environmental conditions, the body does not employ methods of heat dissipation until the elevated set point has been reached.

In hot environments we are able to maintain temporary thermal balance during exercise by virtue of circulatory adjustments and evaporation of sweat. The body gains heat when the air temperature exceeds the temperature of the skin. When humidity is low the evaporation of sweat maintains thermal equilibrium. But when humidity is high and evaporation cannot take place, heat is stored, body temperature rises, and performance is severely impaired. Blood is diverted from muscles to the skin, blood volume is reduced through sweating, and water and electrolytes are lost in the sweat. Stroke volume declines, heart rate increases, and lactic acid may accumulate. Blood may even begin to pool in the large veins, further reducing venous return and cardiac output. The result, an alarming rise in body temperature called hyperthermia, sets the stage for heat stress disorders, heat exhaustion, or even heatstroke, the potentially fatal collapse of the temperature-regulating mechanism (see "Heat Stress," page 333).

Fluid Replacement

In a normal day, we lose and must replace about 2.5 liters of water (1 liter equals 1.057 quarts; 1 quart equals 0.946 liter). Of this water loss, about 0.7 liter comes from the lungs and skin (insensible water loss), 1.5 liters from the urine, 0.2 liter from the feces, and about 0.1 liter through perspiration. During heavy exercise in the heat, the water lost through sweating can exceed 2 liters per hour. Sweat production may amount to as much as 12 liters per day. Because work capacity becomes impaired as water loss progresses, it is essential that the fluid be replaced. Dehydration in excess of 3 to 5 percent of body weight leads to a marked decline in strength, endurance, and work capacity. Estimate 1 liter for each 2-pound (.9-kilogram) weight loss; therefore, if you weigh 150 pounds (68 kilograms) and lose 8 pounds (3.6 kilograms), or more than 5 percent, you will be about 4 liters low on fluid!

> Because work capacity becomes impaired as water loss progresses, it is essential that the fluid be replaced.

The thirst mechanism always underestimates fluid loss during work in the heat and after work ends. Therefore, you should take frequent drinks throughout the work period. If you drink 250 milliliters (about 1 cup) every 15 minutes, you can replace 1 liter per hour. If the sweat rate is higher, you will find it extremely difficult to keep up with fluid needs. Marathon runners are wise to drink as much as possible (up to 500 milliliters) before the event to offset the tremendous water loss and difficulty of replacement. If, during prolonged periods of work in the heat, weight loss exceeds 2 percent (e.g., 3 pounds for a 150-pound person, or 1.4 kilograms for a 68-kilogram person), the person should rehydrate before returning to work or exercise.

You can assess your level of dehydration by observing the color of your urine. When the urine is clear or wheat colored, you are hydrated. When it is dark, you are dehydrated and should begin replacing fluids immediately (Armstrong 2000). Sweating rates and evaporative cooling depend on adequate hydration. Hyperhydration, or excess fluid intake, allows you to sweat more and work with a lower rectal temperature and heart rate, enabling increased work performance in hot work or sporting environments.

Hyponatremia

Excess intake of water during prolonged vigorous effort can lead to a dangerously low concentration of sodium, a condition known as hyponatremia. Symptoms range from weakness, disorientation, seizures, coma, and death. Unfortunately, the early symptoms sometimes lead to even greater water intake. Problems occur when athletes consume 3 or more liters of water per hour in a long event such as a marathon. For prolonged work we recommend a fluid intake of 1 liter per hour. The fluid should contain some electrolytes to replace those lost in the sweat.

Electrolytes

Water replacement will not compensate for the loss of electrolytes (sodium, chloride, and potassium) in the sweat. For each liter of sweat lost, approximately 1.5 grams of salt are lost as well. Because the average meal includes 3 to 4 grams of salt, three meals per day will satisfy most salt needs. For long periods (8 hours or more) of work in the heat, when considerable loss of water and salt will occur, workers and athletes should salt food liberally (8 hours at 1.5 grams of salt per liter equals 12 grams of salt loss). We do not recommend salt tablets for several reasons. They are slow to dissolve and leave the stomach, so they will not provide aid for several hours, and while they are dissolving they take needed water from the bloodstream through osmosis. In addition, excessive salt intake can cause stomach cramps, weakness, high blood pressure, and other problems. Recently developed electrolyte supplements help athletes maintain electrolyte balance during daylong competitions.

You have several choices for replacement of water and salt. You can buy solutions containing the necessary electrolytes as well as some glucose (carbohydrate–electrolyte beverages) but remember that you may have to replace several quarts (liters) of fluid. Replacing water and salt in this way could become expensive. You can save money by using the saltshaker at mealtime, drinking citrus fruit drinks for potassium, and obtaining the balance of fluid needs with water. Alternatively, you can prepare your own solution by adding a bit of salt to a quart of half-strength frozen lemonade. Another approach is to replace some of your fluid needs with tomato juice and the rest with water. When long periods of work in the heat make it necessary to replace electrolytes, use commercially available carbohydrate–electrolyte beverages or add a quarter teaspoon of salt to each quart (liter) of water and be sure to replace potassium during mealtime with citrus fruits or drinks, bananas, or other potassium-rich foods.

Carbohydrate–electrolyte sports drinks may offer several advantages. Their palatability ensures greater fluid intake, they help maintain blood glucose levels and performance during prolonged exertion, and the electrolytes reduce fluid loss through the urine. In addition, the carbohydrate helps maintain immune function (Ruby et al. 2003), and the elevated blood sugar serves to maintain cognitive function (Puchkoff et al. 1998).

Avoid very high glucose levels (over 8 percent) in fluid-replacement solutions while running in the heat; the glucose could retard emptying of the stomach and reduce delivery of essential fluid. In a marathon or other long-duration race, runners should drink cool (40 degrees Fahrenheit, or 4 degrees Celsius) electrolyte solutions that are relatively low in carbohydrate (under 40 to 80 grams per liter, or 4 to 8 percent). Cyclists and cross-country skiers can tolerate higher carbohydrate concentrations during exercise, especially in cool temperatures.

To maintain proper hydration, you should drink before, during, and after vigorous activity.

- Before: Drink 2 to 3 cups (500 to 750 milliliters) before the event.
- During: Drink a cup (250 milliliters) or more of fluid every 15 to 20 minutes, or 1 quart (1 liter) per hour.
- After: Replace fluid and carbohydrate after the event.

> To maintain hydration, you should drink before, during, and after vigorous activity.

After exercise, drink plenty of fluids and begin to replace carbohydrates to replace muscle glycogen. The best postexercise strategy is to eat high-glycemic foods (e.g., sweets, breads, potatoes) in the first 2 hours after exercise, a critical period for glycogen replacement. A four to one carbohydrate to protein ratio may help speed muscle recovery.

Replacing fluids and electrolytes is essential after vigorous exercise in the heat.

Heat Stress

When the body is at rest, metabolic heat production amounts to about 1.2 calories per minute, or 72 calories per hour. Moderate exercise can elevate heat production to 600 calories or more per hour. You can see that exercise, by itself, can create considerable heat. Normally, heat is lost by convection, radiation, or evaporation of sweat. But when exercise is performed in a hot environment or when the humidity is high, metabolic heat cannot be dissipated and the body temperature rises, as does the risk of heat disorders.

- Heat cramps occur when electrolytes are lost in the sweat. Take a sport drink and use stretching and massage to relieve the cramp.

- Heat exhaustion occurs when the heat stress exceeds the capacity of the temperature-regulating mechanism. A person with cold, pale skin; body temperature of 39 to 41 degrees Celsius (102 to 106 degrees Fahrenheit); a weak pulse; and dizziness should be given fluids and allowed to rest in a cool environment.

- Heatstroke means that the temperature-regulating mechanism has failed. The skin is flushed, hot, and dry; sweating stops; and body temperature may rise above 41 degrees Celsius (106 degrees Fahrenheit). Heatstroke can lead to permanent damage of the temperature-regulating center of the brain, or even to death. Heatstroke is a medical emergency! Cool the victim rapidly and administer fluids, if possible, while awaiting transport.

As you may have guessed, we cannot predict heat stress based on air temperature alone. Relative humidity is an important factor in determining how effective sweating will be. If sweat cannot evaporate, if it merely drips from the body, little heat is lost, and the water loss only adds to a circulatory problem. Air movement and radiant heat also are important factors to consider in evaluating the effect of a given environment on human comfort and performance. Even the type and color of clothing affect heat loss. Finally, we must consider metabolic heat production resulting from physical activity, because it is the major heat source.

One way to assess the risk of heat stress is to use the heat stress chart (figure 16.1). This chart is based on the shaded air temperature, moderate radiant heat from the sun, a light breeze, and a moderate work rate. Unfit or nonacclimated people will suffer at lower levels of heat, humidity, or work.

In sport or the workplace the wet bulb globe temperature (WBGT) provides a simple and accurate indication of the effect of environmental factors on active people. The index uses dry bulb and wet bulb thermometers to assess air temperature and relative humidity (see figure 16.2). The black copper globe thermometer indicates radiant heat as well as air movement. The several temperatures are weighted to indicate their relative contribution to the total heat stress. As you can see in the figure, the wet bulb temperature, or relative humidity, is the greatest contributor to heat stress (70 percent of the total).

The U.S. Marine Corps uses the WBGT to determine when to reduce or cancel physical training activities, and many high school and college athletic trainers and coaches use it to determine when to schedule practice sessions or distance runs. Bear in mind that the WBGT does not allow an estimate of the effect of clothing or energy expenditure. Dark or nonporous clothing can increase radiant heating or reduce evaporation. High levels of energy expenditure can create internal heat problems in moderate environments. No simple index tells you everything about heat stress, but for moderate energy expenditures (up to 425 calories per hour), while you are wearing light clothing (in color and weight), the WBGT is an excellent indicator of heat stress.

Heat Stress Chart

When heat and hard work combine to drive the body temperature up, the temperature-regulating mechanism begins to fail and the worker faces serious heat stress disorders. This dangerous—often deadly—combination of circumstances can be avoided by monitoring the environment with simple measurements of temperature and humidity. This chart can help alert individuals to dangerous heat stress conditions.

■ Extreme heat stress conditions. Only heat-acclimated individuals can work safely for extended periods. Take frequent breaks and replace fluids.

□ Watch for changing conditions. Heat-sensitive and nonacclimated individuals may suffer. Increase rest periods and be sure to replace fluids.

□ Little danger of heat stress for acclimated individuals. Lack of air movement, high radiant heat, and hard effort can raise danger.

Figure 16.1 Heat stress chart.
Reprinted from Sharkey, 1997.

Figure 16.2   WBGT Heat Stress Index

WBGT heat stress index						Example				
Wet bulb	=	_____ °F	×	.7	=	_____	80	×	.7	= 56
Dry bulb	=	_____ °F	×	.1	=	_____	90	×	.1	= 9
Black globe	=	_____ °F	×	.2	=	_____	120	×	.2	= 24
			WBGT		= _____ °F			WBGT		= 89° F

The wet bulb indicates humidity, the dry bulb measures the ambient temperature, and the black copper globe measures radiant heat and air movement.

Standards for work or exercise:

　　　Above 80° F—use discretion

　　　Above 85° F—avoid strenuous activity

　　　Above 88° F—cease physical activity*

*Trained people who have been acclimated to the heat can continue limited activity.

Reprinted from Sharkey, 1974.

Heat Acclimatization

On the first day of vigorous exercise in a hot environment, you may experience a near-maximal heart rate, elevated skin and core temperatures, and severe fatigue. But after just a few days of exposure to work in the heat, you can accomplish the same task with a lower heart rate, made possible by improved blood distribution and increased blood volume. Skin and core temperatures are lower, because sweating begins at a lower temperature (Wenger 1988). The loss of water in the urine diminishes, and the salt concentration of the sweat gradually declines. This increase in circulatory and cooling efficiency is called heat acclimatization, and most of the process occurs after 5 to 10 days of work in a hot environment (increases in sweat rate may take longer).

Highly fit people become acclimatized in 4 to 5 days, whereas sedentary subjects take twice as long. The best way to acclimatize is to work in the actual conditions (temperature and humidity) that you'll have to endure. If you live in a cool climate and don't have a heat chamber in which to achieve acclimatization, high-intensity training can get you halfway there, probably because of the heat generated during vigorous effort. Using a nonrubberized sweat suit will increase the temperature close to the skin. Fit people start to sweat at a lower body temperature, and they increase sweat production at a faster rate. Acclimatization helps move the set point for sweating even lower.

> Highly fit people become acclimatized in 4 to 5 days, whereas sedentary subjects take twice as long.

Less fit people should acclimatize using periods of light to moderate activity in a hot environment, alternated with rest periods during which they replace fluid. Electrolytes can be replaced with commercial drinks or the saltshaker at meals, plus potassium-rich citrus fruits or bananas. The vitamin C in the citrus drinks may hasten the acclimatization process.

In summary, the prescription for exercise in a hot, humid environment includes the following advice:

- Wear porous, light-colored, loose-fitting clothing.
- Acclimatize to the expected environment and workload (i.e., do 50 percent the first day, 60 percent the second, and add 10 percent each day until you do 100 percent on the sixth day).
- Take 250 to 500 milligrams a day of vitamin C while acclimatizing.
- Always replace water and electrolytes.
- Find a cool place for rest periods.
- Always work or train with a partner.
- Don't be too proud to quit when you feel the symptoms of heat stress (dizziness, confusion, cramps, nausea, clammy skin).
- Keep a record of body weight during prolonged periods of work or training in the heat. Weigh in before and after exercise to gauge fluid loss. To check for day-to-day rehydration, weigh yourself in the morning, after toilet but before breakfast.
- Maintain aerobic fitness; the enhanced circulatory system and blood volume will help you work better in the heat, acclimate faster, and hold your acclimatization longer.

Follow these suggestions and you can join the "mad dogs and Englishmen" out in the midday sun.

Exercising in the Cold

Because of the metabolic heat generated during exercise, cold temperatures do not pose a threat similar to that posed by hot, humid conditions. But severe exposure to low temperatures and high winds can lead to frostbite, freezing, hypothermia, and even death. Constriction of blood vessels (vasoconstriction) increases the insulating capacity of the skin, but it also results in a marked reduction in the temperature of the extremities. The body almost seems willing to lose a few fingers or toes to save the more important parts. Protective vasoconstriction often leads to severe discomfort in the fingers and toes. To relieve the pain, warm the affected area or raise the core temperature to allow reflexive return of blood to the extremities. Although shivering may cause some increase in temperature, gross muscular activity is far more effective in restoring heat to the troubled area. Because large muscle activity takes considerable energy, the cold-weather enthusiast must maintain a reserve of energy for use in emergencies. Excessive fatigue is the first step toward hypothermia and possible death.

Windchill

Windchill describes the effect of wind speed on heat loss (see figure 16.3). When the wind speed is 20 miles (32.2 kilometers) per hour, a reading of 10 degrees Fahrenheit (minus 12 degrees Celsius) is equivalent to minus 9 degrees Fahrenheit (minus 23 degrees Celsius). Runners, skiers, and skaters can create their own windchill. Skiing at 20 miles per hour on a 10-degree Fahrenheit day is equivalent to minus 9 degrees Fahrenheit. If the skier is moving into a wind, the effect is even worse. When possible, run, ski, or skate away from the wind. If you must face into the wind on a cold day, be sure to cover exposed flesh, including earlobes and the nose, and be on the lookout for frostbite.

Wind chill chart

Temperature (°F)																	
Calm	40	35	30	25	20	15	10	5	0	-5	-10	-15	-20	-25	-30	-35	-40	-45
5	36	31	25	19	13	7	1	-5	-11	-16	-22	-28	-34	-40	-46	-52	-57	-63
10	34	27	21	15	9	3	-4	-10	-16	-22	-28	-35	-41	-47	-53	-59	-66	-72
15	32	25	19	13	6	0	-7	-13	-19	-26	-32	-39	-45	-51	-58	-64	-71	-77
20	30	24	17	11	4	-2	-9	-15	-22	-29	-35	-42	-48	-55	-61	-68	-74	-81
25	29	23	16	9	3	-4	-11	-17	-24	-31	-37	-44	-51	-58	-64	-71	-78	-84
30	28	22	15	8	1	-5	-12	-19	-26	-33	-39	-46	-53	-60	-67	-73	-80	-87
35	28	21	14	7	0	-7	-14	-21	-27	-34	-41	-48	-55	-62	-69	-76	-82	-89
40	27	20	13	6	-1	-8	-15	-22	-29	-36	-43	-50	-57	-64	-71	-78	-84	-91
45	26	19	12	5	-2	-9	-16	-23	-30	-37	-44	-51	-58	-65	-72	-79	-86	-93
50	26	19	12	4	-3	-10	-17	-24	-31	-38	-45	-52	-60	-67	-74	-81	-88	-95
55	25	18	11	4	-3	-11	-18	-25	-32	-39	-46	-54	-61	-68	-75	-82	-89	-97
60	25	17	10	3	-4	-11	-19	-26	-33	-40	-48	-55	-62	-69	-76	-84	-91	-98

Wind (mph)

Frostbite times ▢ 30 minutes ▮ 10 minutes ▮ 5 minutes

Figure 16.3 Windchill index.
Courtesy of the National Oceanic and Atmospheric Administration.

Frostbite

Frostbite is damage to the skin resulting from exposure to extreme cold or windchill. As you can see on the windchill index, the danger of frostbite is minimal at temperatures above 20 degrees Fahrenheit (minus 7 degrees Celsius). A temperature or windchill of minus 20 degrees Fahrenheit (minus 29 degrees Celsius) seems necessary to produce the condition.

At first, frostbite appears as a patch of pale or white skin, because of the constriction of blood vessels in the area. After mild frostbite, the skin appears red and swollen when the blood returns. In severe frostbite, the skin may appear purple or black after it is warmed. Immersion in warm (not hot) water will hasten the return of blood to the area. Do not massage the affected part. Protect the groin and other sensitive areas to avoid the excruciating pain that occurs when circulation returns. If your feet become frostbitten on a winter outing, do not remove your boots to warm your feet. Your feet could swell and prevent you from being able to put your boots back on. Walk or ski out before removing your boots and warming your feet.

If you're worried about freezing the delicate tissues of the lungs during cold-weather exercise, don't. Cold air may make your breathing uncomfortable because it is so dry, but the danger of damage to the tissue is small. The respiratory system has a remarkable ability to warm and humidify air. Humans tolerate air temperatures well below minus 20 degrees Fahrenheit (minus 29 Celsius) without damage. The cold air is warmed to above 32 degrees Fahrenheit (0 degrees Celsius) before it reaches the bronchi. When the temperature goes below minus 20 degrees Fahrenheit, however, you should modify or curtail your exercise plans. The danger to earlobes, nose, fingers, and toes is great, and at much lower temperatures, respiratory tract damage is possible, though unlikely. Very cold air constricts airways and makes vigorous effort difficult. Use a scarf or mask to cover the mouth and nose if effort in very cold temperatures is necessary.

Hypothermia

When your body begins to lose heat faster than it can produce it, you are undergoing exposure. Prolonged exertion leads to progressive muscular fatigue. Shivering and vasoconstriction are attempts to preserve body heat and the temperature of vital organs. Exhaustion of energy stores and neuromuscular impairment lead to the virtual termination of activity. As exposure continues and your body loses additional heat, the cold reaches the brain. You then lose judgment and the ability to reason. Your speech becomes slow and slurred, you lose control of your hands, walking becomes clumsy, and you want to lie down and rest. Don't do it! You are hypothermic. Your core temperature is dropping, and without treatment you will lose consciousness and die.

You may be surprised to learn that most hypothermia cases occur in air temperatures above 30 degrees Fahrenheit (minus 1 degree Celsius). Cold water, windchill, and fatigue combine to set the stage for hypothermia. Avoid the problem by staying dry. If you become wet, dry off as soon as possible. Be aware of the windchill and how wind refrigerates wet clothing. During a cold-weather hike or ski tour, take off layers of clothing before you perspire and put them back on as you begin to cool. Eat and rest often to maintain your energy level. Stop or make camp when you still have energy. Don't wait until the situation is critical.

If someone exhibits the symptoms of hypothermia, transport the victim to a medical facility as quickly as possible. The heart may begin to fibrillate during rewarming, and emergency equipment will be needed. If immediate transport isn't possible, or if the case isn't severe, do the following:

- Get the victim out of the wind and rain.
- Remove all wet clothing.
- Provide dry clothing; warm drinks; and a warm, dry sleeping bag for a mildly impaired victim.
- If the victim is only semiconscious, try to keep the person awake and put him or her, unclothed, in a sleeping bag with another person.
- Build a fire.

Cold-Weather Clothing

Physiologists rate the insulating value of clothing in Clo units, with 1 Clo unit being equivalent to the clothing that will maintain comfort at a room temperature of 70 degrees Fahrenheit, or 21 degrees Celsius (roughly equivalent to a cotton shirt and slacks). Table 16.1 and figure 16.4 illustrate how the insulating requirements change during vigorous activity such as cross-country skiing or hiking (heavy work), light work, and rest. That variation is precisely why it is necessary to dress in layers in cold weather. At 0 degrees Fahrenheit (minus 18 degrees Celsius), a light shirt will be adequate during vigorous effort, whereas you may need 2 inches (5 centimeters) of insulation to maintain comfort at rest, and more for a good night's sleep.

Because perspiration is a major problem during exercise in the cold, you would be smart to buy a set of synthetic undergarments. These fabrics wick perspiration away from the skin so that evaporative cooling won't strip heat from the body. Next should come a wool or fleece layer for warmth. Layers of clothing provide an insulating barrier of air, and you can peel off layers as your temperature rises and put them back on as it falls.

Figure 16.4　Clothing requirements at different energy expenditures in the cold.

Table 16.1　Comfort Data

Effective temperature (° F)	THICKNESS OF INSULATION REQUIRED FOR COMFORT (IN.)		
	Sleeping	Light work	Heavy work
40 (4° C)	1.5 (3.8 cm)	0.8 (2.0 cm)	.20 (0.5 cm)
20 (–7° C)	2.0 (5.0 cm)	1.0 (2.5 cm)	.27 (0.7 cm)
0 (–18° C)	2.5 (6.4 cm)	1.3 (3.3 cm)	.35 (0.9 cm)
–20 (–29° C)	3.0 (7.6 cm)	1.6 (4.1 cm)	.40 (1.0 cm)
–40 (–40° C)	3.5 (8.9 cm)	1.9 (4.8 cm)	.48 (1.2 cm)

These figures are approximate but are a good base for an average healthy person.

A windproof and rainproof slicker should be all the additional clothing that you need during exercise. Invest in a breathable slicker if you can afford one, but don't expect any garment to handle the tremendous moisture load created during vigorous skiing or running. You can carry a down or pile coat in your pack for use at lunch or in camp. Modern, light, synthetic fabrics have several advantages over goose down. They are less expensive, easier to care for, and don't mat and lose insulating qualities when wet.

> With the right clothing you can enjoy outdoor activity in all but the most severe conditions.

Of course, you'll also need a hat and gloves. If you are a hot exerciser try a polypropylene ear band that allows heat loss from the top of the head. When you stop, put on a pile or wool hat to retain body heat. The same goes with gloves. Wear lighter ones during vigorous exercise but be ready to put on warm mitts for extended breaks. With the right clothing you can enjoy outdoor activity in all but the most severe conditions.

Cold Acclimatization

Are we able to adjust to the cold as we are able to acclimatize to hot environments? If so, what are the physiological mechanisms involved? Specific examples of cold acclimatization appear in the research literature (Folk 1974). One mechanism is a metabolic adjustment wherein metabolism increases as much as 35 percent. The female divers (Ama) of the Korean Peninsula evidence this adjustment, as well as improved tissue insulation during the winter months when the water temperature falls to 50 degrees Fahrenheit (10 degrees Celsius). Australian aborigines are able to sleep in cold conditions through a hypothermic response, a lowering of the core temperature from 98.6 degrees Fahrenheit (37 degrees Celsius) to a more easily maintained 95 degrees Fahrenheit (35 degrees Celsius). Of course, natural selection and heredity play important roles in adaptation to cold environments. Large body mass, short extremities, high levels of body fat, and deep routing of venous circulation also help.

Repeated exposure to cold seems to lead to physiological and psychological adjustments that allow one to tolerate and enjoy physical activity in cold environments (Young 1988). We may perceive near-freezing temperatures as bitter in November but balmy in February. The extra calories that we consume in fall and winter lead to extra weight and an increase in the insulating layer of subcutaneous fat. The extra fat may be why we can cross-country ski barehanded at 25 degrees Fahrenheit (minus 4 degrees Celsius) in February!

Finally, let us remind you of the need for hydration during exercise in the cold. The body is perspiring and losing water vapor as you exhale. Plan to carry and use a water bottle or hydration system, and consider a carbohydrate drink and energy snacks to help maintain energy levels.

Exercising at Altitude

More than 40 million people live at altitudes above 10,000 feet (3,000 meters), and some live above 17,000 feet (5,200 meters). No permanent habitations are found above 18,000 feet (5,500 meters), however, indicating that such an elevation may be incompatible with adaptation and long-term survival. Indeed, the upper reaches of 29,000-foot-high (8,840-meter-high) Mount Everest have been called the death zone.

Although arterial oxygen desaturation begins as we move upward from sea level, elevations below 5,000 feet (1,500 meters) have little noticeable effect on otherwise healthy people. But as you ascend to higher elevations to ski, hike, climb, or even to live, barometric pressure declines along with available levels of atmospheric and alveolar oxygen. When this occurs, the arterial blood is unable to become highly saturated, less oxygen is transported, and the tissues are forced to operate with a reduced supply (see table 16.2). Thus, in spite of the heroic efforts of the oxygen intake and transport systems, altitude always leads to a reduction in aerobic fitness and associated endurance performance.

Table 16.2   Altitude and Oxygen

Altitude (ft)	Barometric pressure (mmHg)	PO_2 in air (mmHg)	PAO_2 alveoli (mmHg)	Resting arterial O_2 saturation (%)	Aerobic fitness (% of sea level max)
0	760	159	105	97	100
3,200 (980 m)	680	142	94	96	
6,500 (1,980 m)	600	125	78	94	90
10,000 (3,050 m)	523	111	62	90	
14,100 (4,300 m)	450	94	51	86	75
18,400 (5,600 m)	380	75	42	80	
23,000 (7,000 m)	305	64	31	63	50
29,141 (8,800 m)	230	48	19	30	

In this age of easy travel, you can quickly ascend to a national park or ski resort located above 5,000 feet (1,500 meters). When you arrive, you'll have to adjust cardiac output for a given workload. The heart rate is higher, but the stroke volume may be lower because of diminished oxygen supply to the heart muscle. You bring more air into the lungs each minute, and this hyperventilation leads to increased carbon dioxide exhalation and the acid–base disturbances associated with mountain sickness. The symptoms—headache, shortness of breath, rapid heartbeat, loss of appetite—appear at 8,000 feet (2,400 meters) or above. Work capacity declines at altitude, as does the motivation to perform hard work.

Does a high level of physical fitness provide some advantage to the newcomer? On arrival, the conditioned person maintains his or her sea-level advantage over the unfit person, but no more. The trained person will be able to do less than he or she could at sea level and is just as likely as others are to suffer mountain sickness. At very high elevations, some highly trained endurance athletes have been found to be "nonresponders" whose respiration fails to adjust adequately to the added demands of the altitude (Jackson and Sharkey 1988).

Altitude Acclimatization

Profound changes occur soon after one ascends to a higher elevation. Pulmonary ventilation increases, so more air can be moved into the lungs. This increase doesn't take more energy, because the air is less dense at higher elevations. Oxygen transport gradually improves through increases in red blood cells, hemoglobin, and blood volume. Above 15,000 feet (4,600 meters) the red blood cells increase from 5 million

Exercise more slowly or for a shorter distance when training at altitude.

per cubic millimeter to 6.6 million, and hemoglobin rises from 15 grams per 100 milliliters to above 20. These changes make the blood more viscous, but that isn't a problem because the hypoxia (lower oxygen tension) of altitude serves to vasodilate or relax the arterioles. Altitude exposure may cause an increase in lung and muscle capillaries, and myoglobin, the molecule that serves to store oxygen in muscles, also is increased at higher elevations (Smith and Sharkey 1984).

A good adjustment to higher elevation occurs in about 3 weeks, or about 1 week for each 1,000 feet (300 meters) above 5,000 feet (1,500 meters). Once acclimated, your oxygen intake and transport systems will be better able to supply oxygen to the working muscles. These adjustments reduce but never eliminate the effect of altitude on aerobic fitness. Endurance performance will always decline at altitude, regardless of your state of acclimatization. Unfortunately, these hard-earned changes (they occur only when you work at altitude) are reversible; they return to prealtitude values within weeks after you leave the mountains.

Altitude Training

Because of the reduced ability to take in oxygen at altitudes above 5,000 feet (1,500 meters), your usual pace will be more anaerobic than usual. You have several options. You can do your usual distance but go more slowly, go at your usual pace but for shorter distances, or (our favorite) slow down and enjoy the view. Go sightseeing and forget about distance or pace. If you are training to compete at altitude, you should realize that the slower pace may cause your speed to slip a little. Occasional shorter but faster runs should help avoid that problem (athletes sometimes drop to lower elevations for speed work).

For years, coaches and athletes have sought the ultimate training stimulus at a moderate altitude of 5,000 to 10,000 feet (1,500 to 3,000 meters). They believe that reduced availability of oxygen to muscles (hypoxia) is the stimulus that causes changes in aerobic fitness, and that exercise at moderate altitude ensures extreme tissue hypoxia. So they travel to a training site at 6,000 to 9,000 feet (1,800 to 2,700 meters) to train for several weeks or months before returning to sea level for a major event such as the Olympic Games. Unfortunately, the effort may not be worth it for all athletes. One study showed that a small benefit resulted from altitude training on return to sea level, but the study did not use a control group. A replication of the study with a control group found that altitude training was no more effective than equally arduous sea-level training. The subjects were highly trained middle-distance runners, 17 to 23 years old, who trained for 3 weeks either at sea level or at 7,500 feet (2,300 meters) (Adams et al. 1975). Arduous effort at sea level also leads to tissue hypoxia.

Live High, Train Low

The benefits of altitude training do not seem to help all athletes equally. A study helps explain why some respond and others do not. Male and female collegiate runners participated in a 28-day live-high, train-low investigation (2,500 meters and 1,250 meters, respectively, or 8,200 feet and 4,100 feet) of the effects of altitude. Those who improved in performance (in a 5,000-meter run) were called responders; those who did not were labeled nonresponders. Responders displayed a significant increase in erythropoietin (Epo), a compound that stimulates production of red blood cells in bone marrow. The authors concluded that the improvement in performance depended, in part, on *(a)* living high enough to increase Epo, red blood cell volume, and $\dot{V}O_2$max; and *(b)* training low enough to maintain interval-training velocity near sea-level values (Chapman, Stray-Gunderson, and Levine 1998). A recent development has been the use of altitude tents to simulate sleeping at higher elevations. Preliminary results suggest that the hypoxia of altitude chambers can lead to improvements in the oxygen-carrying capacity of the blood.

Casual observers of sport may be quick to conclude that an athlete's performance is due to his or her residence at high altitude. Several outstanding African athletes have emerged to perpetuate the practice of altitude training. The athletes live above 7,000 feet (2,100 meters), but many observers forget that the athletes were born there and lived there most of their lives. Their parents were born there, as were their grandparents. So the benefit that these observers identify as resulting from training at altitude is, in reality, a product of natural selection combined with long-term residence at a higher elevation, not just a few weeks of altitude training.

Avoiding the Effects of Air Pollution

Long-term exposure to respirable particulate has been associated with heart and lung disease; ozone exposure has been associated with lung and heart problems; and carbon monoxide exposure is associated with central nervous system and heart problems. Do we have to check the local air pollution index before going outside to exercise? In some cities children's school recesses and sporting events are canceled when pollution rises. If you fly over any major city in the United States, you'll see the pall of pollution that daily diminishes the quality of our lives. Although some forms of pollution are most dangerous for old or weak people, young children, and those with respiratory and cardiac problems, other forms attack physically active people. Exercise increases the volume of air taken into the lungs each minute. Because pollution-related respiratory disorders often are related to the degree of exposure, avoiding or reducing exercise in polluted atmospheres seems wise.

We are beginning to recognize the many sources of air pollution as threats to the quality of life and to life itself. Efforts are under way to lower carbon monoxide, dust, and soot (respirable particulate); sulfur dioxide; and other pollutants. Some pollutants are relatively harmless by themselves, but in combination with others they can exert potent biological effects.

The biological effects of air pollution include the following:

- Deadening of ciliary action
- Reduction of oxygen-transport capacity (because carbon monoxide competes for space on hemoglobin molecules)
- Suppression of the immune system
- Chronic obstructive pulmonary disease, including alveolar breakdown in emphysema, irritation of airways in chronic bronchitis, and loss of diffusing surfaces in pulmonary fibrosis
- Lung and other cancers
- Heart disease

> Studies have shown that smoking contributes to depression and impotence, and it has been associated with musculoskeletal and low-back problems and with long-term disability.

Although many forms of industrial, urban, and automotive pollution are troublesome, nauseating, or even fatal, no single source of pollution is as deadly as the cigarette, which causes most of the biological effects just listed. Smoking can irritate the bronchial tubes; deaden ciliary action and make the smoker more susceptible to infection, chronic bronchitis, and emphysema; reduce oxygen transport; and cause lung cancer and heart disease. In the United States, cigarette smoking is responsible for 400,000 deaths annually! Studies have shown that smoking contributes to depression and impotence, and it has been associated with musculoskeletal and low-back problems and with long-term disability (Amoroso et al. 1996).

To gain a perspective on the risks of smoking versus industrial pollution and the extreme risk of combining the two, consider the risks of dying from lung cancer. Although an asbestos worker has a lung cancer mortality rate 5 times that of the general population, a smoker's rate is 10 times greater, and the asbestos worker who smokes has a rate 87 times greater than that of the population (USDHEW 1979).

We must continue the fight for clean air so that we don't have to regulate our activities in accordance with the air pollution index or see our enjoyment of physical activity decline because of humankind's mistreatment of the environment. In the meantime, you should avoid exercise in obviously dangerous areas (along expressways, near industrial pollution) and when air pollution warnings are in effect. That recommendation doesn't mean that you shouldn't exercise; you just need to find a way to avoid the pollution. Be sure to add your voice to the growing fight against all forms of pollution, including the worst of all, the cigarette.

Summary

In this chapter we've outlined the problems encountered in different environments and provided practical advice on how to minimize the problems and maximize performance and enjoyment. Solutions range from improving fitness and acclimatization to dressing properly and maintaining hydration and energy. Fitness, although especially important in the heat, improves performance in all environments. Acclimatization is necessary for heat and altitude and useful in the cold. Fluid replacement is critical in the heat, but it is also extremely important in the cold and at altitude, where breathing causes the loss of considerable fluid. Maintaining energy levels is essential to prolonged performance in all environments. Finally, proper clothing is required to cope with the demands of the environment.

But what about air pollution? What can we do to minimize its effects? The answers are simple. Minimize exposure and maintain your immune system with regular exercise, rest, and good nutrition. Include immune-friendly foods in your diet (see chapter 11). If your diet is inadequate, consider antioxidant supplements to counter the free radicals found in pollutants. Minimize exposure by exercising where or when pollution levels are lowest. If you are particularly sensitive to pollutants or allergens, you may want to use a dust mask to filter particles or a mask impregnated with activated charcoal to absorb pollutants. Unfortunately, simple masks do not remove carbon monoxide, so avoid high-traffic areas during exercise.

Part VI

Vitality and Longevity

The prevailing view of aging is a dreary one, depicting a life of limits and ailments, a vicious cycle with loss of function, frailty, and failure. Fortunately, you do not have to accept this tragic opera as your script. If you are willing to adopt the appropriate lifestyle, you will be able to take command of your role, to write and perform an epic that features a long and satisfying life.

The final chapters of this book are designed to help you develop the daily habits, psychosocial skills, and other behaviors that contribute to a happy, healthy, and vigorous life. Daily habits are an indispensable part of your life, and the appropriate habits contribute to health and the quality of life. Psychosocial skills are necessary for a full and complete life. Chapter 18 provides ways to use psychology to help motivate and maintain your commitment to regular, moderate physical activity.

The goal is to be vigorous and fully involved throughout life, to live each stage to the fullest. In return for your efforts you will retain the vitality and mobility needed for a full, independent life, and you may even live longer. But the most compelling outcome of the active life is that you'll add life to your years, not just years to your life. Stated simply, you'll extend the prime of life.

Age, Activity, and Vitality

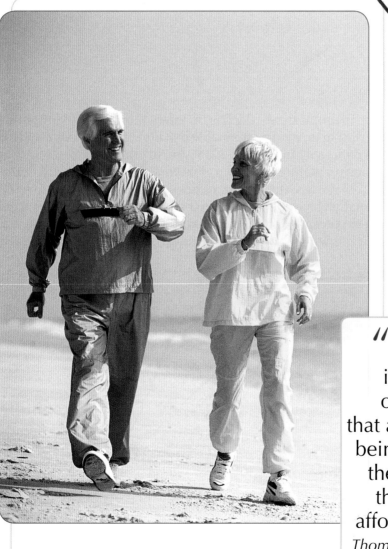

"Time is really the only capital that any human being has, and the one thing that he can't afford to lose."

Thomas Alva Edison

Age tells little about your health, your appearance, your fitness, or your ability to perform. Although aging inevitably leads to death, it does so at different rates for different people, depending on heredity and on personal decisions about how you choose to age.

Sometime after the peak reproductive years, when the direct evolutionary advantage has passed, virtually all tissues and organs begin to age. Parents remain important, at least until the child becomes a young adult, and grandparents serve to pass on wisdom or assist the parents. But when a person reaches the 70s, biological justification to continue life diminishes, and indeed, life expectancies range from 78 to 79 for women and 73 to 74 for men. But life expectancies, which have risen throughout the past century, tell only part of the story.

This chapter will help you

- differentiate life expectancy from life span,
- understand how activity and other habits influence longevity,
- appreciate how fitness influences your physiological age, and
- understand how activity and fitness extend the prime of life.

Life Span

Life expectancy has gone up in proportion to declines in infant mortality and infectious diseases. But the attainable life span, the age attainable in a life free of serious accident or illness, has not changed noticeably in the past 200 years. In other words, we are not living longer; we are avoiding premature death. Survival curves point to a theoretically attainable life span of about 85 years, with a standard deviation of 4 years (figure 17.1). Thus 68 percent of the population have the potential to live between 81 and 89 years (85 plus or minus 4 years), and 95 percent of deaths from natural causes would fall between 77 and 93 years (85 plus or minus two standard deviations, or 8 years). Rare indeed

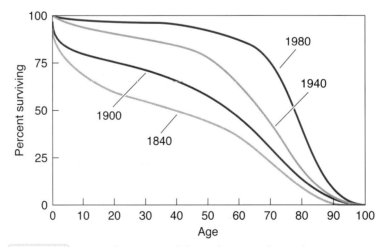

Figure 17.1 Survival curves. With less infant mortality and trauma (accidental death), more people survive to the attainable life expectancy, 85 years. With good health habits, more are able to postpone chronic debilitating illness, to remain vigorous until the last years or months of life.
Adapted from National Center for Health Statistics, 1977.

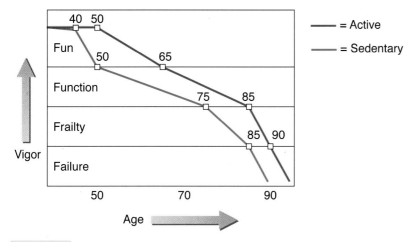

Figure 17.2 Vigor and the active life. Active living extends the periods of fun and function and shortens the time of frailty and failure.

are people who live beyond 97 years, more than three standard deviations above the mean. The oldest documented life spans are in the neighborhood of 120 years (Fries and Crapo 1981).

Postponement of chronic illness has extended the period of adult vigor, so life remains physically, emotionally, and intellectually vigorous until shortly before its close (figure 17.2). Appropriate behaviors can modify many of the factors believed to be associated with age, including heart and lung function, bone density, blood pressure, and cholesterol. People who choose not to age rapidly can reduce morbidity and extend the vigorous years by living an active, healthy life (Fries and Crapo 1981). On the other hand, those who decide to age rapidly are destined to become a burden on family, health care, and community support systems.

> Activity adds life to your years as well as years to your life! Unfortunately, as some have said, the years you add all come at the end.

Earlier we quoted studies that indicate an increase in longevity for those who lead the active life. Activity adds life to your years as well as years to your life! Unfortunately, as some have said, the years you add all come at the end. And some have suggested that the years you add are about equal to the time that you spent in exercise. Can that be true? One study found at least a 2-year increase in life expectancy associated with activity. If you exercise 1 hour every day for 40 years, you'll spend 14,560 hours engaged in exercise. Divide that number by 24 hours per day, and you get 607 days, or 1.67 years, somewhat less than the 2 years or more that you'll earn. Of course, you will enjoy the time you spend in exercise, recreation, and sport, and you will extend the years of fun and function, the prime of life.

Theories of Aging

Theories of aging are many, including those dealing with gene defects or chromosomal damage, errors in protein synthesis, and limits to the number of cell divisions (the Hayflick limit). Other factors associated with aging include caloric intake, inherited factors, free radicals, and stress.

- **Caloric restriction.** Animal studies have shown that eating fewer calories (up to 40 percent less) can extend survival time dramatically (28 percent in one study) when adult animals were put on a low-protein diet (Miller and Payne 1968). Some researchers have felt that the most important factors determining life span were those that influenced body fatness. Animals fed fewer calories also had a lower tumor incidence and less chronic disease (Comfort 1979). When Alexander Leaf studied healthy old people in three remote parts of the world, he found their diets low in calories and fat (1973). Leaf believed that the low-calorie diet, combined with regular activity and a productive and respected role in society, contributed to good health and long life.

Activity helps you extend the physically and mentally vigorous years of your life.

■ **Inherited factors.** People with exceptional longevity and their offspring have significantly larger low-density lipoprotein (LDL) cholesterol particles, which are associated with lower prevalence of hypertension, cardiovascular disease, and metabolic syndrome. This genetic variation is favorable because the larger LDL is less likely to adhere to artery walls. Although genes probably determine this favorable particle size, studies suggest that exercise can enlarge the LDL particles (Barzalai et al. 2003).

■ **Free radicals.** One theory of aging holds that so-called free radicals (reactive molecules with one or more unpaired electrons) prove toxic to vulnerable tissues. In the biologic world, life span is inversely related to metabolic rate. Exercise produces free radicals that can harm the body. But moderate activity enhances antioxidant protection and the immune system. Chronic heavy exertion may produce an excess of free radicals, raise the risk of heart disease, and depress the immune response (Demopoulos et al. 1986). The role of free radicals in exercise and aging requires more study. In the meantime, vitamins C and E and other antioxidants are believed to provide some protection against these potentially toxic by-products of oxidative metabolism.

■ **Stress.** Working in a stressful job is associated with a doubling of the risk of death from cardiovascular disease. Workers with the greatest disparity between effort and reward and those with high job strain and perceived lack of control over their jobs were more than twice as likely to die from heart disease compared with those with a better balance between these factors (Kivimaki et al. 2002).

In terms of aging, studies of women caring for the chronically ill or children suggest that stress or the perception of stress is linked to aging. Researchers studied telomeres, DNA protein complexes that cap the ends of chromosomes and promote genetic stability. As cells divide a portion of the telomere is lost, and after considerable loss, the cell stops dividing. The oxidative stress of continuous care was linked with shortening of the telomeres of the cells, equivalent to a decade of additional aging when compared with women under low stress (Epel et al. 2004).

> What is surprising is the realization that the rate of decline or senescence is not fixed but variable, subject to considerable modification.

At present no single theory explains the decline that occurs with age. What is surprising is the realization that the rate of decline or senescence is not fixed but variable, subject to considerable modification. A list of changeable aspects of aging has emerged, markers that are subject to changes brought about by one's personal decisions and behaviors (Fries and Crapo 1981) (table 17.1).

A definite pattern emerges from a consideration of the changeable aspects of aging, a pattern that points to the importance of daily habits as the way to improve your health span, your active life expectancy.

Table 17.1 Changeable Aspects of Aging

Aging marker	Personal decision or behavior
Cardiac output	Exercise
Glucose tolerance	Exercise, diet, weight control
Osteoporosis	Weight-bearing exercise, diet
Pulmonary function	Exercise, nonsmoking
Blood pressure	Exercise, diet, weight control
Endurance and strength	Exercise
Reaction time	Training, practice
Cholesterol	Diet, weight control, exercise
Arterial wall rigidity	Diet, exercise
Intelligence and memory	Training, practice
Skin aging	Avoid sun

Several factors affected by aging appear to be nonmodifiable. These include graying and thinning of hair, elasticity of skin, kidney reserve, and degeneration of the eyes including cataracts and macular degeneration.

Adapted from Fries and Crapo, 1981.

Health Habits

Since 1962, researchers at the Human Population Laboratory of the California Department of Health have studied the relationship of health to various behaviors or habits. Health and longevity are associated with the following:

- Adequate sleep (7 to 8 hours per day)
- A good breakfast
- Regular meals—avoid snacks
- Weight control
- Not smoking cigarettes
- Moderate alcohol consumption
- Regular exercise

The study found that men could add 11 years to their lives and women 7 years, just by following six of the habits (Breslow and Enstrom 1980). Let's examine each practice to see whether it fits your current lifestyle. Then you can decide if changes are in order.

SLEEP When men or women sleep 6 hours or less per night, they are not as healthy as when they sleep 7 or 8 hours. Those who sleep 9 hours or more are slightly below average in health. Thus 7 to 8 hours of sleep is most favorable, and, as you might expect, too little sleep is more of a problem than too much.

Sleep is characterized by alternating stages. One stage involves rapid eye movements (REM) and changes in heart rate, blood pressure, and muscle tone. This stage may serve as a rest period for the inhibitory nerve cells of the brain. It usually is accompanied by dreams, and if it is interrupted we become anxious and irritable. This REM sleep constitutes about 20 percent of the total for the night. Deeper or quieter periods provide the rest necessary for recovery from fatigue. If you miss some sleep one night, the body will not make any serious attempt to recover the sleep deprivation. But if a substantial amount of the loss is REM sleep, more REM sleep will occur on subsequent nights (figure 17.3). Going without sleep seems to impair cre-

Figure 17.3 The stages of sleep.

ative capabilities, which suggests that another function of sleep is to restore a cerebral cortex fatigued by consciousness.

Moderate physical activity seems to enhance the ability to fall into deep sleep without altering the time spent in REM sleep. Too little or too much exercise appears to result in sleep disturbance, and significant sleep loss seems to suppress the immune system.

BREAKFAST   In the California study, those who ate breakfast almost every day experienced better health than those who ate breakfast some of the time (Breslow and Enstrom 1980). Furthermore, a good breakfast may be a prerequisite to good performance in work and sport. Breakfast often comes 12 hours after the evening meal, so you can see why it is important for energy and cellular metabolism. A few researchers suggest that breakfast should be the largest and most important meal of the day, and everyone agrees that it should include more than a cup of coffee and a doughnut.

REGULAR MEALS   Erratic eaters have poorer health than those who eat regular meals. Those who seldom or never eat between meals have better health than those who regularly eat between meals. Unfortunately, this study did not compare the health status of those who eat smaller but more numerous nutritious meals, but it does indicate the effects of erratic eating behavior and snacking. We can only guess at the content of the between-meal snacks, but chances are that they were toxic foods, high in simple sugars and saturated fat and low in nutrients (Breslow and Enstrom 1980).

WEIGHT CONTROL   When weight is more than 20 percent above, or more than 10 percent below, the desirable weight, health status declines. For example, if your desirable weight is 150 pounds (68 kilograms), your health status is most favorable when you maintain your weight between 135 pounds (61.2 kilograms; minus 10 percent) and 180 pounds (81.6 kilograms; plus 20 percent), a broad margin of error indeed. An interesting study would be to compare the effects on health of low body weight (more than 10 percent below desirable) because of malnutrition, illness, or smoking with the effects of low body weight resulting from habitual, vigorous exercise. Personal observation indicates that low body weight associated with vigorous exercise and good nutrition is at least as healthy as being at or above the desirable weight.

SMOKING   Smoking remains the leading modifiable cause of death in the United States (435,000 deaths in 2000). But factors associated with overweight and obesity—poor diet and physical inactivity—may soon overtake tobacco as the leading cause of death (400,000 deaths) (Mokdad et al. 2004). If you don't smoke, don't start.

If you do smoke, stop. Quitting could be the best thing that you ever did for yourself. If you can't stop for your own health, think of loved ones, especially children, who are exposed to your habit.

Secondhand tobacco smoke is responsible for asthma and respiratory problems, not to mention lung cancers, for many thousands of children. Is quitting worth the trouble? Data from numerous studies show that quitting has many benefits, including better oxygen-carrying capacity, lower blood pressure, improved night vision, and increased effectiveness of prescription drugs. Although some tobacco-related diseases, such as emphysema, cannot be reversed, others seem to repair with time. Repair time for smoking-induced illnesses include 10 years for heart disease and 10 to 15 years for cancer. Quit today and help make the nation smoke free.

ALCOHOL   Poor health is associated with heavy alcohol consumption (five or more drinks at one sitting). Those who never drink and those who drink moderately (one to two drinks a day for men, one to three per week for women) enjoy the same level of good health. The French paradox ponders why the French seem to tolerate rich foods without an increase in heart disease. The answer may lie in regular consumption of wine. Some studies show that those who drink one or two alcoholic drinks daily have a lower risk of heart disease, perhaps because alcohol is associated with higher levels of HDL cholesterol (Gaziano et al. 1993). You should not construe this finding as a broad endorsement of alcohol consumption. Some level of alcohol consumption, if continued for a sufficient period, may lead to degenerative effects on the liver, even when nutrition is adequate. The best advice is to drink moderately (one to two drinks per day for men, one every other day for women) or to avoid drinking altogether. And no, you cannot save your daily drinks for a weekend binge.

REGULAR ACTIVITY   Researchers in the California study compared the health benefits of five types of activity: active sports, swimming or long walks, garden work, physical exercises, and hunting and fishing. Only hunting and fishing (seasonal and infrequent) were not associated with improved health. For all the other activities, those who participated most often experienced the best physical health. The best health was associated with active sports, followed by swimming or walking, physical exercise, and gardening. The lowest death rates occurred among those who were often active in sports, and the highest death rates were for those who chose not to engage in any exercise.

In summary, physical health, longevity, and the rate of aging are associated with your daily health habits and your lifestyle. These health habits have more to do with your health and longevity than all the influences of medicine. The California study indicated that a man 55 years old who follows all seven health habits has the same health status as a person 25 to 30 years younger who follows fewer than two. Moreover, the researchers found a positive relationship between physical and mental health (Breslow and Enstrom 1980). You know that an association or relationship between variables does not imply cause and effect, that good physical health doesn't necessarily cause good mental health, but you are probably familiar with psychosomatic illnesses and should realize that the opposite effects are possible. A healthy body is an important aid to good mental health, and you can help maintain physical health by following the recommended health habits.

> Your daily health habits and your lifestyle have more to do with your health and longevity than all the influences of medicine.

Longevity

One key to longevity, to what it takes to live well beyond normal life expectancy, is your lifestyle. Observations of healthy older people (aged 75 years and over) provide intriguing insights into the personality traits and living habits associated with long-term survival. The following characteristics are associated with longevity:

- **Moderation.** Moderation is a common denominator in all phases of life, including diet, vices, work, and physical activity. Long-term survival in a footrace or the human race depends on pacing.

- **Flexibility.** Psychological flexibility implies the ability to bend but not break, to accept change, to avoid rigid habits.

- **Challenge.** Accept challenges. Create them if necessary. Don't allow life to become too easy. But when a challenge becomes too great, say so, and seek an alternative.

- **Health habits.** A relaxed attitude toward health characterizes long-term survival. Older "survivors" are unconcerned and not obsessive about health habits. They eat a variety of foods and are not terribly concerned about avoiding items such as cholesterol. They are moderate in their use of alcohol, and some even smoke now and then. These people demonstrate the need for balance and moderation and in general lead healthy lifestyles.

- **Relationships.** Older citizens enjoy other people. They maintain an interest in and continuous contact with friends and family. They enjoy their marriages.

Regular involvement in activity is one key to longevity.

- **Outlook.** Healthy elders maintain a positive outlook. They recognize the effects of advancing age and plan to enjoy each phase of life. They realize that long life means growing old, and they are prepared to enjoy both.
- **Active life.** Of course, those who age successfully are engaged in daily routines that require activity. They find reasons to be socially and physically active. Involvement in daily chores provides the purpose, rhythm, and activity that everyone needs.

The active life can benefit you in a number of ways, including the following:

- **Health.** Regular activity enhances both physical and mental health.
- **Mobility.** Regular aerobic activity, supplemented with resistance exercises, retains or restores mobility and the capacity for a free and independent life.
- **Economy.** To save money, walk, jog, or ride a bike. Cross-country skis are cheaper than a snowmobile and better for you.
- **Ecology.** The active life, with emphasis on muscle-powered sport and recreation, helps conserve limited energy supplies. Physically active people have less effect on the environment than do their sedentary counterparts who use energy-consuming recreational vehicles and leaf blowers.
- **Adaptability.** The active person retains the ability to adapt to changes in life, the economy, or the environment.
- **Survival.** Older people are survivors. Along the way they accumulate wisdom and insights that have value to coming generations. The axiom in nature applies to the human race as well: The fittest survive. When fitness is measured and subjects are followed for years, the data supporting the concept of survival of the fittest are strong and compelling (Balady 2002).

Active people view each moment as one to be lived. They avoid people who depress them. When they feel moody or depressed, they do something. They take risks, engage in life, and enjoy it. They don't waste the present with moods, worry, or immobilizing thoughts about the future. Depression, worry, guilt, and anger can lead to (or be caused by) subtle changes in brain chemistry and hormone levels. Physical activity can directly affect moods and the chemistry of behavior, and it can divert attention and provide enjoyment and a sense of self-satisfaction that minimizes or eliminates self-defeating behavior.

You are free to think, feel, and act as you desire. Circumstances, biorhythms, behavior traits, genetics, or deep-seated psychological problems do not control you. You can create the life that you desire, if you really want to. Don't fall back on excuses like "I haven't got the time," "I'll start next week (month, year)," "I'm too busy right now, but when the kids are a little older . . ."

Finally, consider the factors that characterize the "happy–well" group in a longitudinal study (Vaillant 2001). Six factors, measured at age 50, predicted the most successful group at age 80: a stable marriage, a mature adaptive style, no smoking, little alcohol, maintenance of normal weight, and regular exercise.

Age and Performance

As we've said, chronological age is a poor predictor of health or performance. Health is a function of your habits, heredity, environment, and previous illness. Performance in work or sport is a function of physiological age, not chronological age.

Physiological Age

Physiological age (also called biological or functional age) is a composite of health, physiological capacity, and performance measures. The best single measure of physiological age is probably the aerobic fitness score. That number tells you about the health and capacity of the respiratory, circulatory, and muscular systems. Moreover, a considerable body of evidence shows an inverse relationship between aerobic fitness and a number of risk factors. Thus a 55-year-old may have the health and performance capability of the average 25- to 30-year-old. This fact has considerable relevance when it comes to changing our society's view of aging and its consequences, such as age discrimination in hiring. Age does not ensure a rapid decline in performance, and when physical performance is important, physiological age is a more accurate predictor of performance potential than chronological age (Sharkey 1987).

Other indicators of physiological age include your family history; health habits; measures such as blood pressure and cholesterol (see the health risk analysis in chapter 3); and measures of strength, reaction time, vision, hearing, and other variables.

Aerobic Fitness and Age

Cross-sectional studies show that aerobic fitness declines at the rate of 8 to 10 percent per decade. But among moderately active people, the decline is 4 to 5 percent, and among trained people, the rate of decline can be 2 percent or less. Figure 17.4 depicts the decline of people who begin with an aerobic fitness of 50 (milliliters per kilogram per minute). Imagine the differences that occur with a very fit athlete (70 milliliters per kilogram per minute) who continues to train versus an unfit person (40 milliliters per kilogram per minute) who remains sedentary. In 10 years the athlete drops 2 percent to 68.6, whereas the inactive person declines 10 percent to 36. Avoiding gains in body weight and fat minimizes the rate of decline in fitness. Increased body fat, less training, and reduced muscle mass accounts for a significant portion of the decline in fitness and performance that occurs with age.

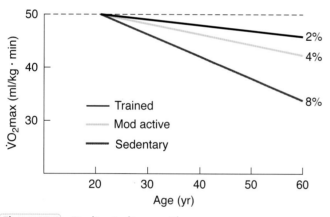

Figure 17.4 Decline in fitness with age.

Eventually, most highly active people cut back on training. Some gain weight, thereby increasing the rate of decline in fitness. The rate of decline in $\dot{V}O_2$max after 50 years of age in endurance-trained individuals was related to a decline in training volume (Pimentel et al. 2003). If you increase your level of activity and maintain the higher level, you can slow the rate of decline until the sixth or seventh decade of life.

The beneficial effects of exercise and weight control on fitness, performance, and health are clear. The quality of life depends on the ability to pursue a variety of activities. Negative factors that affect this capacity for activity, such as excess body fat, should receive attention before irreversible physiological deterioration occurs. A reduction in body fat allows and promotes a more active life and minimizes the decrease in fitness and performance previously blamed on increasing age.

Vicious Cycle

Excess fat restricts exercise capacity, causing a decline in fitness, which further reduces activity, resulting in additional fat accumulation—a vicious cycle indeed. Additionally, sedentary behavior decreases lean body mass, further reducing resting metabolism, thus pushing the energy balance toward ever increasing fat storage. As caloric intake greatly exceeds expenditure, a person's ability to internally adjust resting metabolism to maintain a constant weight is overcome and internal set-points for weight appear to increase, making future weight loss more difficult. Compounding the problem, aerobic fitness is calculated per kilogram of body weight. Thus, even if a person is able to maintain muscle mass, a rise in weight and fat equates to a decline in fitness and functional capacity.

Strength and Age

Strength declines rather slowly with age until the fifth decade, when the rate of decline increases. This loss of muscle mass has been called sarcopenia, or vanishing flesh. Sarcopenia is an important component of frailty in older people, contributing to a loss of strength, increased falls, and fractures (Welle 2002). It has been linked to other afflictions of aging, osteoporosis, insulin resistance, and arthritis. Sarcopenia results from loss of muscle fibers and fiber atrophy, because of lack of use, decreased muscle-building hormones (testosterone), and possibly an increase in catabolic hormones and other agents that accelerate the rate of muscle wasting in older people (Deschenes 2005). People who use their strength regularly retain muscle function much longer. Evidence suggests that very old men and women (average age 87 years) can counter muscle weakness and frailty with resistance training (Fiatarone et al. 1994). Activities of daily living such as gait velocity, stair-climbing power, and spontaneous physical activity all improved in the resistance-training group. Muscle mass increased as well, in contrast to a decline for the inactive control group. Indeed, this study, along with others, suggests that maintenance of strength throughout the life span may reduce the prevalence of functional limitations (Brill et al. 2000).

Summary

We're all concerned about saving enough and investing wisely during our working years to ensure financial security in retirement. Fiscal fitness is important, but that is only part of the story. To ensure a vigorous and independent retirement, you need to invest in physical fitness as well. In personal finance, the sooner you start to invest the better, so that you can enjoy the fruits of compound interest. The same is true with fitness. You'll achieve maximum gains with an early start. The best time to begin the active life is when you are young. The second best time to start is now.

In many ways, the active life and fitness represent money in the bank, by reducing future medical costs, minimizing the need for long-term care, and eliminating future burdens on family, friends, and society. The active life represents an investment in vitality and vigor that will pay off many times over in your retirement years. In crass financial terms, the several years of extended life are like a greater starting balance in your retirement fund, giving you an extended return on your annuities and social security. But the greatest return is having the vigor and independence to pursue life to the fullest, all the days of your life.

Activity and training maintain fitness and other measures of performance that normally decline with age. Tennis players and other avid sports participants maintain reaction and movement times, which typically slow with age. The body doesn't wear out; it rusts out. So the old adage "Use it or lose it" is worth noting. Humans were not designed for a sedentary life. With good genetics and a sensible diet, you may live a long life. Would you rather spend the final years of your life in a nursing home, or living independently, traveling, and enjoying the active life? The choice is yours.

Psychology of Activity

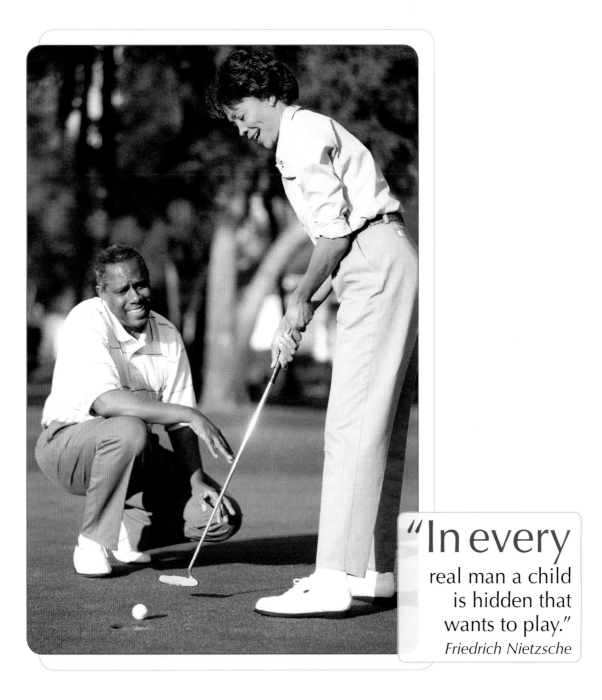

"In every real man a child is hidden that wants to play."

Friedrich Nietzsche

We can safely say that from a health standpoint, the people likely to benefit the most from regular, moderate physical activity seem most resistant to adopting or maintaining the behavior. As teachers and researchers we have devoted our careers to the proposition that increased knowledge concerning the health benefits of activity and fitness will lead to increased participation. Unfortunately, for the majority, this has not been the case. Indeed, feelings related to well-being, enjoyment, and pleasure seem more important in initiating and maintaining activity than concerns about health or factual knowledge. So we must journey beyond the comfortable landscape of physiology into the realm of psychology in search of answers to questions of motivation and adherence to regular, moderate physical activity.

This chapter presents ways to help you begin and maintain a healthy, active life. It deals with motivation, the reasons to become involved in regular activity, and adherence, how to sustain that involvement throughout life. Central to the discussion will be the concepts of enjoyment, pleasure, satisfaction, and having fun. The active life is not a monastic existence, an exercise in asceticism. Rather, it is a vital, vigorous, and joyful life, replete with satisfactions, healthy pleasures, and even thrills.

This chapter will help you

- understand the importance of enjoyment, pleasure, and satisfaction in activity and other life choices;
- appreciate the role of motivation, goal setting, and feedback in the initiation and adherence to the active life;
- identify your current involvement in physical activity;
- plan systematic changes in your activity plan;
- learn to visualize yourself as you would like to be; and
- develop a reinforcement schedule to reward new behaviors.

Motivation

What motivates people to engage in regular activity? Is it to look or feel good, for weight control, or to improve and maintain health? Far fewer than half of all Americans follow the health recommendation of the Centers for Disease Control and Prevention (CDC) and the American College of Sports Medicine (ACSM) that every adult should accumulate 30 minutes or more of moderate-intensity physical activity on most, preferably all, days of the week (Pate et al. 1995). Fewer still follow the Institute of Medicine recommendation to engage in activity for 60 minutes a day. Among those who do 30 minutes of activity, fewer than 20 percent do so in a way that will bring about improvements in fitness. The rest lack the interest or motivation necessary to ensure regular participation. Let's examine the psychology of motivation in hopes of finding ways to motivate ourselves, family members, and friends. Motivation involves the arousal, direction, and persistence of behavior.

SELF-TEST FOR MOTIVATION

What reasons have you given for your lack of participation in regular, moderate physical activity?

Interested, but haven't taken action:

- ❏ Can't afford the time; too busy right now
- ❏ Lack of opportunity
- ❏ Not convenient
- ❏ Too expensive
- ❏ Don't know how to start

Not interested:

- ❏ Low priority at this point in my life
- ❏ Concerned about my health
- ❏ Don't want to be embarrassed
- ❏ Bad childhood experiences
- ❏ Never have enjoyed it

What would you say to motivate a family member or friend who expressed one of these reasons for not participating in regular activity?

Arousal

Physiological motives or drives are triggered by basic biological needs such as food, water, elimination, and sex. Safety and health needs are next in the hierarchy of human motives or needs—to be safe from threat, to be secure. Then come love and belonging—needs involving genuine affection and a place in one's group. Next in the hierarchy are the esteem needs—to be liked and respected and to respect oneself. At the top of the hierarchy is the need for self-actualization, to realize one's potential (Maslow 1954). Any of these needs may serve to arouse a person to action (see figure 18.1).

Figure 18.1 Hierarchy of needs.

Directing Behavior

The direction of behavior—that is, where and how one behaves when aroused—is a complex study involving a multitude of learned behaviors and their interaction with ever-varying situations. Kenyon (1968) categorized the reasons that people engage in physical activity:

- Social reasons—to meet or be with people or part of a group
- Pursuit of vertigo—the thrill of speed and change of direction while remaining in control
- Aesthetic reasons—the beauty of movement
- Catharsis—relief from stress and tension
- Ascetic reasons—self-denial, discipline, training
- Health and fitness

Many forms of activity can satisfy a person's needs. One could walk, jog, run, swim, or cycle for health and fitness. Or a person could climb, kayak, ski, mountain bike, or windsurf in pursuit of vertigo. The direction chosen will depend on several factors, including the level of arousal, previous exercise experiences, opportunity, the physical and social environment, and a bit of chance.

Before Brian moved to Montana some 40 years ago, he had never seen a pair of skis, let alone a real mountain. Yet he was motivated to try skiing, probably because friends and coworkers were skiers (social reason). Before long he realized that skiing was for him. Soon he was skiing not to belong or for esteem, but because it was exciting (pursuit of vertigo), because it felt good, because he wanted to test himself and find his potential. He became hopelessly hooked, positively addicted to the sport.

Type T

Type T (for thrill) is a personality type that describes people who are hooked on excitement, risk, and tempting fate. Jack, a physician friend, is the quintessential type T. Over the years he has raced motocross, climbed mountains, kayaked rivers, and sailed a catamaran. He mastered downhill skis, moved on to Telemark skis, and is now a board skier. His latest passion, windsurfing, takes him to the Columbia River, the mecca for the sport. Type Ts fit Kenyon's category pursuit of vertigo, defined as the thrill of speed and change in direction while remaining in control. Some find pleasure and satisfaction in pushing the limits, in gaining mastery, in flirting with danger while remaining in control, if just barely. People have said that type Ts get high on their own hormones. Certainly this behavior can become addictive, leading to tougher climbs and more challenging descents. Or it can become somewhat less dangerous, taking the form of inline skating, scrambling up peaks, or even caving. Following the thrills to an untimely end isn't necessary. A person can channel the addiction into demanding but safer pursuits, compatible with the needs of family and career.

It strikes us that Kenyon's list of reasons that people engage in physical activity needs to be updated. A study of runners indicated additional reasons that people participate, including challenge, centering, afterglow, and because it feels good (Johnsgard 1985). What a surprise—people engage in physical activity because it feels good and brings them enjoyment. Another reason for participation is to improve or enhance appearance. For some this means losing weight or fat, toning muscles, developing a "six pack" set of abdominal muscles, looking slim and svelte. Wow, exercise not only feels good, contributes to vitality, and brings enjoyment but also improves health and appearance!

Pleasure Principle

In their book *Healthy Pleasures*, Ornstein and Sobel (1989) describe the pleasure principle and its role in the motivation of behavior. Pleasurable sensations reverberate in the nervous system, releasing endorphins and other opiate-like chemicals. These chemicals find their way to receptors and satisfy physiological needs. The authors reason that the human desire for enjoyment evolved to enhance survival. They cite eating, reproductive behavior, and caring for others as examples of pleasures that are good for health and survival of the species. And they suggest that measurable, pleasurable benefits of physical activity may be as close, as easy, and even as enjoyable as a walk in the park. Their advocacy of natural pleasures, of things that feel good, is consistent with the active life. Exercise doesn't have to hurt to be good; it only has to be regular and moderate to bestow the benefits and healthy pleasures.

> You must be willing and able to delay gratification if you are to experience the pleasure and relief that comes with completion of a difficult task.

Even so, not all healthy pleasures are easy or immediately gratifying. Pleasure is synonymous with enjoyment and satisfaction. Some of the hardest things we have ever done are the most satisfying, such as running or cross-country skiing a marathon, climbing a mountain, or completing a triathlon. The training is always satisfying and usually enjoyable. But you must be willing and able to delay gratification if you are to experience the pleasure and relief that comes with completion of a difficult task.

> "It is impossible to live pleasurably without living wisely, well, and justly, and impossible to live wisely, well, and justly without living pleasurably."
>
> *Epicurus*

Intrinsic Motivation

Intrinsic or self-directed goals are more effective in long-term motivation and adherence to exercise. Extrinsic or external sources of motivation may arouse and direct efforts to win a prize, medal, trophy, or scholarship or to gain social acceptance, but the motivation necessary to persist, to ensure lifelong participation in the active life, must come from within, from the upper reaches of the hierarchy of human needs (self-respect, self-actualization), and from the pleasure principle. Consider the former athletes who lose interest in their sport when the glory fades and the medals tarnish. Then look at your habitually active friends, the hikers, runners, tennis and racquetball players, and skiers. What keeps them going? Do they seek health, a trophy, or a championship? They go out each day because they must, because they are addicted, and because being active feels good. They go out to be themselves, and in the process they come closer to their potential.

Compulsion

An addiction can be nothing more than a habit. Of course, some of us are compulsive, prone to carrying things to extremes. Compulsive exercise behavior shares similarities with anorexia nervosa. Both groups include hard-working achievers who employ an ascetic approach to their problems. Do compulsive runners and those with anorexia nervosa share an obsessive–compulsive disorder? Probably not, but the discussion serves to reinforce the old-fashioned but ever applicable admonition for moderation in all things.

Persistence

Defined as the ability to go on resolutely or stubbornly in spite of difficulties, persistence is the key to success in physical activity and in life. Calvin Coolidge summed up its importance in the following lines:

> "Nothing in the world can take the place of persistence. Talent will not; nothing is more common than unsuccessful men with talent. Genius will not; unrewarded genius is almost a proverb. Education will not; the world is full of educated derelicts. Persistence and determination alone are omnipotent."

We need persistence to meet fitness, performance, weight-control, or other goals, especially on cold, windy, or rainy days. Persistence implies faith in the eventual outcome, the ability to delay gratification, and confidence in our ability to cope with adversity. Without it we could never leave our cozy homes and venture forth in cold and snow. Persistence helps us sustain effort over a prolonged period to reach a goal. It is the foundation of adherence.

Adherence to Activity

To adhere means to maintain loyalty, to stick fast, to cling. Why do some stick with the active life while others slip away? We define dropouts as those who begin an exercise program and then cease participation. Exercise program dropout rates range from 20 percent to more than 50 percent. People most often cite lack of time as the reason for dropping out, as well as for not starting in the first place. Family, career, or other responsibilities make it difficult for many who say they are just too busy. We think of our recent presidents when we hear this excuse. They found time for physical activity in their schedules. Effective time management is one of the hallmarks of success, as is involvement in the active life. Other reasons for dropping out include having no place to exercise, fatigue, inadequate information, inconvenience, and lack of willpower.

Studies have shown that factors associated with dropping out include a sedentary youth and previous unfavorable exercise experience, which underscores the need for enjoyable activity experiences, for having fun in school physical education and youth sports programs. Education and income have also been linked positively with adherence; more education means more income, and both have been associated with adherence. In personality tests, adherers were found to exhibit more self-confidence and emotional stability than dropouts did. Cigarette smoking is usually linked with

Find the environment that will help you stay active.

a higher rate of dropping out of exercise (Willis and Campbell 1992). Family and peer support enhances adherence, and excessive work demands hinder it.

A number of factors that influence continued participation have been identified. Some relate to individual participation, and others pertain to exercise programs. Some folks thrive in an individual program, whereas others enjoy group participation and supervision. One local company's wellness program provides for both types, offering both individual time-share programs (in which employees match their personal exercise time with an equal amount of company-paid time), and fitness club memberships that provide group or individual programs. Convenience, good facilities, likable leadership, and social support are factors related to adherence in group programs. Another determinant is how well the program meets participants' needs. Finally, we return to the pleasure principle. Programs that are enjoyable and foster a sense of achievement and satisfaction are more likely to encourage adherence.

> Programs that are enjoyable and foster a sense of achievement and satisfaction are more likely to encourage adherence.

Drill Instructors?

Several years ago my old friend Dr. Paul Davis initiated an unusual exercise program in Washington, D.C., called the Sergeant's Program. Former drill instructors staffed the program and led participants through a grueling program of calisthenics and running. The instructors used salty speech, derisive comments, and epithets to motivate the group of young male and female lawyers, MBAs, and bureaucrats. To everyone's surprise, the program was a great success.

Group cohesion is defined as a dynamic process reflected by the tendency of a group to stick together and remain united in the pursuit of its objectives and for the satisfaction of its members' needs. Increased group cohesion leads to an increase in adherence to an exercise program. Indeed, a recent summary of research concluded that people who hold strong beliefs about the cohesiveness of their exercise group will

- attend more classes,
- be on time,
- be less likely to drop out,
- be resistant to disruptions,
- experience more positive effects,
- have improved attitudes toward exercise, and
- achieve confidence in their ability to successfully carry out actions to satisfy situational demands (self-efficacy) (Estabrooks 2000).

Climate for Adherence

With maturation comes the satisfaction of lower-order needs and the opportunity to seek self-actualization. The self-actualized person is free to determine his or her lifestyle and personal goals and to pursue them without anxiety and without the necessity to conform, except superficially, to society's conventions and restraints. Self-actualized people seek to be, not to become. They enjoy their lives as they seek to realize their capacity. They require neither the attention nor the adulation of the crowd, only a personal sense of satisfaction and achievement.

Even self-actualized people sometimes find it difficult to make the necessary sacrifices. Pursuing any goal is hard when those around you are not supportive. Fitness studies have shown that the emotional climate created by significant others is highly related to the participant's adherence to the program. When wives, husbands, and loved ones offer encouragement and support, the participant is likely to continue. Why would anyone deprecate a loved one's efforts in a fitness or sports training program? Spouses may complain about the amount of time involved, the cost, and upset schedules and vacations. Of course, some may complain because, secretly, they envy their spouse's dedication and satisfaction, or they fear losing their rejuvenated loved one or the loss of shared experiences.

To avoid emotional conflicts, discuss your interests and goals with loved ones. Realize how your participation may affect them and try to minimize adverse effects. Invent new shared experiences to replace those lost as a result of your personal quest for excellence. A supportive emotional climate is certain to prevail when both husband and wife are happily involved in the active life. Both need not be involved in the same activity, although there are many such cases. If both seek excellence in tennis, they do not necessarily have to play mixed doubles. What matters are that each understands how important participation is to the other and that the emotional climate they create influences enjoyment and adherence.

Climate and geography can enhance or detract from the enjoyment of participation. When young women performed aerobic exercise in a naturalistic environment, the activity was associated with decreases in state anxiety and increases in tranquility, positive engagement, and revitalization (Focht and Hausenblas 2001). In some cases the environment can preclude certain activities. For example, skiing isn't available in some parts of the country—if you want to participate regularly, you'll have to move or take expensive vacations. The answer, often ignored, is to move to where climate and geography suit your interests. Ridiculous, you say? Perhaps, but we've met hundreds of people who have done just that—left high-paying jobs amid urban sprawl to seek a better way. We've met them by mountain lakes, on ski lifts, running in the desert, and skiing in the wilderness. Do they have any regrets? Perhaps. Decide on your goals, your priorities, the kind of life you want to live, and then give it your best effort. In time, if you feel the need to change, do it. It's all a part of the process of achieving your potential.

With 85 years at your disposal, you have time to try out several careers and locations. Don't lament time that you must spend away from a favored environment. Enjoy yourself as much as possible and realize that future careers and locations await you. Active, creative lives are available everywhere, not just at distant holiday resorts. Adapt to the environment that you are in and use it to learn new skills, not to regret the ones that don't fit the setting. But never give up on the dream that unites vocation, avocation, and location. One of our dreams has been to live where we can cross-country ski on groomed tracks right outside the backdoor. We haven't quite achieved the dream, but we are close—within a mile.

Improving Adherence

We've considered some of the reasons that people drop out and the factors associated with adherence to the active life. We've discussed the emotional climate and the importance of pleasure and having fun. Now let's turn our attention to psychological concepts that shed light on ways to enhance adherence. One concept is the therapeutic use of physical activity as a means of coping with moods, stress, anxiety, depression, and other problems. As part of a daily schedule the activity becomes preventive, an inoculation against moods that interfere with life satisfaction. For more on adherence consult Weinberg and Gould's *Foundations of Sport and Exercise Psychology* (2003).

Internals Versus Externals

The psychological construct called locus of control separates people into internals, those who believe that they can control outcomes in their lives, and externals, who believe that chance or others control their lives. Internals are more likely to adhere to healthy behaviors than externals are. Which better fits your view of life? Can you modify your locus of control to enhance adherence to healthy behaviors, such as regular activity? We believe that you can.

Self-Efficacy

The theory of self-efficacy suggests that coping behaviors such as physical activity are influenced by the perception of acquiring mastery in that area. Perception of mastery influences performance, and theory suggests that positive experience alters this perception. Thus successful experience may reinforce an activity, leading to continuation of the behavior. Although judgments of efficacy are situation specific, it has even been suggested that enhanced self-efficacy in one behavior may generalize to others. Research indicates that self-efficacy plays a prominent role in the early adoption and adaptation stages of exercise programs but is less potent in the maintenance stage. Self-efficacy takes on renewed importance when structured programs end and a person must rely on his or her own resources to develop an exercise program (McAuley and Blissmer 2000).

If the perception of mastery reinforces behavior, perhaps we can influence that perception with affirmative statements, positive reinforcements of progress and performance. Elite athletes use affirmative statements to build confidence and aid performance, part of the positive internal dialogue that leads to success, in sport and in life. If it works for athletes, you too can use positive self-talk to reinforce your sense of success, thereby enhancing adherence. Recognize your sacrifices, your progress, and your achievements. Celebrate your epic adventures. At the same time, you must eliminate negative self-talk. Extol your virtues, and you'll boost self-esteem, adherence, and possibly performance.

> Extol your virtues, and you'll boost self-esteem, adherence, and possibly performance.

Internal Dialogue

The first step toward a positive internal dialogue is to eliminate negatives, irrational thinking, and cognitive distortions from your internal dialogue. Stop blaming yourself, focusing on negatives, overgeneralizing, magnifying, and minimizing. Don't undervalue your accomplishments. Change the negative "I look flabby" into the positive "I need to improve muscle tone." Then select positive affirmations to reinforce your behavior. Add simple statements such as "I can do this," "I'm making progress," "I'm looking good," and "I'm achieving my goals." Use them regularly and you'll feel better about yourself and your program.

Goal Setting

A goal is an aim or a purpose, what a person seeks to accomplish. Goals serve to help focus and regulate behavior, thus affecting both motivation and adherence. Goal setting has a beneficial influence on the performance of a task. Although most folks use goals to a certain extent, few take full advantage of their influence on the motivation for and adherence to physical activity. By using short- and long-term goals, you can devise a strategy to achieve the desired result.

Goal setting works best by using process-oriented goals. For instance, a process-oriented goal is to work up gradually to 30 miles (48.2 kilometers) of running per week, or to complete a 10-kilometer (6.2-mile) race. An outcome-oriented goal would be to run the 10-kilometer race in less than 40 minutes, an outcome that might be very difficult to achieve. Outcome-oriented goals have their place, but they need to be reasonable and adaptable. If the day of the 10-kilometer race is hot and humid, you'll need to adjust your goal.

We use goals to prepare for upcoming events and adventures, such as our annual winter ski trip in Yellowstone Park. In fall we engage in muscular fitness training to build strength and endurance in skiing muscles. As soon as the snow flies we begin training so that we'll be able to keep up with our partners in February. Of course, we thoroughly enjoy every phase of the preparation, particularly the sense of accomplishment at the end of a long, hard trail. Set long-term goals as targets and short-term goals to help attain them. Write down your goals and keep records as you progress. Back when Brian considered himself a serious runner, he set training targets and recorded daily mileage on the calendar. At the end of the week he'd add the total to see whether he was on target to reach the goal.

Set realistic goals, such as 30 minutes of moderate physical activity most days of the week. When the goal becomes too easy and loses its motivational effect, set a new, more challenging goal. Challenging goals get better results than easy ones. Use specific goals; don't just plan to "work hard." Finally, keep the list simple. Don't set too many goals. As you achieve success you may expand the list. But for now begin with one or two long-term targets and some short-term steps to guide progress toward the targets (Locke and Latham 1985). When you achieve a significant long-term goal, celebrate!

When Steven was coaching the U.S. Nordic Combined Team, the team had a sports medicine advisory group that included a sport psychologist, our publisher, Dr. Rainer Martens. One skill that Rainer taught was the exceptionally helpful tool of visualization. After athletes had defined their short- and long-term goals, Rainer helped them visualize themselves accomplishing those goals. "Treat yourself as you would like to be and you will become that person." To be a champion, you have to see yourself as a champion and all that it includes. Visualization is a powerful tool to change behavior, self-beliefs, actions, sport technique, and self-image. "Change the action in the mind and the mind will control the body."

To begin an exercise program you need to think of yourself as a person who lives the active life. See yourself achieving the goals that you would like to achieve and slowly but surely you will move to the new reality.

Behavioral Change

This section outlines important steps in the initiation and maintenance of regular physical activity. It begins with a sincere intention to change behavior, perhaps the best indicator of success. We then look at the early stages of behavior change, followed by factors associated with program maintenance or adherence. Finally, we review behavior therapy as a strategy to aid the initiation and maintenance of the activity program.

Intention to Change

A number of factors influence one's intention to adopt a new behavior, including information, role models, authoritative figures (e.g., physician), previous experience, and social pressure. A person may need time to move from disinterest to being ready to change. The status of exercise behavior model (SOEB) includes six stages of change:

> One of the best indicators of future success is a person's readiness to change. If people say they are ready, they probably are.

1. Precontemplative—not considering activity
2. Contemplative—thinking about it
3. Preparation—exhibiting some activity
4. Action—fully engaged in activity
5. Maintenance—active for months
6. Adoption—activity internalized as part of lifestyle (Stone and Klein 2004)

One of the best indicators of future success is a person's readiness to change. If people say they are ready, they probably are.

Initiating Behavior

Early success is associated with reasonable expectations and goals, gradual change, appropriate reinforcement, social support, and cognitive strategies (relaxation, dissociation). Relax during activity by focusing on your breathing.

Relaxation

Sit in a comfortable chair in a quiet room and repeat a simple sound (mantra) such as "easy" each time you exhale. Concentration on the breathing and the mantra masks disturbing thoughts, and the body begins to relax. As you become more proficient with the technique, you may achieve a transcendent state of relaxation, clear thought, imagery, well-being, and openness. In time you'll be able to use the skill during activity and sport. Meditation is not a substitute for exercise; it will not induce the many physiological changes that result from regular activity. On the other hand, some find activity to be as effective as meditation in the achievement of relaxation.

Dissociation involves diverting attention from how you feel during exercise by focusing on other topics or conversation with a partner. For some people, the first 20 minutes of activity are the hardest, until pain-killing endorphins kick in. Similarly, the first few weeks of a new program are the toughest. So it helps to have ways to cope until appreciable changes become evident or until you become addicted. Behavior therapy seems to work for difficult cases.

Behavior Therapy

According to the stages of change model, people move through five behavioral strategies as they adopt and maintain a new habit: substituting alternatives, participating in activity while under stress, enlisting social support, rewarding themselves, committing themselves, and reminding themselves (Marcus and Forsyth 2003). This section provides a way to identify the desired behavior and make progress toward its acquisition. The essentials are threefold:

1. Identify the behavior that you wish to modify (e.g., physical activity) and maintain an accurate record of your current behavior. Maintain a weeklong record of all your physical activity (figure 18.2). Include the intensity and duration of your involvement, and complete the cognitive question for fitness training and recreational activities.

2. Analyze your current behavior and then plan needed modifications. Do you need to burn more calories, increase intensity, or do specific training (e.g., muscular fitness)? Plan appropriate modifications to meet your needs and interests. For example, you could increase your activity to meet the Centers for Disease Control and American College of Sports Medicine activity guideline (30 minutes of physical activity most days of the week).

3. Develop a contract with specific goals and a schedule of rewards to reinforce the new behavior (figure 18.3). Use activity benchmarks such as minutes or miles (or kilometers) per day or week, weight loss, or other indicators of successful adoption of the new activity. A tangible, universally accepted reward such as money seems to work for most of us. Spend the reward immediately or save it for something that you

Figure 18.2   Daily Activity Log

Date _____

Time	Place	Exercise	Intensity	Duration	What were your thoughts during exercise?

Note: Include all forms of physical activity, including work, walking, and household chores.

Score	Intensity	Score	Duration
5	Sustained heavy breathing and perspiration	4	Over 30 min
4	Intermittent heavy breathing and perspiration—as in tennis	3	20 to 30 min
3	Moderately heavy—as in recreational sports and cycling	2	10 to 20 min
2	Moderate—as in volleyball, softball	1	Under 10 min
1	Light—as in fishing, walking		

From *Fitness and Health, Sixth Edition* by Brian J. Sharkey and Steven E. Gaskill, 2007, Champaign, IL: Human Kinetics.

really want but might otherwise not buy. Don't worry about the expense. The new behavior will save more than the cost of the reward in medical and other expenses. In time the behavior will become a healthy habit, and you will be able to focus on new goals or new behaviors (e.g., weight control, time management).

Maintenance

Adherence to a newly adopted behavior can be difficult; 50 percent of participants drop out of exercise programs within the first year. Certain strategies help improve the odds of success (Taylor and Miller 1993). People continue activity if

- it meets a need,
- it is fun,
- they have social support, and
- they see evidence of change.

To ensure lifelong participation, the person must move from extrinsic to intrinsic motivation; become self-sufficient, independent of the instructor and the setting; and develop strategies to deal with factors that threaten continued participation. Work, illness, or family crises may interrupt but must never terminate participation in regular, moderate activity.

Develop a network of support systems to ensure your adherence. Support is available from family and friends, interest groups, professionals, clubs, programs, publications, and organizations.

Figure 18.3 Activity Reinforcement Schedule

Date	Activity	Distance or time	Reward*
	Weekly total		
	Weekly total		
	Weekly total		
	Weekly total		
	Total for month		

Note: Daily reward—for meeting activity goal (e.g., 2 mi, or 3 km); weekly reward—for meeting activity goal (e.g., 12 mi, or 18 km); monthly reward—for meeting activity goal (e.g., 50 mi, or 80 km; improved fitness score). Adjust goals as fitness improves.

*Rewards: daily—a small monetary award (e.g., $1) or a cool drink; weekly—a larger monetary reward (e.g., $5) or a special favor (e.g., movie); monthly—a substantial monetary reward (e.g., $20) or a very special favor (e.g., concert, dinner out). Rewards can be saved for a special purpose (e.g., new warm-up outfit, tennis racket).

From *Fitness and Health, Sixth Edition* by Brian J. Sharkey and Steven E. Gaskill, 2007, Champaign, IL: Human Kinetics.

- **Family.** Spouses provide support by taking a sincere interest in each other's activity, and when possible, participate together. Family members often select gifts to encourage or enhance participation. Trips may revolve around a shared experience, such as hiking, canoeing, skiing, or golf.

- **Friends.** Most of our longtime friends share our interests. The shared interests are the foundation of the relationship, the glue that holds it together. Their presence gets us out and keeps us going. Together we do more than any of us would do alone.

- **Interest groups.** We all have access to hiking, skiing, and running clubs, and more. Our local canoe-racing group welcomes neophytes to join their Wednesday evening training sessions. If you can't find a group with your interests, start one.

- **Professionals.** From personal trainers to fitness and sport instructors, a wide array of help is available. Seek out experts for advice and motivation. Get professional instruction to improve your performance and enjoyment of tennis, skiing, or other recreational sports.

- **Clubs.** By joining a health and fitness club you'll gain access to equipment, instruction, and an added bonus, the social support of fellow members. Club-based programs often succeed when home-based programs fail because of social and psychological support.

- **Programs.** Take advantage of your workplace wellness program and become involved in new activities. The wellness program at our university has provided us with weightlifting, swimming, inline skating, ski clinics, and many other classes. Our campus recreation program has welcomed us on winter ski trips and in canoe and kayak classes.

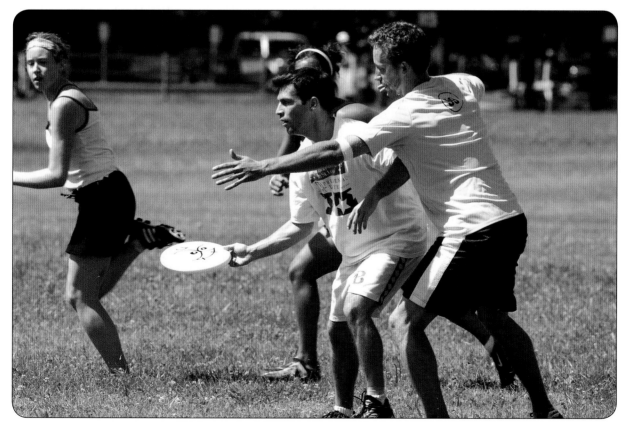

Joining an organization or a recreational league can help you maintain a fitness routine.

- **Publications.** Many books are available to help you maintain or expand your interests. Magazines cater to general *(Outside)* or specific interests *(Backpacker)*. Videos and computer programs provide instruction in everything from golf to mountain biking.

- **Organization.** The American College of Sports Medicine (ACSM) provides information and publications on fitness, exercise science, and sports medicine. ACSM also publishes position papers on a wide range of topics (www.acsm.org). Sport organizations such as the United States Tennis Association provide sport-specific pamphlets, instruction, and tournaments.

Sometimes a new piece of equipment will generate or revive interest in an activity. For example, adjustable ski poles increase interest in and enjoyment of backcountry hiking. The poles aid uphill travel, relieve aging knees on the downhills, and provide balance in crossing logs and streams. Sporting goods stores and equipment catalogs provide ways to make activity more pleasurable. Take advantage of these and other support systems to ensure lifelong involvement in physical activity.

Relapse

Participants often relapse, slipping back to inactivity after an initial change for the better. Relapse occurs for many reasons, ranging from emotional and social to physical. Because the event is so common, if it happens you should not let it bother you. Relapse is part of the process of change, for athletes as well as newcomers. In dieting, relapse is par for the course. The question is, what can you do to prevent or recover from relapse? One approach calls for a planned relapse, just to test the reaction when instructor support is still available. To date, most relapse prevention programs have been labor intensive, teaching how to anticipate and cope with relapse, using strategies that we have already discussed, such as behavior therapy and goal setting. Most have yielded modest results.

Our suggestion is to search for intrinsic motivation and to strive for internal control. Free yourself from the need for external validation from fitness instructors. Their responsibility is to lead you to a level of independence so that you will no longer rely on them for information or encouragement. Wean yourself from dependence on their motivation and control. Then develop your own approach to relapse prevention. Build the social support and emotional climate you need to keep going. Don't depend on one activity; be ready to adapt in the event of injury or chronic illness. When relapse comes, and it will, return to your goals, to behavior therapy, and to your support systems. Study your schedule and find opportunities for activity. Set new goals, avoid negative messages, and focus on your strengths (Blair, La Monte, and Nichaman 2004). People who develop behavioral or cognitive strategies, such as positive self-talk, are more successful at coping with relapse (Willis and Campbell 1992). By devising your own solution you'll be better prepared for the future.

Get a Dog

What are the secrets of long-term participation in physical activity? Studies of lifelong participants show that a number of factors are associated with their persistence. They are higher in self-motivation and self-efficacy and lower in negative barriers than those less persistent. They cite fitness, well-being, and energy as reasons to continue. They enjoy activity and make it a priority (Stone and Klein 2004). Morgan (2001) argues for the importance of purposeful or meaningful physical activity. In his study of long-term adherents, he found two meaningful categories of activity—transportation and dog walking. Those of us with dogs understand how they enjoy their time out and how that walk is good for us as well as for them.

The Active Personality

Do activity and improved fitness influence personality, or are some personality types more likely to be active? Personality is a frame of reference that psychologists use in the study of behavior. More than a mask but less than reality, personality is a product of heredity and the environment, usually studied with paper-and-pencil tests or in-depth interviews, but never really defined or measured.

Cattell suggests that one's personality indicates what he or she will do when in a given mood and placed in a given situation. He developed the Cattell 16 Personality Factor Questionnaire, a personality test used widely by researchers (Cattell, Eber, and Tatsuoka 1970). The test, typical of the paper-and-pencil approach, scores the subject on each of 16 factors, or personality traits (aloof–sociable, emotional–calm, timid–adventurous, confident–insecure). Assuming that this approach is valid, let's use it to consider how activity and personality are related.

Studies of the personalities of middle-aged men have shown that highly fit subjects are more unconventional, composed, secure, easygoing, emotionally stable, adventurous, and higher in intelligence than low-fitness subjects are. The most pronounced personality differences were those related to emotional stability and security. The presence of differences between high- and low-fitness groups, however, does not prove that the differences are due to fitness. Emotionally stable and secure men may be more likely to engage in a fitness program. When researchers studied the effects of a 4-month fitness program on these subjects, they noted little personality change in the low-fitness group, in spite of a conspicuous improvement in fitness. The researchers reasoned that it takes years to become fit or unfit, and that a few months of activity is insufficient to bring about significant personality changes (Ismail and Young 1977). Longitudinal studies are necessary to confirm or reject the hypothesis that personality improves with activity or fitness.

Perception: Listen to Your Body

Years ago, we researchers felt that perceptions were too subjective, too prone to error and variation. When an athlete said that he was too tired to go on, we doubted his motivation. But Swedish psychologist Dr. Gunnar Borg changed all that when he developed and validated his ratings of perceived exertion (RPE; see table 6.2 on page 103). Borg (1973) realized that the brain integrated sensory stimuli generated during physical effort into a perception of effort. The brain perceives and evaluates stimuli from muscles, respiratory distress, pain, and the sensation of a pounding heart. Subsequent studies have shown that these subjective estimates of effort are highly related to workload, heart rate, oxygen consumption, and even lactic acid and hormones. In other words, our subjective estimate of work intensity provides a rather accurate gauge of the load itself, as well as the internal factors affected by the work. Of course, our subjective perception of effort is also closely tied with the pleasure that we derive from participation.

Because we are able to judge our effort accurately in an exercise such as cycling or running, and because the heart rate and metabolic cost of the effort are closely related to those ratings, we should listen to our bodies during exercise. If the exercise feels too difficult, it probably is. The use of the heart rate training zone in exercise prescription is an attempt to employ important physiological criteria in the determination of a safe and effective dose of exercise. You may find that running at your training heart rate feels "somewhat hard." Thereafter, you can use that sense of difficulty to guide your exertion. If high temperatures cause your heart rate to rise, your perception of effort will adjust your pace to a more prudent level. Eventually this sense of effort is all that you need to gauge exercise intensity.

While we're on the subject of perception, let us spend a moment on the concept of preferred exertion. When subjects participated in a low- or high-preference activity, fatigue and psychological distress were higher in the low-preference condition, and positive well-being was higher and perceived exertion lower in the high-preference activity, even though work rate remained constant across conditions (Parfitt and Gledhill 2004).

In another area of preference, experienced exercisers seem to require a certain level of exertion to be satisfied. If the exertion is too easy, their sense of satisfaction diminishes. Training increases the preferred exertion, whereas inactivity lowers it. People who have been involved in highly competitive sports often have learned to prefer a high level of exertion. Some erroneously believe that exercise has to hurt to be good (it docs not), or they subscribe to the maxim "No pain, no gain" (also untrue). Therefore, when they resume activity after a prolonged layoff, they overdo it and end up with soreness or injury.

The preference for exertion is learned. For most Americans, the learned preference consists of the minimum, of walking to and from the car. This circumstance could be different. If parents, schools, and community leaders demonstrate and encourage sensible and inexpensive exercise habits, more kids will grow up with a predisposition to regular activity. If parents become involved, the kids will make physical activity a family affair. Elementary, high school, and even college students should be encouraged to participate in healthful activities. Community organizations can sponsor activities for which participation is the major goal. The objective is to raise preferred exertion to the level required to achieve the health benefits of regular, moderate physical activity.

Summary

This chapter has looked at motivation and adherence to help you initiate and maintain involvement in enjoyable, lifelong physical activity. We've learned that motivation involves the arousal, direction, and persistence of behavior and that intrinsic motivation is more persistent than extrinsic motivation. We've also learned that internals, those who feel in control of their lives, are more likely to adhere to healthy behaviors than are externals, those who believe that chance or others control their lives. We've seen that success or the perception of mastery reinforces participation and aids adherence. The chapter provides a way to identify current activity patterns, establish realistic goals for new behaviors, and use reinforcement to help ensure attainment of those goals.

Throughout this book we have advocated realistic goals, minor adjustments, and gradual change as a proved approach to improvements in activity and other health behaviors. Research and common sense support this approach. Most people won't need a radical change if they just stick with minor adjustments, such as taking daily walks or substituting low-fat foods for high-fat foods. But one school of thought suggests that moderate changes are hard to measure and easy to ignore, making a slip back into bad habits more likely. Gradual change may not provide the results and positive feedback required to reinforce the behavior, whereas big changes in health behaviors are more likely to yield big results. If you think that you might prefer this second approach, set lofty goals, such as running a marathon or making major changes in diet and body weight. Make a major commitment and see what happens. Use the approach that works for you.

A Project

To complete her senior project, Steven's youngest daughter decided to take on a formidable challenge. She had read about the Border-to-Border ski across Finland, an event requiring use of traditional cross-country technique to cover 28 to 52 miles (45 to 84 kilometers) per day for 7 days to traverse the 278-mile (450-kilometer) distance across Finland from Russia to Sweden. Because Steven thought that the trip would be fabulous, he agreed to join her and they began training to develop the technique and endurance that they would need. Having the major goal motivated their training and made it more enjoyable. Because Heidi had never been to Finland, he helped her imagine the rolling landscape near the Arctic Circle. Visualizing the benefits, the sauna at the end of each day, and the feeling of accomplishment helped to sustain the hours of gentle skiing that preceded the trip.

Active people seem better able to cope with the problems of life. These hardy people share several characteristics: a sense of being in control, a sense of involvement and purpose, and the flexibility to adapt to challenges and opportunities (Kobasa 1979). Robust good health and resistance to illness don't absolutely require regular, moderate activity, not if you are blessed with superb genes. But if you are like most of us, activity provides a coping mechanism that contributes to health, adaptability, and resistance to stress. And more important, it's fun.

It's been said, "Begin; the rest is easy." Of course, that isn't true—the rest isn't easy. But unless you begin, you'll never know how easy or hard the road may be. Life is a journey, not a destination.

Activity and the Quality of Life

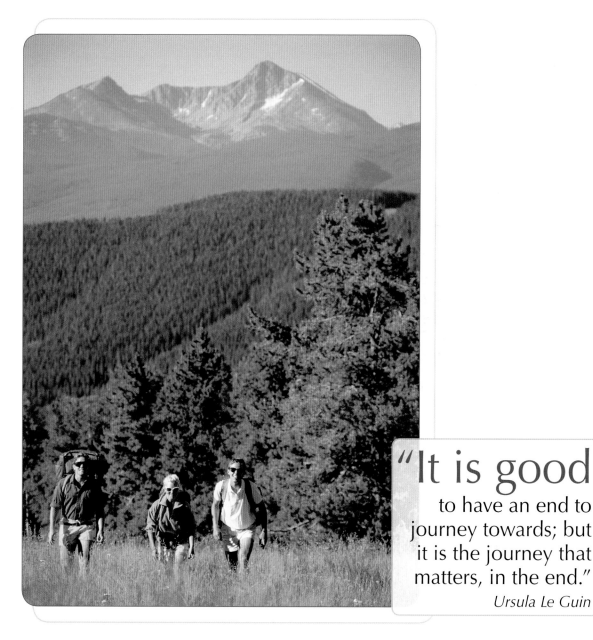

"It is good to have an end to journey towards; but it is the journey that matters, in the end."

Ursula Le Guin

What began with a catalog of physical and mental health benefits associated with the active life now concludes with a consideration of the contribution of physical activity to an elusive concept, the quality of life. We'll begin with a consideration of quality and ways to measure it, as well as success in life. Then we'll consider how the definition of success shifts with the seasons of life. We'll conclude with an invitation to action, a challenge to maintain and improve the quality of life in your family and community.

This chapter will help you

- construct your definition of quality and success in life,
- understand how the definitions change at different stages of life,
- find ways to influence the quality of your experiences,
- understand your responsibility to maintain and improve the quality of life, and
- appreciate the dimensions of the active life.

Quality of Life

Quality of life, quality time—just what is this quality thing all about? The dictionary definition of quality includes "degree of excellence" and "a distinguishing attribute." Quality is necessarily a subjective, personal response, not an absolute. We can easily distinguish quality from quantity. For example, for competitive runners, quantity of training simply refers to the miles (kilometers) run, whereas quality refers to the race-pace training that leads to improvement in performance. Similarly, although some find quality in a difficult mountain climb, others prefer the tranquility of a hike in the forest below.

Objective measurement of this subjective concept has just begun. Research has provided some insights into the relationship between physical activity and the quality of life. Active people have better health, more stamina, more positive attitudes toward work, and greater ability to cope with stress. Active older adults report greater life satisfaction, less dependence on others, and better overall health (Weinberg and Gould 2003). The health care debate has prompted discussion of quality-of-life issues in reference to treatment decisions, such as surgery, chemotherapy, radiation, or drugs. Will surgery or some other therapy improve the quality of life? Removal of the prostate gland may excise a cancer, but it often comes at a terrible cost (incontinence, impotence).

You make quality-of-life decisions daily. Be certain that you understand the options and factors that contribute to your personal definition of quality. Do you value family or friends above wealth and fame, excitement over tranquility, sociability above privacy? Try to be certain that your decisions are consistent with the things that you value. To do this, you'll have to arrive at your own definition of what constitutes a successful life.

Quality Time

A recent addition to the lexicon of pop psych, *quality time*, or *QT*, usually refers to time spent with loved ones. The idea of QT reminds us to do the obvious: spend time with those whom we value. But QT means more than just spending time; it means being there in mind as well as body. Put aside work or diversions; turn off the cell phone, pager, and TV; and become fully engaged in the moment. Play games with the kids, walk and talk with your significant other, or simply sit and watch the sunset. Don't wait for an accident, heart attack, or some other disaster to remind you of the things that really matter in life.

Success

Definitions of success differ among people and may change as one ages. Many people set out to be successful in business or a profession, or to earn wealth and fame. In time one may modify the definition to include financial security and spending more time with family and friends. Consider the things that you associate with success.

"Fame—if you win it, comes and goes in a minute."

Remember the lyric "Fame—if you win it, comes and goes in a minute." You don't need fame, status, power, or a pile of money to be successful, just a favorable or satisfactory outcome or result. Few of us look back and wish we had spent more time working or acquiring wealth, whereas many of us wish that we had spent more time with family and friends, or in healthy pursuits. Your definition of success may have a lot to do with how you view the quality of life.

The inane bumper sticker "He who has the most toys wins" describes the credo of the motorized recreationist, owner of powerboat, jet ski, all-terrain vehicle, motorcycle, and snowmobile. Although these methods of transportation have a legitimate purpose—access to recreation or work—they have become an end instead of a means. One loud, polluting machine can spoil the tranquility of lake or forest, ruining the quality of experience for human-powered paddlers, hikers, and cross-country skiers. Worse yet is the realization that this lifestyle is being handed down to the next generation of overweight, underactive kids.

Healthy, Wealthy, and Wise

For years we have known that physical activity is associated with education and income. Does that mean that becoming active will increase your intelligence or your income? Probably not, but a recent study that compared the connection between health and success among leaders of some of America's top 100 corporations to the average American citizen found that the corporate execs weighed 12 pounds (5.4 kilograms) less; ate more fish and salad; consumed less coffee, alcohol, or tobacco; and stayed married longer. And they named exercise as their number-one form of stress management (Edstrom 1999).

Perception of Quality

Psychologists and sensory physiologists long have known how to measure the quantity of stimulus (e.g., sound, light, exertion). Assessing the quality of an experience is far more difficult, yet the quality of an exercise experience is what provides pleasure and brings us back for more. If you ask someone to rate the quality of an exercise experience, he or she will respond with a long-winded evaluation of the physical environment, weather, companions, personal sensations, expectations. The quality of an exercise experience involves many factors.

A creek-side run on a tree-shaded path amid the beauty of the mountains is an experience to be savored and long remembered. Covering the same distance on a short, crowded running track or along a busy city street becomes an ordeal, unless, of course, you are with company you enjoy or glad for the chance to get away from the office. You can control the factors that enhance the quality of your exercise experiences. If you abhor noisy, crowded public tennis courts and are bothered by players who don't know or won't practice the etiquette of the sport, build your own court, join a private club, play before the crowds arrive, or encourage the city recreation department to teach court etiquette. Your exercise experiences will be more enjoyable if you follow these guidelines:

- **Be flexible.** Don't depend on one activity, time, or place for satisfaction.
- **Plan ahead.** Plan your participation, your companions, the time of day, the place. If the afternoon winds diminish the quality of tennis, plan to play in the morning.

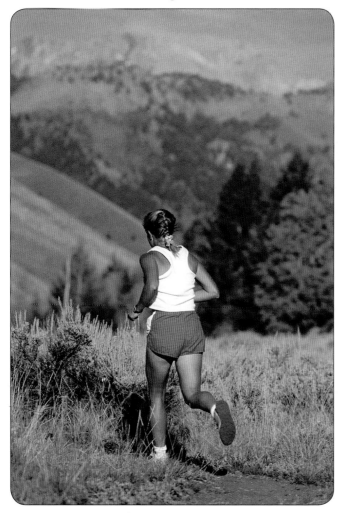

Manage the quality of your exercise experiences to ensure adherence.

- **Set realistic goals.** If you set out to run 10 miles (16 kilometers) on a hot, humid day and don't finish, you may feel that you've failed, but you haven't. You just set an unrealistic goal.
- **Recognize your moods.** We all get depressed, concerned, worried. Sometimes exercise can help you calm down when you're too excited or pick you up when you're depressed, but a really foul mood can ruin the experience for you and your companion.
- **Be prepared.** Keep your equipment in good condition, get adequate rest, eat sensibly, bring extra food or drink if you may need it, and have first aid supplies, tools, and extra parts available.
- **Learn to relax.** Sit in a quiet room and focus on your respiration. Think "easy" with each exhale. Practice daily. When you become proficient, start using the technique in your sport, while driving in traffic, or whenever the need arises.

You are responsible for ensuring the quality of your exercise experiences. If your daily activity is satisfying, it may bubble over and affect other phases of life. If it isn't, you may feel cheated, lose interest in the activity, and quit. In that case, you will be the loser.

Seasons and Stages of Life

Physical activity should be spontaneous and enjoyable. Excessive planning can inhibit spontaneity and induce the kind of drudgery found in many fitness programs. On the other hand, a well-conceived plan can contribute to the flow of life, helping one season melt into the other. Why not give your physical life the same attention that you give to work, finances, education, or travel? We'll look first at the seasons of the year and then at the stages of life.

Annual Plan

Once a year take time to outline the activities in which you intend to participate during the coming year. Fill in the sports or recreational activities that you enjoy each season. When you come upon a blank season, consider a new activity, a supplement, or preparation for an upcoming season (figure 19.1). This brief exercise will show you how one activity can blend into the next, removing the need for extensive physical preparation. Arm endurance developed in swimming transfers to cross-country ski poling and then to paddling a canoe. Year-round activity is the ideal way to maintain a desired level of fitness; it minimizes the discomfort associated with the first few days of exercise, maintains fitness, and optimizes energy balance. Of course, most of us remain active because we enjoy the experiences.

Figure 19.1   Seasonal Activity Planner

	Winter	Spring	Summer	Fall
Major activities				
Minor activities				
Supplements				

From *Fitness and Health, Sixth Edition* by Brian J. Sharkey and Steven E. Gaskill, 2007, Champaign, IL: Human Kinetics.

Stages of Life

Each of us is engaged in a lifelong search for meaning. The seasons of our lives are marked by an ebb and flow of purpose and confidence, periods of satisfaction followed by doubt. Our goals shift as the stages unfold.

- **Young adult.** This stage usually requires severing ties, acquiring an education, finding a mate, establishing a career, and perhaps starting a family. So it isn't surprising to find definitions of success framed in educational, financial, and material terms.

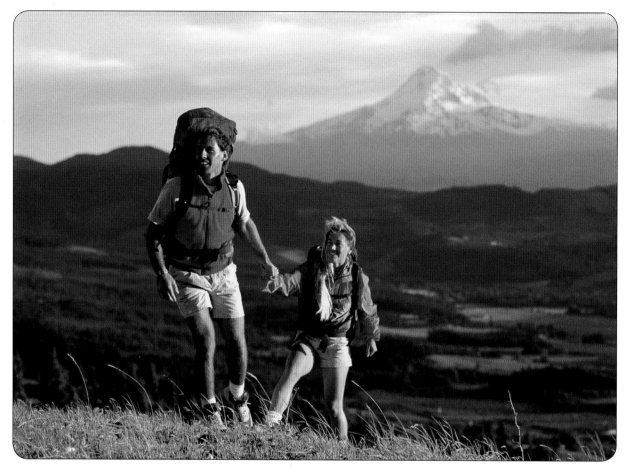

Each stage of your life presents opportunities for new activities.

- **Adult.** By avoiding divorce and major career changes, the 30-something adult may be able to buy a home and put down roots. But uncertainties in the workplace or economy often threaten achievement of that goal. This period sometimes brings the midlife crisis, a realization that time to reach goals is running out.

During the decade from 45 to 55 years, what some call middle age, we begin to accept ourselves and our lives, and to redefine our goals for success and the quality of life. Thereafter we may be refreshed or resigned, facing the best time of life if we let go of old roles and definitions and find a renewal of purpose (Sheehy 1976).

- **Senior.** Sometimes called the golden years, the senior stage may be the best of all, finally providing the time and resources to fulfill personal goals. Limited resources won't diminish satisfaction if goals are qualitative rather than quantitative.

- **Elder.** Sometime after the age of 80 folks say they begin to slow down but not stop. Many artists and musicians continue to create and perform. In spite of crippling rheumatoid arthritis, Brian's independent mother continued to play the piano in musical programs until shortly before her death at age 84. Gardening and swimming helped maintain the physical vitality that she needed to pursue her passion for music. Steven's indefatigable 78-year-old mother continues to be an on-site driving force behind the development and maintenance of the 458-mile Colorado Trail, a high-altitude hiking route.

> Give some thought to activities that you want to take up in the future, when you'll have time to enjoy them.

Are you too busy to do all the things that you want to do? Only the young should attempt some activities, such as football, whereas other activities are perfectly suited for adults, seniors, and even elders. People in any stage of life can enjoy activities such as fishing, sailing, or golf. So relax. You have time for everything that you want to do. Give some thought to activities that you want to take up in the future, when you'll have time to enjoy them.

As you advance in years you will find new challenges and new adventures, and although you may temporarily put aside favorite activities, you'll never forget well-learned skills. Competition becomes more difficult as you approach the top of an age group, but when you enter a new age category, it's like being a kid again. Eventually, most of us seek less competition and more cooperation. We discover the quiet world of sailing, the solitude of wilderness, or companionship in golf and tennis. For everything there is a season. By keeping active, you'll find time to enjoy the seasons and stages of life.

Dimensions of the Active Life

This book began with a physiological analysis of the active life and its benefits. Eventually it dealt with less measurable but no less meaningful aspects of psychology and their relationship to fitness and health. As we approach the end of the book we want you to know about another dimension of exercise and fitness, a dimension that provides meaning far beyond the measurable. We refer to the transcendent, peak, or even mystical experiences frequently reported by those who regularly engage in exercise and sport.

These moments of perfection are characterized by total involvement, control, concentration, ease of movement, and a sense of flow, described as a smooth sequence of movement without conscious effort. These rare moments can occur in training or competition, in individual or team sports, and at all levels of ability. They are more likely to occur when you are relaxed and nonjudgmental rather than when you are critical or dissatisfied. When they come they impart meaning and satisfaction that transcend the physiological benefits of physical activity and fitness.

So as you pursue the pleasures and values of the active life, remain open to peak experiences and flow. Don't become preoccupied with time, distance, or heart rates. Set aside a time during each exercise session where you just let it happen. Ignore form so that you can enjoy sensations. Forget time so that you can experience the timelessness of flow. Once you do, you will come back day after day to repeat the experience. Activity will become an integral part of your life.

Complementary Themes

The active life is not a stand-alone philosophy. Complementary themes surround and support it. Some of them may appeal to you.

Simplicity

A modern version of a timeless theme, simplicity is a reaction to the mindless quest for material possessions, sometimes called affluenza.

"We are spending money we don't have, to buy things we don't need, to impress people we don't like."

Anonymous

Hallmarks of the simplicity movement are frugality, the concept that less is more; energy conservation; recycling; low-cost transportation (walking, bicycling); and self-sufficiency. People committed to the movement ignore advertising and the throwaway society and concentrate on things that matter, things that last. Converts find that when they don't have to work long hours to buy the latest styles or gadgets, they have more time to spend with family and friends, more time to pursue hobbies and the active life. You may find that when you spend less, you seem to have more.

> You may find that when you spend less, you seem to have more.

Individual Responsibility

An underlying theme of this book has been individual responsibility. You are responsible for your health, your actions, and your behaviors. Your doctor can't ensure your health. Only you can control your food intake; avoid smoking and excess alcohol consumption; use seat belts, ski helmets, and bicycle helmets; and engage in regular, moderate activity. Similarly, you are responsible for your actions and behaviors, and you shouldn't blame others for your mistakes. For example, if you smoke cigarettes for 30 years, who is at fault when you become ill with heart disease or lung cancer? More important, who should pay for your mistakes? If you elect to ride a motorcycle without a helmet and are involved in an accident, should others be responsible for your long-term care in a rehabilitation facility? Should people who practice moderation pay the bills for those who do not? Failure to make individuals responsible for their behaviors teaches the wrong lesson. Your behavior has consequences, and you should be willing to accept them.

Part of the blame for the loss of personal responsibility belongs to a legal system that sues others for our mistakes. When a drunk wanders into a railroad yard in the dark and is injured, the family sues the railroad. When someone spills hot coffee in a moving car and gets burned, she sues the restaurant that sold the coffee. This lack of personal responsibility threatens the world of physical activity. Trampolines are no longer used in schools, and diving boards are fast disappearing from swimming pools. Wilderness users are suing for injuries sustained in dangerous pursuits. When a backcountry skier died in an avalanche, the family sued the government for failing to provide adequate warning to the skier. If we don't take responsibility for our actions, the cost of living will rise and the quality of life will decline.

A Challenge

If you're still with us this late in the book, you've probably accepted the importance of the active life and the positive health habits it fosters. No doubt you are engaged in regular, moderate activity, and you practice healthy habits most of the time. You are taking responsibility for your behaviors and your health. If so, you are ready for a new challenge.

Working to improve your health and the quality of life is not enough. You must strive to do the same for family, friends, and the community. As you become convinced of the contribution and potential of the active life, you will appreciate your responsibility to extend the message and the opportunity to others. We need to redirect a society caught in a cycle of inactivity and overindulgence; of energy-wasting, polluting, motorized recreation; of declining health and vitality. This effort is important if we are to reduce disease and disability and gain control of spiraling health care and worker's compensation costs. We need to restore the sense of personal responsibility for our health and our actions. Also essential is the need to preserve the physical, emotional, and social environments that we want for our children and our children's children.

Improve Your Quality of Life

What can you do to reverse the trend toward inactivity? You can start by acting locally. Begin with little acts of kindness to family and friends. Find the time to acquaint others with the pleasures of the active life. Invite a friend for a walk. Plan a hike with the family. Give gifts that encourage activity and then find ways to make certain that they are used. When his grandson wanted another video game for Christmas, Brian presented him with cross-country skis, boots, and poles. Then one sunny day he took the boy skiing, masking the effort with drinks and snacks. Fortunately, the two of them didn't have to go far to find good ski trails.

Happy Trails

Gordon, an avid cross-country skier, came to our community as a graduate student and stayed on to pursue a career and raise his family. He used his term as president of the Nordic Ski Club to improve our local ski trails. Because of his efforts, the work of club volunteers, and the cooperation of local agencies and ski shops, we now have a fine network of trails located minutes from town. Other trailblazers helped create a local wilderness area, with trails for hikers, runners, skiers, mountain bikers, and horses. We have been blessed with river walks, hillside trails, and other pathways to the active life, all because people made the effort.

If you believe, as we do, that the quality of life is closely tied to the environment, then you may accept our challenge and work to preserve and improve the features you enjoy. Brian served as a member of our community Air Quality Advisory Council. Our mountain valley traps pollutants during the air inversions common in winter months. Wood-burning stoves, automobiles, and industrial pollution contribute pollutants to the air shed. But with health department efforts and citizen cooperation, the community has seen substantial improvement in air quality. New regulations control wood-burning stoves, automobiles have improved pollution-control systems, industrial pollution has diminished, and air quality has improved dramatically, in spite of a substantial increase in population.

With some thought and attention, you'll find dozens of ways to promote activity, enhance the environment, and improve the quality of life. You could help start a worksite wellness program or work to improve the one that you have. You could join the PTA and work for improved programs and facilities for the kids and the community. For additional ideas consult the guide *Promoting Physical Activity: A Guide for Community Action*, prepared by agencies of the U.S. Department of Health and Human Services (USDHHS 1999). To improve your environment and quality of life, be a volunteer in local causes and clean-up efforts, or write letters to policy makers and agencies to encourage better use of the environment, limits on motorized recreation,

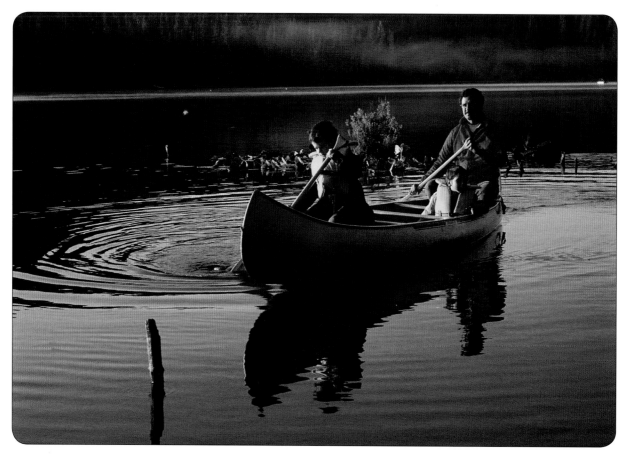

Work to encourage activity and improve the quality of life in your community.

and preservation of open space. Vote for bond issues that are designed to preserve open spaces or improve the environment, and contribute to the work of organizations that share your goals.

Influence Public Policy

Public policy influences health behavior. Local, state, and national laws and policies should encourage healthy behavior, such as walking (Librett, Yore, and Schmid 2003). People are more likely to quit smoking when it is banned in the workplace, in public buildings, in restaurants, and on airline flights. On the other hand, people are more likely to participate in sedentary, energy-consuming, polluting activities (using snowmobiles, motorboats, all-terrain vehicles) when they are allowed or even encouraged in local, state, and national parks. Sometimes the contrasts are perplexing, as when Yellowstone National Park grooms trails for snowmobile use but bans mountain bikes and arrests runners who use park trails for races. The contrast is even more puzzling when you learn that Glacier National Park bans the snowmobile and Crater Lake National Park conducts an annual marathon. Based on the acknowledged contribution of physical activity to health, Congress and the Public Health Service should endeavor to make participation in physical activity and other healthy behaviors a high priority in decision making for all government agencies. Just as land-use policies require environmental impact analyses before changes in land use can occur, we should require health impact analyses before approval of all laws and policies.

An array of environmental and policy determinants, particularly those related to the physical environment, are associated with physical activity and should be taken into account in the design of activity interventions (Brownson et al. 2002). The prevalence of physical activity varies by degree of urbanization and geographic region of the United States. Those living in Northeast metro and large urban areas and in Midwestern areas were more likely to be inactive than those residing in Western metro and urban areas (Reis et al. 2004). Areas with walkable green spaces positively influenced the longevity of older urban citizens. Urban planning should emphasize greenery-filled public areas that promote walking (Takano, Nakamura, and Watanabe 2003). Residents of highly walkable neighborhoods had more activity and less obesity than did residents of neighborhoods in which walking was not easy. Surprisingly, walkable areas were associated with higher residential density, as well as street connectivity, aesthetics, and safety (Saelens et al. 2003). Is walking important? Walking can reduce the rate of mental decline, the onset of dementia and Alzheimer's disease. Long-term regular physical activity such as walking is associated with significantly better cognitive function and less decline in seniors and elders (Weuve et al. 2004). Encourage your local, state, and national legislators and bureaucrats to consider the effect of public policy on health and the quality of life.

As you pursue your cause, be patient, be positive, but be persistent. Employ persuasion, avoid confrontation, and seek mutually beneficial solutions. By keeping a sense of humor, you'll be more likely to achieve results and enjoy the experience. Good luck. We look forward to hearing of your successes.

Reverse the Cost of Sloth

By now you know that physical inactivity comes at a cost. Inactivity is responsible for major health and economic costs. Inactivity may be responsible for somewhere between 250,000 and 365,000 deaths annually and is a major contributor to heart disease, diabetes, osteoporosis, and some forms of cancer. In spite of this burden, our society is doing little to reverse the shuffle toward inactivity, sloth, and obesity. What can we do? Here are a few ideas:

Children and Adolescents

- Restore school physical education programs
- Train and test for fitness
- Institute weight management programs
- Eliminate school-based fast food and soft drinks
- Restore after-school programs
- Initiate community-based and club programs
- Foster involvement in lifetime sports

Families

- Discuss, plan, and engage in active recreation
- Emphasize muscle-powered activities
- Take active vacations
- Plan activities for every season
- Limit high-calorie desserts, snacks, and soft drinks

Adults

- Make time for physical activity and sport
- Exercise outdoors when possible
- Use health and fitness clubs
- Participate in worksite employee health (wellness) programs
- Identify activities for every season

Older adults

- Continue activities in every season
- Engage in aerobic and muscular fitness training
- Use community and health club resources
- Train to travel—walk and weight train
- Participate with children and grandchildren

Elders

- Walk for physical and mental health
- Do muscular fitness training to maintain mobility and independence

Summary

The stages of life provide many challenges and opportunities. We need an arsenal of activities and coping strategies to help us through the lows as we regain confidence and establish new goals. Although faith, family, and friends provide the major sources of support, the active life serves by providing vitality, discipline, challenge, and time for reflection. We hope that this book helps you improve your health, enhance the quality of life, and experience and appreciate all the dimensions of the active life, including the spiritual.

"Know ye not that your body is the temple of the Holy Spirit?"

Corinthians 6:19

"The human body is the best picture of the human soul."

Ludwig Wittgenstein

Glossary

acclimatization—Adaptation to an environmental condition such as heat or altitude.

accommodating resistance—Resistance that adjusts to meet the changing force capabilities of the contracting muscles during resistance training.

actin—Muscle protein that works with the protein myosin to produce movement.

adenosine triphosphate (ATP)—High-energy compound formed from oxidation of fat and carbohydrate and used as energy supply for muscle and other body functions; the biological energy currency.

adipose tissue—Tissue in which fat is stored.

aerobic—In the presence of oxygen; aerobic metabolism utilizes oxygen.

aerobic capacity—Maximal oxygen intake in liters per minute (L/min).

aerobic fitness—Maximum ability to take in, transport, and utilize oxygen.

agility—Ability to change direction quickly while maintaining control of the body.

altitude sickness—Symptoms related to ascending to altitudes above 8,000 feet (2,400 meters), which include headache, shortness of breath, rapid heartbeat, loss of appetite.

alveoli—Tiny air sacs in the lungs where oxygen and carbon dioxide exchange takes place.

amino acids—Chief components of proteins; different arrangements of the 22 amino acids form the various proteins (muscles, enzymes, hormones).

anaerobic—In the absence of oxygen; nonoxidative metabolism.

anaerobic threshold—More properly called the lactate threshold, the point at which lactic acid produced in muscles begins to accumulate in the blood; defines the upper limit that can be sustained aerobically.

angina pectoris—Chest pain (also called necktie pain) associated with narrowed coronary arteries and lack of oxygen to heart muscle during exertion.

anorexia nervosa—An eating disorder characterized by excessive dieting and subsequent loss of appetite.

antioxidants—Compounds such as vitamins C and E or beta-carotene that can trap free radicals. Free radicals are highly reactive compounds formed during oxidative energy production that can damage tissues.

arrhythmia—Irregular rhythm or beat of the heart.

asymptomatic—Without symptoms.

atherosclerosis—Narrowing of coronary arteries by cholesterol buildup within the walls.

ATP—*See* adenosine triphosphate.

atrophy—Loss of size of muscle.

balance—Ability to maintain equilibrium while in motion.

behavior therapy—A system of record keeping and motivation designed to help change a behavior (e.g., overeating).

blood pressure—Force exerted against the walls of arteries.

blood volume—The amount of blood in the vascular system; blood volume increases with endurance training.

body composition—The relative amounts of fat and lean tissue.

body mass index—A common method using weight and height to estimate overweight, obesity, and risk for chronic diseases such as heart disease, stroke, hypertension, hyperlipidemia, and diabetes. The index is calculated as weight in kilograms divided by height in meters squared (kg/m^2).

bronchiole—Small branch of airway; sometimes undergoes spasm, making breathing difficult, as in exercise-induced asthma.

buffer—Substance in blood that soaks up hydrogen ions to minimize changes in acid–base balance (pH).

bulimia—An eating disorder characterized by alternate bouts of gorging and purging.

C-reactive protein (C-RP)—An indicator of inflammatory activity that is associated with increased risk of heart attack.

calisthenics—An exercise method including a wide range of body-weight resistance exercises including push-ups, chin-ups, jumping jacks, and sit-ups. Calisthenics are often used when the strength-training prescription calls for high resistance and low repetitions.

caloric cost—The energy expenditure in calories of an activity. Usually measured in calories per minute.

calorie—Amount of heat required to raise 1 kilogram of water 1 degree Celsius; same as kilocalorie.

capillaries—Smallest blood vessels (between arterioles and venules) where oxygen, foods, and hormones are delivered to tissues and carbon dioxide and wastes are picked up.

carbohydrate—Simple (e.g., sugar) and complex (e.g., potatoes, rice, beans, corn, and grains) foodstuff that we use for energy; stored in liver and muscle as glycogen, while excess can be stored as fat.

carbohydrate loading—A procedure that elevates muscle glycogen stores before an endurance event.

cardiac—Pertaining to the heart.

cardiac output—Volume of blood pumped by the heart each minute; product of heart rate and stroke volume.

cardiorespiratory endurance—Synonymous with aerobic fitness or maximal oxygen intake.

cardiovascular system—Heart and blood vessels.

central nervous system (CNS)—The brain and spinal cord.

cholesterol—Fatty substance found in nerves and other tissues; excessive amounts in blood have been associated with increased risk of heart disease.

circuit weight training—A system of weight training in which a person rotates through one set of a number of different exercises before repeating the exercises two or more times. This training is generally used with lighter weights or body resistance training.

Clo units—The insulating value of clothing.

concentric—Contraction that involves shortening of the contracted muscle.

conduction—The removal of body heat through direct contact with or flow through other material.

contraction—Development of tension by muscle; under tension, concentric muscle shortens and eccentric muscle lengthens; static contractions are contractions without change in length.

convection—The removal of body heat by air flow or water flow over the surface of the skin.

cool-down—Postperformance exercise used to dissipate heat, maintain blood flow, and aid recovery of muscles.

core training—Training abdominal, back, chest, shoulder, and hip muscles that control the core of the body.

coronary arteries—Blood vessels that originate from the aorta and branch out to supply oxygen and fuel to the heart muscle.

coronary prone—Having several risk factors related to the development of heart disease.

cortisol—Stress hormone secreted by adrenal gland.

creatine phosphate (CP)—Energy-rich compound that backs up ATP in providing energy for muscles.

defibrillator—Device that applies a strong electric shock to stop irregular heart action and restore normal heart rhythm.

dehydration—Loss of essential body fluids.

delayed-onset muscle soreness (DOMS)—Muscle soreness that peaks 24 to 48 hours after unfamiliar exercise or vigorous eccentric contractions.

deoxyribonucleic acid (DNA)—The source of the genetic code housed in the nucleus of the cell.

detraining—Cessation of training; used to observe the decline of important measures (e.g., blood volume) associated with performance.

diastolic pressure—Lowest pressure exerted by blood in an artery; occurs during the resting phase (diastole) of the heart cycle.

dietary fiber—The portion of ingested plant material that is indigestible.

dieting—Eating according to a prescribed plan.

duration—Distance or length of time (or calories burned, in the case of the exercise prescription).

early competitions—Training period that involves a build-up to the important part of the season, the peak performance period.

eccentric—Contraction that involves lengthening of a contracted muscle.

electrocardiogram (ECG)—A graphic recording of the electrical activity of the heart.

electrolyte—Solution of ions (sodium, potassium) that conducts electric current.

endurance—The ability to persist or to resist fatigue.

energy balance—Balance of caloric intake and expenditure.

energy expenditure—The energy consumed by metabolism. The three main areas of energy expenditure are **activity expenditure** to allow movement, **resting expenditure** to maintain basic cell function and life, and **digestive and absorptive expenditure** to digest and absorb food. The sum of these is total energy expenditure.

enzyme—An organic catalyst that accelerates the rate of chemical reactions.

epinephrine (adrenaline)—Hormone from the adrenal medulla and nerve endings of the sympathetic nervous system; secreted during times of stress and to help mobilize energy.

ergometer—A device, such as a bicycle, used to measure work capacity.

evaporation—Elimination of body heat when sweat vaporizes on the surface of the skin; evaporation of 1 liter of sweat yields a heat loss of 580 calories.

exercise—Means structured physical activity, but usually denotes any form of physical activity, exertion, effort, and so forth.

Fartlek—Swedish term meaning "speed play"; a form of training in which participants vary speed according to mood as they run through the countryside.

fast glycolytic fiber (FG)—Fast-twitch muscle fiber with limited oxidative capabilities; easily fatigued.

fast oxidative glycolytic fiber (FOG)—Fast-twitch fiber with oxidative and glycolytic capabilities.

fast-twitch muscle fibers—Muscle fibers that contract quickly. Includes both fast oxidative glycolytic and fast glycolytic fibers.

fat—Important energy source; stored for future use when excess calories are ingested.

fatigue—Diminished work capacity, usually short of true physiological limits; real limits in short, intense exercise are factors within muscle (muscle pH, calcium); in long-duration effort, limits are glycogen depletion or central nervous system fatigue caused, in part, by low blood sugar.

fibrillation—Rapid and uncoordinated contractions in the heart that can be life threatening.

first lactate threshold—The early rise in blood lactic acid associated with long-term endurance or sustainable fitness.

FIT—The FIT principle of training refers to the frequency, intensity, and duration (time) of training.

fitness—A combination of aerobic capacity and muscular strength and endurance that enhances health, performance, and the quality of life.

flexibility—Range of motion through which the limbs or body parts are able to move.

frequency—Number of times per day or week (in the case of the exercise prescription).

free radicals—Reactive molecules with one or more unpaired electrons that can damage biological tissues.

free weights—Weights that are free of machinery, such as dumbbells, bars with attached weights, or even ankle and wrist weights.

gender-specific fat—Also called essential fat, this fat is necessary for cell membranes, organs, protection, and reproductive organs. In general, it is reported as 3 to 6 percent in males and 12 percent in females. The additional fat specific to reproductive organs in females is referred to as gender-specific fat.

glucose—Basic carbohydrate energy source transported in blood; essential energy source for brain and nervous tissue.

glycemic index—A measure of how rapidly a carbohydrate is digested and absorbed into the blood.

glycogen—Storage form of glucose; found in liver and muscles.

heart attack—Death of heart muscle tissue that results when atherosclerosis blocks oxygen delivery to heart muscle; also called myocardial infarction.

heart rate—Frequency of contraction, often inferred from pulse rate (expansion of artery resulting from beat of heart).

heart rate range—The difference between the resting and maximal heart rates.

heat stress—Combination of temperature and humidity that leads to heat disorders such as heat cramps, heat exhaustion, or heatstroke.

hemoglobin—Iron-containing compound in red blood cells that forms a loose association with oxygen.

high-density lipoprotein (HDL) cholesterol—A carrier molecule that takes cholesterol from the tissue to the liver for removal; inversely related to heart disease risk.

hyperthermia—An alarming rise in body temperature that sets the stage for heat stress disorders.

hypertrophy—An increase in muscle mass and cross-sectional area because of the increase in the size of individual muscle fibers.

hypoglycemia—Low blood sugar (glucose).

hyponatremia—Low sodium concentrations generally resulting from excess fluid intake or excess sweating without sodium replacement.

hypothermia—Life-threatening heat loss brought on by rapid cooling, energy depletion, and exhaustion.

hypoxia—Low oxygen.

inhibition—Opposite of excitation in the nervous system.

insulin—Pancreatic hormone responsible for getting blood sugar into cells.

insulin resistance—A condition in which people produce adequate, or excess, insulin but have insulin receptors on muscle cells that have become insensitive to insulin and no longer stimulate muscle cells to take up glucose from the blood.

intensity—The relative rate, speed, or level of exertion.

interval training—Training method that alternates short bouts of harder effort with periods of active rest.

ischemia—Lack of blood to a specific area such as heart muscle.

isokinetic—Contraction against resistance that maintains a fixed speed throughout range of motion.

isometric—Contraction against an immovable object (static contraction).

isotonic—Contraction against a constant resistance.

lactate threshold—**first lactate threshold (LT1)**—The intensity of aerobic exercise at which blood lactate begins to increase; associated with long-term (more than 3 hours) endurance. **second lactate threshold (LT2)**—The point at which lactate and respiration rise rapidly; associated with performance in events lasting 30 to 120 minutes.

lactic acid—A by-product of glycogen metabolism that also transports energy from muscle to muscle and from muscle to the liver; high levels in muscle poison the contractile apparatus and inhibit enzyme activity.

lean body weight—Body weight minus fat weight.

leptin—A hormone produced by fat cells that helps regulate body weight and metabolism.

lipid—Fat.

lipoprotein—A fat–protein complex that serves as a carrier in the blood (e.g., high-density lipoprotein cholesterol).

lipoprotein lipase (LPL)—An enzyme in adipose tissue (also found in muscle). Its activity has been found to increase in the fat cells of obese people who lose weight.

low-density lipoprotein (LDL) cholesterol—The cholesterol fraction that accumulates in the lining of the coronary arteries and causes atherosclerosis and ischemia.

maximal oxygen intake (consumption)—Aerobic fitness; measure of fitness with implications for health; synonymous with $\dot{V}O_2$max and cardiorespiratory fitness.

metabolic equivalent (MET)—Unit of measure; 1 MET is resting metabolism.

metabolic rate—Also called resting metabolic rate, this is the energy expenditure rate that occurs during quiet sitting and rest. It is estimated at 3.5 milliliters of oxygen per kilogram of body weight each minute (about 1.25 calories each minute for a 155 pound [70kg] person) but varies slightly within and between individuals.

metabolic syndrome—A clustering of metabolic abnormalities including elevated blood pressure, triglycerides, and blood glucose, with central adiposity (waist circumference greater than 40 inches, or 100 centimeters) and low HDL cholesterol.

metabolism—Energy production and utilization processes, mediated by enzymatic pathways.

mitochondria—Tiny organelles within cells; site of all oxidative energy production.

motor area—Portion of cerebral cortex that controls movement.

motor neuron—Nerve that transmits impulses to muscle fibers.

motor unit—Motor neuron and the muscle fibers that it innervates.

mountain sickness—*See* altitude sickness.

muscle fiber types—Fast-twitch fibers are fast contracting but fast to fatigue; slow-twitch fibers contract somewhat more slowly but are fatigue resistant.

muscular endurance—The ability to sustain muscular contractions.

muscular fitness—The strength, muscular endurance, and flexibility needed to carry out daily tasks and avoid injury.

myocardium—Heart muscle.

myofibril—Contractile threads of muscle composed of the proteins actin and myosin.

myogenic—Training that influences the muscles.

myosin—Muscle protein that works with actin to produce movement.

neurogenic—Training that influences the nervous system.

neuron—Nerve cell that conducts an impulse; basic unit of the nervous system.

nutrition—Provision of adequate energy (calories) as well as needed amounts of fat, carbohydrate, protein, vitamins, minerals, and water.

obesity—Excessive body fat (more than 20 percent of total body weight for men, more than 30 percent for women).

occupational physiology—The study of work physiology specific to occupations.

off-season—The period of the year when training is nonspecific and foundational; far from the competitive season.

osteoporosis—Weakening of bones through loss of bone minerals.

overload—A greater load than normally experienced; used to coax a training effect from the body.

overtraining—Excess training that leads to staleness, illness, or injury.

oxidation—The process of breaking down fuels (carbohydrate, fat, and protein) in the presence of oxygen to produce energy (ATP and heat) plus carbon dioxide (CO_2) and water (H_2O).

oxygen debt—Postexercise oxygen intake that exceeds resting requirements; used to replace the oxygen deficit incurred during exercise.

oxygen deficit—Lack of oxygen in early moments of exercise.

oxygen intake—Oxygen used to provide energy through oxidative pathways.

peaking—The process of preparing for best possible performances; *see also* peak performance period and taper.

peak performance period—The period designed to produce peak performances; involves a decrease in training volume, an increase in training intensity, and sufficient rest to allow complete recovery.

perceived exertion—Subjective estimate of exercise difficulty.

performance threshold—Current race speed (usually measured in meters per minute).

periodization—The process of planning systematic variations of work and rest in the training program that may be programmed at several levels—daily, weekly, seasonal, and career.

peripheral nervous system—Parts of the nervous system not including the brain and spinal cord.

pH—Acidity or alkalinity of a solution; below 7 is acid, and above 7 is alkaline.

Phosphocreatine (PCr)—Another name for creatine phosphate (CP), a high-energy compound stored in muscle.

physical fitness—The state of energy (aerobic) fitness or muscular (strength and power) fitness.

physiological age—Also called functional age, as contrasted to chronological age; defines a person's ability to perform physically.

plaque—A growth of cellular debris and low-density lipoprotein cholesterol that impedes blood flow in the arteries.

plyometrics—A form of power training that uses vigorous contractions with resistance.

power—The rate of doing work.

preload—Often called elastic recoil. A short eccentric contraction preceding a forceful concentric contraction.

progression—The training concept that states that the training overload must increase as a person becomes more fit to elicit continuing improvements.

progressive resistance—Training program in which the resistance is increased as the muscles gain strength.

protein—Organic compound formed from amino acids; forms muscle tissue, hormones, and enzymes.

psychoneuroimmunology—A field of study that explores links between the brain and nervous system and the immune system, or between thoughts and emotions and sickness and health.

pulse—The wave that travels down the artery after each contraction of the heart; *see also* heart rate.

purposeful physical activity—Physical activity with a purpose, such as walking a dog or walking to the store.

radiation—The removal or addition of heat to the body through radiant energy.

rapid eye movement (REM)—A stage of sleep associated with dreams.

recovery—Time between intervals to rest. Time between training sessions to allow training adaptations to take place. Period at the end of a training year during which an athlete relaxes and does nonspecific training.

relative fitness—The percentage of maximal aerobic capacity that a person can sustain.

relaxation response—Proven method to achieve relaxation.

repetitions—The number of times that a person repeats a strength exercise before resting.

repetition maximum (RM)—The maximum number of times that a person can lift a given weight (1RM is the most that a person can lift one time).

respiration—Intake of oxygen (from the atmosphere into the lungs and then to the blood and to the tissues) and exhalation of carbon dioxide (from tissues to the blood, to the lungs, and to the atmosphere).

resting metabolic rate—*See* metabolic rate.

ribonucleic acid (RNA)—A cellular compound that carries messages from the nucleus (DNA) to the rest of the cell (messenger RNA) or transfers amino acids to the ribosome for protein synthesis (transfer RNA).

ribosome—A cellular organelle that synthesizes protein from amino acids.

risk factors—Factors associated with a higher risk for a certain disease (e.g., coronary risk factors).

sarcomere—The contractile unit of the muscle.

sarcopenia—Loss of muscle with age and inactivity.

set point theory—A theory that the body has a preferred weight range that it tries to maintain based on current weight. The term *set point* also refers to homeostasis, the body's effort to maintain a constant internal environment such as temperature, fluid volume, and so on.

slow-twitch muscle fibers—Muscle fibers that contract more slowly than fast-twitch fibers but are more resistant to fatigue.

somatotype—Body type; ectomorph is linear or thin, mesomorph is muscular, and endomorph is fat.

specificity—A principle of training that states that the type of training undertaken must relate to the desired results.

speed of movement—The sum of reaction time (time from stimulus to start of movement) and movement time (time to complete the movement).

strength—Ability of muscle to exert force.

stroke volume—Volume of blood pumped from the ventricle during each contraction of the heart.

subcutaneous fat—Fat layers located just below the skin.

submaximal aerobic fitness—Ability to sustain an aerobic workload for extended periods.

synapse—Junction between neurons.

systolic pressure—Highest pressure in arteries that results from contraction (systole) of the heart.

taper—A reduction in training volume lasting from several days to 2 weeks before an important competition to allow complete recovery and the best possible performance.

tendon—Tough connective tissue that connects muscle to bone.

tension—The condition of being strained or stretched.

testosterone—An anabolic (tissue building) hormone found in higher concentrations in males.

threshold—The minimal level required to elicit a response or a transition point (training threshold).

tonus—Muscle firmness in absence of a voluntary contraction.

training plateau—When fitness no longer improves as a result of a training stimulus.

training stimulus—The type of exercise that elicits the desired adaptation to training.

training zone—The heart rate or work intensity or speed within which training is likely to produce the desired effect.

triglyceride—A fat consisting of three fatty acids and glycerol.

Valsalva maneuver—Increased pressure in abdominal and thoracic cavities caused by breath holding and extreme effort.

variable (or accommodating) resistance—A machine or system that matches resistance across a range of motion to the capability of the muscle group.

velocity—Rate of movement or speed.

ventilation—The amount of air inhaled per minute; the product of tidal volume and breathing frequency.

ventricle—Chamber of the heart that pumps blood to the lungs (right ventricle) or to the rest of the body (left ventricle).

warm-up—A preexercise activity used to increase muscle temperature and rehearse skills.

weight training—Progressive resistance exercise using weight for resistance.

wellness—A conscious and deliberate approach to an advanced state of physical, psychological, and spiritual health.

wind chill—Cooling effect of temperature and wind.

work—Product of force and distance.

work capacity—The ability to achieve work goals without undue fatigue and without becoming a hazard to oneself or coworkers; also referred to as sustainable work capacity.

References

Achten, J., M. Gleeson, and A. Jeukendrup. 2002. Determination of the exercise intensity that elicits maximal fat oxidation. *Medicine and Science in Sports and Exercise* 34:92–97.

Adams, W.C., E.M. Bernauer, D.B. Dill, and J.B. Bomar Jr. 1975. Effect of equivalent sea level and altitude training on $\dot{V}O_2$max and running performance. *Journal of Applied Physiology* 39:262–268.

Ainsworth, B., W. Haskell, A. Leon, D. Jacobs Jr., H. Montoye, J. Sallis, and R. Paffenbarger. 1993. Compendium of physical activities: Classification of energy costs of human physical activities. *Medicine and Science in Sports and Exercise* 25:71–80.

Alderman, B., and D. Landers. 2004. The influence of cardiorespiratory fitness and hostility on cardiovascular reactivity in mental stress. *Medicine and Science in Sports and Exercise* 36:S91.

Amako, M., T. Oda, K. Masuoka, H. Yokoi, and P. Campisi. 2003. Effects of static stretching on prevention of injuries for military recruits. *Military Medicine* 168:442–446.

American College of Sports Medicine (ACSM). 2005. *ACSM guidelines for exercise testing and prescription.* 7th ed. Baltimore: Williams and Wilkins.

Amoroso, P., K. Reynolds, J. Barnes, and D. White. 1996. *Tobacco and injury.* Natick, MA: U.S. Army Research Institute for Environmental Medicine, Technical Report 91–96.

Anderson, T., and J. Kearney. 1982. Effects of three resistance training programs on muscular strength and absolute and relative endurance. *Research Quarterly for Exercise Science and Sport* 53:1–7.

Ardell, D. 1984. *The history and future of wellness.* Pleasant Hills, CA: Diablo Press.

Armstrong, L. 2000. *Performance in extreme environments.* Champaign, IL: Human Kinetics.

Armstrong, R. 1984. Mechanisms of exercise-induced delayed-onset muscular soreness: A brief review. *Medicine and Science in Sports and Exercise* 16:529–538.

Asahina, S., K. Asano, H. Horikawa, T. Hisamitsu, and M. Sato. 2003. Enhancement of beta-endorphin levels in rat hypothalamus by exercise. *Japanese Journal of Physical Fitness and Sports Medicine* 52:159–166.

Åstrand, P.O., and K. Rodahl. 1970. *Textbook of work physiology: Physiological bases of exercise.* 2nd ed. New York: McGraw-Hill.

Avins, A., and J. Neuhaus. 2000. Do triglycerides provide meaningful information about heart disease risk? *Archives of Internal Medicine* 160:1937–1944.

Baechle, T., R. Earle, and D. Wathen. 2000. Resistance training. In *Essentials of strength training and conditioning,* ed. T. Baechle and R. Earle. Champaign, IL: Human Kinetics.

Balady, G. 2002. Survival of the fittest—more evidence. *New England Journal of Medicine* 346:852–854.

Balady, G., B. Chaitman, D. Driscoll, C. Foster, E. Froelicher, N. Gordon, R. Pate, J. Rippe, and T. Bazzarre. 1998. Recommendations for cardiovascular screening, staffing, and emergency policies at health/fitness facilities. *Medicine and Science in Sport and Exercise* 30:1009–1018.

Balke, B. 1963. *A simple field test for the assessment of physical fitness.* Report no. 63-66. Oklahoma City: Civil Aeronautic Research Institute, Federal Aviation Agency.

Barham, J. 1960. A comparison of the effectiveness of isometric and isotonic exercise when performed at different frequencies per week. Unpublished doctoral dissertation, Louisiana State University, Baton Rouge.

Barnard, R.J., G.W. Gardner, N. Diaco, and A.A. Kattus. 1972. Ischemic response to sudden strenuous exercise. Paper presented at the annual meeting of the American College of Sports Medicine, Philadelphia.

Barton-Davis, E., D. Shoturma, and H. Sweeney. 1999. Contribution of satellite cells to IGF-I induced hypertrophy of skeletal muscle. *Acta Physiologica Scandinavica* 167:301–305.

Barzalai, N., G. Atzmon, C. Schecter, E. Schaefer, A. Cupples, R. Lipton, S. Cheng, and A. Shuldiner. 2003. Unique lipoprotein phenotype and genotype associated with exceptional longevity. *Journal of the American Medical Association* 290:2030–2040.

Bauer, D., I. Varahram, G. Proest, and U. Halter. 2001. Benefits from aerobic exercise in patients with major depression: A pilot study. *British Journal of Sports Medicine* 35:114–117.

Baun, W., M. Baun, and P. Raven. 1981. A nomogram for the estimate of percent body fat from generalized equations. *Research Quarterly* 52:382.

Beck, B., and C. Snow. 2003. Bone health across the lifespan: Exercising our options. *Exercise and Sports Science Reviews* 31:117–122.

Bell, G., D. Syrotuik, T. Martin, R. Burnham, and H. Quinney. 2000. Effects of concurrent strength and endurance training on skeletal muscle properties and hormone concentrations in humans. *European Journal of Applied Physiology* 81:418–427.

Benson, H. 1975. *The relaxation response*. New York: Harper and Row.

Blair, S. 2000. Benefits of physical activity and fitness in high risk populations. Paper presented at the annual meeting of the American College of Sports Medicine, Indianapolis, June 2.

Blair, S., and H. Kohl. 1988. Physical activity or physical fitness: Which is more important for health? *Medicine and Science in Sports and Exercise* 20:S8.

Blair, S., H. Kohl, C. Barlow, R. Paffenbarger, L. Gibbons, and C. Macera. 1995. Changes in physical fitness and all-cause mortality: A prospective study of healthy and unhealthy men. *Journal of the American Medical Association* 273:1093–1098.

Blair, S., H. Kohl, R. Paffenbarger, D. Clark, K. Cooper, and L. Gibbons. 1989. Physical fitness and all-cause mortality: A prospective study of healthy men and women. *Journal of the American Medical Association* 262:2395–2401.

Blair, S., M. LaMonte, and M. Nichaman. 2004. The evolution of physical activity recommendations: How much is enough? *American Journal of Clinical Nutrition* 79:913–920.

Blaschke, F., D. Bruemmer, F. Yin, Y. Takata, W. Wang, M. Fishbein, T. Okura, J. Higaki, K. Graf, E. Fleck, W. Hsueh, and R. Law. 2004. C-reactive protein induces apoptosis in human coronary vascular smooth muscle cells. *Circulation* 110:579–587.

Blomqvist, C.G., and B. Saltin. 1983. Cardiovascular adaptations to physical training. *Annual Review of Physiology* 45:169–185.

Blumenthal, J., A. Sherwood, E. Gullette, M. Babyak, R. Waugh, A. Georgiades, L. Craighead, D. Tweedy, M. Feinglos, M. Appelbaum, J. Hayano, and A. Hinderliter. 2000. Exercise and weight loss reduce blood pressure in men and women with mild hypertension. *Archives of Internal Medicine* 160:1947–1958.

Boileau, R., B. McKeown, and W. Riner. 1984. Cardiovascular and metabolic contributions to the maximal aerobic power of the arms and legs. *International Journal of Sports Cardiology* 4:67–75.

Booth, F., and M. Chakravarthy. 2002. Cost and consequences of sedentary living: New battleground for an old enemy. *President's Council on Physical Fitness and Sports Research Digest*, 3rd ser., no. 16.

Booth, F., S. Gordon, C. Carlson, and M. Hamilton. 2000. Waging war on modern chronic diseases: Primary prevention through exercise. *Journal of Applied Physiology* 88:774–787.

Borensztajn, J. 1975. Effect of exercise on lipoprotein lipase activity in rat heart and skeletal muscle. *American Journal of Physiology* 229:394–400.

Borg, G. 1973. Perceived exertion: A note on history and methods. *Medicine and Science in Sports and Exercise* 5:90–93.

Borg, G. 1985. *An introduction to Borg's RPE scale*. Ithaca, NY: Mouvement Publications.

Bouchard, C., P. An, T. Rice, J. Skinner, J. Wilmore, J. Gagnon, L. Perusse, A. Leon, and D. Rao. 1999. Familial aggregation of $\dot{V}O_2$max response to exercise training: Results from the Heritage Family Study. *Journal of Applied Physiology* 87:1003–1008.

Bouchard, C., M. Boulay, J. Simoneau, G. Lorrie, and L. Pierrise. 1988. Heritability and trainability of aerobic and anaerobic performance: An update. *Sports Medicine* 5:69–73.

Bouchard, C., W. Holimann, H. Venrath, G. Herkenrath, and H. Schlussel. 1966. Minimal amount of physical training for the prevention of cardiovascular disease. Paper presented at the 16th World Conference for Sports Medicine, Hanover, Germany.

Bravata, D., L. Sanders, J. Huang, H. Krumholz, I. Olkin, C. Gardner, and D. Bravata. 2003. Efficacy and safety of low-carbohydrate diets: A systematic review. *Journal of the American Medical Association* 289:1837–1850.

Bray, G. 1983. The energetics of obesity. *Medicine and Science in Sports and Exercise* 15:32–40.

Breslow, L., and J. Enstrom. 1980. Persistence of health habits and their relationship to mortality. *Preventive Medicine* 9:469–483.

Brill, P., C. Macera, D. Davis, S. Blair, and N. Gordon. 2000. Muscular strength and physical function. *Medicine and Science in Sports and Exercise* 32:412–416.

Brooks, G., N. Butte, W. Rand, J. Flatt, and B. Cabellaro. 2004. Chronicle of the Institute of Medicine physical activity recommendation: How a physical activity recommendation came to be among dietary recommendations. *American Journal of Clinical Nutrition* 79:921–930.

Brown, R., and C. Cox. 1998. Effects of high fat versus high carbohydrate diets on plasma lipids and lipoproteins in endurance athletes. *Medicine and Science in Sports and Exercise* 30:1677–1683.

Brownell, K. 1995. Exercise and obesity treatment: Psychological aspects. *International Journal of Obesity* 19:S122–125.

Brownell, K., M. Greenwood, E. Stellar, and E. Shrager. 1986. The effects of repeated cycles of weight loss and regain in rats. *Physiology and Behavior* 38:459–464.

Brownell, K., and J. Rodin. 1994. Medical, metabolic, and psychological effects of weight cycling. *Archives of Internal Medicine* 154:1325–1330.

Brownson, R., E. Baker, R. Housemann, L. Brennan, and S. Bacak. 2002. Environmental and policy determinants of physical activity in the United States. *American Journal of Public Health* 91:1995–2003.

Brynteson, P., and W. Sinning. 1973. The effects of training frequencies on the retention of cardiovascular fitness. *Medicine and Science in Sports and Exercise* 5:29–33.

Bussau, V., T. Fairchild, A. Rao, P. Stelle, and P. Fournier. 2002. Carbohydrate loading in human muscle: An improved 1 day protocol. *European Journal of Applied Physiology* 87:290–295.

Calle, E., C. Rodriquez, K. Walker-Thurmond, and M. Thun. 2003. Overweight, obesity, and mortality from cancer in a prospectively studied cohort of U.S. adults. *New England Journal of Medicine* 348:1625–1638.

Calle, E., M. Thun, J. Petrelli, C. Rodriguez, and C. Heath. 1999. Body mass index and mortality in a prospective cohort of U.S. adults. *New England Journal of Medicine* 341:1097–1105.

Campbell, W., M. Crim, V. Young, and W. Evans. 1994. Increased energy requirements and changes in body composition with resistance training in older adults. *American Journal of Clinical Nutrition* 60:167–175.

Carey, T., J. Garrett, A. Jackman, C. McLaughlin, J. Fryer, D. Smucker, P. Curtis, J. Darter, G. DeFriese, A. Evans, N. Hadler, G. Hunter, J. Joines, W. Kalsbeek, T. Konrad, R. McNutt, T. Rickets, and D. Taylor. 1995. The outcomes and cost of care for acute low-back pain among patients seen by primary-care practitioners, chiropractors, and orthopaedic surgeons. *New England Journal of Medicine* 333:913–917.

Carpenter, D., and B. Nelson. 1999. Low back strengthening for the prevention and treatment of low back pain. *Medicine and Science in Sports and Exercise* 31:18–24.

Cattell, R.B., H.W. Eber, and M.M. Tatsuoka. 1970. *Handbook for the sixteen personality factor questionnaire.* Champaign, IL: Institute for Personality and Ability Testing.

Centers for Disease Control. 2002. *National Vital Statistics Reports*, www.cdc.gov.

Chang, P., D. Ford, L. Meoni, N. Wang and M. Klag. 2002. Anger in young men and subsequent premature cardiovascular disease. *Archives of Internal Medicine* 162:901–906.

Chapman, R., J. Stray-Gunderson, and B. Levine. 1998. Individual variation in response to altitude training. *Journal of Applied Physiology* 85:1448–1456.

Choi, H., K. Atkinson, W. Karlson, W. Willett, and C. Curhan. 2004. Purine-rich foods dairy and protein intake, and the risk of gout in men. *New England Journal of Medicine* 350:1093–1103.

Christensen, E.H., and O. Hansen. 1939. Arbeitsfähigkeit und shrnährung [Working capacity and diet]. *Scandinavian Archives of Physiology* 81:160–172.

Coggan, A., and B. Williams. 1995. Metabolic adaptations to endurance training: Substrate metabolism during exercise. In *Exercise metabolism*, ed. M. Hargraves, 177–210. Champaign, IL: Human Kinetics.

Colditz, G.A. 1999. Economic costs of obesity and inactivity. *Medicine and Science in Sports and Exercise* 31(11):S663–667.

Comfort, A. 1979. *The biology of senescence.* New York: Elsevier.

Consolazio, C.F., R.E. Johnson, and L.J. Pecora. 1963. *Physiological measurements of metabolic functions in man.* New York: McGraw-Hill.

Cooper, K. 1968. *Aerobics.* New York: Bantam Books.

Cooper, K.H., J.G. Purdy, S.R. White, M.L. Pollock, and A.C. Linnerud. 1975. Age-fitness adjusted maximal heart rates. In *The role of exercise in internal medicine,* ed. D. Brunner and E. Jokl. Vol. 10 of *Medicine and sport.* Basel, Switzerland: Karger.

Cordes, K., and B. Sharkey. 1995. Physiological comparison of protective clothing variations. *Medicine and Science in Sports and Exercise* 27:S153.

Cotman, C., and C. Engesser-Cesar. 2002. Exercise enhances and protects brain function. *Exercise and Sports Science Reviews* 30:75–79.

Coyle, E. 1995. Substrate utilization during exercise in active people. *American Journal of Clinical Nutrition* 61:S968–979.

Coyle, E., M. Hemmert, and A. Coggan. 1986. Effects of detraining on cardiovascular responses to exercise: Role of blood volume. *Journal of Applied Physiology* 60:95–99.

Crews, D., M. Lochbaum, and D. Landers. 2004. Aerobic physical activity effects on psychological well-being in low-income Hispanic children. *Perceptual and Motor Skills* 98:319–324.

Cureton, T.K. 1969. *The physiological effects of exercise programs upon adults.* Springfield, IL: Charles C Thomas.

Danesh, J., J. Wheeler, G. Hirschfield, S. Eda, G. Eirksdottir, A. Rumley, G. Lowe, M. Pepys, and V. Goudnason. 2004. C-reactive protein and other circulating markers of inflammation in the predictin of coronary heart disease. *New England Journal of Medicine* V350:1387-1397.

Dansinger, M., J. Gleason, J. Griffith, H. Selker, and E. Schaefer. 2005. Comparison of the Atkins, Ornish, Weight Watchers, and Zone diets for weight loss and heart disease risk reduction. *Journal of the American Medical Association* 293:43–53.

Davis, P., and A. Starck. 1980. Age and performance in a police population. *Law Enforcement Bulletin.* Washington, DC: Federal Bureau of Investigation, 15–21.

DeLorme, T., and A. Watkins. 1951. *Progressive resistance exercise.* New York: Appleton-Century-Crofts.

Demopoulos, H., J. Santomier, M. Seligman, D. Pietrogro, and P. Hogan. 1986. Free radical pathology: Rationale and toxicology of antioxidants and other supplements in sports medicine and exercise science. In *Sport, health, and nutrition: 1984 proceedings of the Olympic Scientific Congress,* ed. F. Katch, 139–189. Champaign, IL: Human Kinetics.

Department of Health, Education, and Welfare - Vital Statistics of the United States. 1977. *National Center for Health Statistics, DHEW Publication* PHS 80-1104 (vol. 2, sec. 5).

Despres, J. 2004. Visceral fat and the metabolic syndrome: Effect of activity intervention. Paper presented at the annual meeting of the American College of Sports Medicine, Indianapolis.

Deschenes, M. 2005. Effects of aging on muscle fiber type and size. *Sports Medicine* 34:809–824.

deVries, H.A., and G.M. Adams. 1972. Electromyographic comparison of single doses of exercise and meprobromate as to effects on muscular relaxation. *American Journal of Physical Medicine* 51:130–141.

deVries, H., and T. Housh. 1994. *Physiology of exercise.* Madison, WI: Brown and Benchmark.

Dintiman, G., and R. Ward. 2003. *Sportspeed,* 3rd ed. Champaign, IL: Human Kinetics.

Docktor, R., and B.J. Sharkey. 1971. Note on some physiological and subjective reactions to exercise and training. *Perceptual and Motor Skills* 32:233–234.

Dotson, C., D. Santa Maria, and P. Davis. 1976. *Development of a job-related physical performance examination for firefighters.* Washington, DC: U.S. Department of Commerce, National Fire Prevention and Control Administration.

Drygas, W., T. Kostka, A. Jegier, and H. Kunski. 2000. Long-term effects of different physical activity levels on coronary heart disease risk factors in middle-aged men. *International Journal of Sports Medicine* 21:235–241.

Edstrom, K. 1999. *Healthy, wealthy and wise.* Los Angeles: Soft Stone.

Ehrlich, N. 1971. Acquisition rates of competitors and performers: A note on the theory of athletic performance. *Perceptual and Motor Skills* 33:10–66.

Eichner, R. 1995. Contagious infections in competitive sports. *Sports Science Exchange* 8(3):1–4.

Enos, W.F., J.C. Beyer, and R.H. Holmes. 1955. Pathogenesis of coronary disease in American soldiers killed in Korea. *Journal of the American Medical Association* 158:912–917.

Epel, E., E. Blackburn, J. Lin, F. Dhabhar, N. Alder, J. Morrow, and R. Cawthon. 2004. Accelerated telomere shortening in response to life stress. *Proceedings of the National Academy of Sciences* 101:17312–17315.

Ernst, E. 1993. Regular exercise reduces fibrinogen levels: A review of longitudinal studies. *British Journal of Sports Medicine* 27:175–176.

Esparza, J., C. Fox, I. Harper, L. Schulz, M. Valencia, and E. Ravussin. 2000. Daily energy expenditure in Mexican and USA Pima Indians: Low physical activity as a possible cause of obesity. *International Journal of Obesity* 24:55–59.

Estabrooks, P. 2000. Sustaining exercise participation through group cohesion. *Exercise and Sports Science Reviews* 28:63–67.

Evans, W. 2000. Vitamin E, vitamin C, and exercise. *American Journal of Clinical Nutrition* 72:S647–652.

Ferreira, I., J. Twisk, W. VanMechelen, H. Kemper, and C. Stehouwer. 2002. Amsterdam growth and health longitudinal study. *European Journal of Clinical Investigation* 32:723–731.

Fiatarone, M., E. O'Neill, N. Doyle Ryan, K. Clements, G. Solares, M. Nelson, S. Roberts, J. Kehayias, L. Lipsitz, and W. Evans. 1994. Exercise training and nutritional supplementation for physical frailty in very elderly people. *New England Journal of Medicine* 330:1769–1775.

Fleck, S., and W. Kraemer. 1997. *Designing resistance training programs.* Champaign, IL: Human Kinetics.

Flegal, K., M. Carroll, C. Ogden, and C. Johnson. 2002. Prevalence and trends in obesity among U.S. adults, 1999–2000. *Journal of the American Medical Association* 288:1723–1727.

Focht, B., and H. Hausenblas. 2001. Influence of quiet rest and acute aerobic exercise performed in a naturalistic environment on selected psychological responses. *Journal of Sports and Exercise Psychology* 23(2):108–121.

Folk, G.E. 1974. *Environmental physiology.* Philadelphia: Lea & Febiger.

Fontaine, K., D. Redden, C. Wang, A. Westfall, and D. Allison. 2003. Years of life lost due to obesity. *Journal of the American Medical Association* 289:187–193.

Food and Nutrition Board. 1989. *Recommended daily allowances.* 7th ed. Washington, DC: National Academy of Sciences.

Foster, C., L. Hector, R. Welsh, M. Schrager, M. Green, and A. Snyder. 1995. Effects of specific versus cross-training on running performance. *European Journal of Applied Physiology and Occupational Physiology* 70:367–372.

Foster, G., H. Wyatt, J. Hill, B. McGukin, C. Brill, B. Mohammed, P. Szapary, D. Rader, J. Edman, and S. Klein. 2003. A randomized trial of a low carbohydrate diet for obesity. *New England Journal of Medicine* 348:2082–2090.

Foster-Powell, K., and J. Miller. 1995. International tables of glycemic index. *American Journal of Clinical Nutrition* 62:S871–890.

Frederick, E.C. 1973. *The running body.* Mountain View, CA: World Publications.

Friedenreich, C., K. Courneya, and H. Bryant. 2001. Influence of physical activity in different life periods on the risk of breast cancer. *Epidemiology* 12:604–612.

Friedenreich, C., S. McGregor, K. Courneya, S. Angyalfi, and F. Elliott. 2004. Case-control study of lifetime total physical activity and prostate cancer risk. *American Journal of Epidemiology* 159:740–749.

Friedman, M., and R. Rosenman. 1973. Instantaneous and sudden death. *Journal of the American Medical Association* 22:1319–1328.

Fries, J., and L. Crapo. 1981. *Vitality and aging.* San Francisco: W.H. Freeman.

Frisch, R., G. Wyshak, N. Albright, T. Albright, I. Schiff, K. Jones, J. Witschi, E. Shiang, E. Koff, and M. Marguglio. 1985. Lower prevalence of breast cancer and cancers of the reproductive system among former college athletes compared to non-athletes. *British Journal of Cancer* 52:885–891.

Froelicher, V.F. 1984. *Exercise testing and training.* Chicago: Year Book Medical.

Frontera, W., and X. Bigard. 2002. The benefits of strength training in the elderly. *Science and Sports* 17:109–116.

Gaskill, S., R. Serfass, D. Bacharach, and J. Kelly. 1999. Responses to training in cross-country skiers. *Medicine and Science in Sports and Exercise* 31:1211–1217.

Gaskill S., A. Walker, C. Bouchard, T. Rankinen, D. Rao, J. Skinner, J. Wilmore, and A. Leon. 2005. Rating of perceived exertion is a stable marker of exercise intensity during training in previously sedentary individuals: The HERITAGE Family Study. Northwest American College of Sports Medicine Proceedings, 3:4.

Gaskill, S., A. Walker, R. Serfass, C. Bouchard, J. Gagnon, D. Rao, J. Skinner, J. Wilmore, and A. Leon. 2001. Changes in ventilatory threshold with exercise training in a sedentary population: The HERITAGE Family Study. Abstract. *Medicine and Science in Sports and Exercise* 33:S3.

Gaziano, J., J. Buring, J. Breslow, S. Goldhaber, B. Rosner, M. Vandenburgh, W. Willett, and C. Hennekens. 1993. Moderate alcohol intake, increased levels of high-density lipoprotein and its subfractions, and decreased risk of myocardial infarction. *New England Journal of Medicine* 329:1829–1834.

Gaziano, J.M., and C.M. Gibson. 2006. Potential for drug-drug interactions in patients taking analgesics for mild-to-moderate pain and low-dose aspirin for cardioprotection. *American Journal of Cardiology* 97(9A):23–29.

Gill, J., and A. Hardman. 2000. Postprandial lipemia: Effects of exercise and restriction of energy intake compared. *American Journal of Clinical Nutrition* 71:465–471.

Glasser, W. 1976. *Positive addiction*. New York: Harper and Row.

Gledhill, N., D. Warburton, and V. Jamnik. 1999. Haemoglobin, blood volume, cardiac function, and aerobic power. *Canadian Journal of Applied Physiology* 24:54–65.

Glowacki, S., S. Martin, A. Maurer, W. Baek, J. Green, and S. Crouse. 2004. Effects of resistance, endurance, and concurrent exercise on training outcomes in men. *Medicine and Science in Sports and Exercise* 36:2119–2127.

Going, S. 1996. Densitometry. In *Human body composition*, ed. A. Roche, S. Heymsfield, and T. Lohman, 3–24. Champaign, IL: Human Kinetics.

Gordon, E.E. 1967. Anatomical and biochemical adaptations of muscle to different exercises. *Journal of the American Medical Association* 201:755–758.

Gordon, P., J. Senf, and D. Campos-Outcalt. 1999. Is the annual complete physical examination necessary? *Archives of Internal Medicine* 159:909–910.

Graham, T., and K. Adamo. 1999. Dietary carbohydrate and its effect on metabolism and substrate stores in sedentary and active individuals. *Canadian Journal of Applied Physiology* 24:393–415.

Greenleaf, J.E., C.J. Greenleaf, D. VanDerveer, and K.J. Dorchak. 1976. *Adaptation to prolonged bedrest in man: A compendium of research*. Washington, DC: National Aeronautics and Space Administration.

Griffin, K. 2004. Health report: No more knife guys. *AARP The Magazine*, Nov–Dec:32–98.

Gruber, J. 1986. Physical activity and self-esteem development in children: A meta-analysis. *American Academy of Physical Education Papers* 19:30–48.

Grundy, S., J. Cleeman, C. Bairey Merz, H. Brewer, L. Clark, D. Hunninghake, R. Pasternak, S. Smith, and N. Stone. 2004. Implications of recent clinical trials for the National Cholesterol Education Program adult treatment panel III guidelines. *Circulation* 110:227–239.

Gwinup, G. 1970. *Energetics*. New York: Bantam.

Hale, B., and J. Raglin. 2002. State anxiety responses to acute resistance training and step aerobic exercise across 8-weeks of training. *Journal of Sports Medicine and Physical Fitness* 42:108–112.

Haltom, R., R. Kraemer, R. Sloan, E. Herbert, K. Frank, and J. Tryniecki. 1999. Circuit weight training and its effects on excess postexercise oxygen consumption. *Medicine and Science in Sports and Exercise* 31:1613–1618.

Hass, C., L. Garzarella, D. DeHoyos, and M. Pollock. 2000. Single verses multiple sets in long-term recreational weightlifters. *Medicine and Science in Sports and Exercise* 32:235–242.

Hays, N., R. Starling, X. Liu, D. Sullivan, T. Trappe, J. Fluckey, and W. Evans. 2004. Effects of an ad libitum low fat, high carbohydrate diet on body weight, body composition, and fat distribution in older men and women: A randomized controlled trial. *Archives of Internal Medicine* 164:210–217.

Hendrix, W., and R. Hughes. 1997. Relationship of trait, Type A behavior, and physical fitness variables to cardiovascular reactivity and coronary heart disease risk potential. *American Journal of Health Promotion* 11:264–271.

Hettinger, T., and E.A. Müller. 1953. Muscle strength and training. *Arbeitsphysiologie* 15:111–126.

Hickson, R. 1980. Interference of strength development by simultaneously training for strength and endurance. *Journal of Applied Physiology* 45:255–263.

Hill, J., and E. Melanson. 1999. Overview of the determinants of overweight and obesity: Current evidence and research issues. *Medicine and Science in Sports and Exercise* 31:S515–621.

Hill, S.R., F.C. Goetz, and H.M. Fox. 1956. Studies on adrenocortical and psychological responses to stress in man. *Archives of Internal Medicine* 97:269–298.

Holloszy, J.O. 1967. Biochemical adaptations in muscle: Effects of exercise on mitochondrial oxygen uptake and respiratory enzyme activity in skeletal muscle. *Journal of Biological Chemistry* 242:2278–2282.

Holloszy, J.O., G. Dalsky, P. Nemeth, B. Hurley, W. Martin, and J. Hagberg. 1986. Utilization of fat as a substrate during exercise: Effect of training. In *Biochemistry of exercise IV*, ed. B. Saltin, 183–190. Champaign, IL: Human Kinetics.

Hood, D., M. Takahashi, M. Connor, and D. Freyssenet. 2000. Assembly of the cellular powerhouse: Current issues in muscle mitochondrial biogenesis. *Exercise and Sports Science Reviews* 28:68–73.

Hulver, M., and J. Houmar. 2003. Plasma leptin and exercise: Recent findings. *Sports Medicine* 33:473–482.

Ikai, M. 1970. Training of muscle strength and power in athletes. Paper presented at Fédération Internationale de Médecine du Sport Congres, Oxford, England.

Ikai, M., and A.H. Steinhaus. 1961. Some factors modifying the expression of human strength. *Journal of Applied Physiology* 16:157–163.

Institute of Medicine. 2002. Dietary reference intakes for energy, carbohydrate, fiber, fat, fatty acids, cholesterol, protein, and amino acids (macronutrients). National Academy of Sciences. www.iom.edu, 936 pages.

Ismail, A.H., and R.J. Young. 1977. Effects of chronic exercise on the personality of adults. In *The marathon*, ed. P. Milvy. New York: New York Academy of Sciences.

Issekutz, B., and H. Miller. 1962. Plasma free fatty acids during exercise and the effect of lactic acid. *Proceedings of the Society of Experimental Biology and Medicine* 110:237–239.

Ivy, J., W. Goforth, W. Damon, T. McCauley, E. Parsons, and B. Price. 2002. Early post-exercise muscle glycogen recovery is enhanced with a carbohydrate-protein supplement. *Journal of Applied Physiology* 93:1337–1344.

Ivy, J., T. Zderic, and D. Fogt. 1999. Prevention and treatment of non-insulin-dependent diabetes mellitus. In *Exercise and sports science reviews*, Vol. 27, ed. J. Holloszy, 1–36. Indianapolis: American College of Sports Medicine.

Jackson, C., and A. Dickinson. 1988. Adaptations of skeletal muscle to strength or endurance training. In *Advances in sports medicine and fitness*, ed. W. Grana, J. Lombardo, B. Sharkey, and J. Stone, 45–59. Chicago: Year Book Medical.

Jackson, C., and B. Sharkey. 1988. Altitude training and human performance. *Sports Medicine* 6:279–284.

Jackson, J., B.J. Sharkey, and L.P. Johnston. 1968. Cardiorespiratory adaptations to training at specified frequencies. *Research Quarterly* 39:295–300.

Jacobson, E. 1938. *Progressive relaxation.* Chicago: University of Chicago Press.

Janssen, I., P. Katzmarzyk, and R. Ross. 2002. Body mass index, waist circumference, and health risk. *Archives of Internal Medicine* 162:2074–2079.

Jenkins, D., R. Taylor, and T. Wolever. 1982. The diabetic diet, dietary carbohydrate and differences in digestibility. *Diabetologia* 23:477–485.

Jensen, M., M. Brant-Zawadzki, N. Obuchowski, M. Modic, D. Malkasian, and J. Ross. 1994. Magnetic resonance imaging of the lumbar spine in people without back pain. *New England Journal of Medicine* 331:69–73.

Johnsgard, K. 1985. The motivation of the long distance runner. *Journal of Sports Medicine* 25:135–143.

Jones, A. 2002. Running economy is negatively related to sit-and-reach test performance in international-standard distance runners. *International Journal of Sports Medicine* 23:40–43.

Kanehisa, H., and M. Miyashita. 1983. Specificity of velocity in strength training. *European Journal of Applied Physiology* 52:104–110.

Kang, J., J. Hoffman, H. Walker, E. Chaloupka, and A. Utter. 2003. Regulating intensity using perceived exertion during extended exercise periods. *European Journal of Applied Physiology* 89:475–482.

Kanter, M. 1995. Free radicals and exercise: Effects of nutritional antioxidant supplements. In *Exercise and sports science reviews*, ed. J. Holloszy. Baltimore: Williams & Wilkins.

Kemi, O., P. Haram, U. Wisloff, and O. Ellingsen. 2004. Aerobic fitness is associated with cardiomyocyte contractile capacity and endothelial function in exercise training and detraining. *Circulation* 109:2897–2904.

Kemmler, W., D. Lauber, J. Weineck, J. Hensen, W. Kalender, and K. Engelke. 2004. Benefits of 2 years of intense exercise on bone density, physical fitness, and blood lipids in early postmenopausal women. *Archives of Internal Medicine* 164:1084–1091.

Kempen, K., W. Saris, and K. Westerterp. 1995. Energy balance during an 8-week restricted diet with and without exercise in obese women. *American Journal of Clinical Nutrition* 62:722–729.

Kenrick, M.M., M.F. Ball, and J.J. Canary. 1972. Exercise and fat loss in obese patients. Paper presented at the annual meeting of the American Academy of Physical Medicine and Rehabilitation, San Juan, Puerto Rico.

Kenyon, G. 1968. Six scales for assessing attitudes toward physical activity. *Research Quarterly* 37:566–574.

Keul, J. 1971. Myocardial metabolism in athletes. In *Muscle metabolism during exercise*, ed. B. Pernow and B. Saltin. New York: Plenum.

Kivimaki, M., P. Leino-Arjas, R. Luukkonen, H. Riihimaki, J. Vahtera, and J. Kirjonen. 2002. Work stress and risk of cardiovascular mortality. *British Medical Journal* 325:857–860.

Klein, S., L. Fontana, V. Young, A. Coggan, C. Kilo, B. Patterson, and B. Mohammed. 2004. Absence of an effect of liposuction on insulin action and risk factors for coronary heart disease. *New England Journal of Medicine* 350:2549–2557.

Kline, G., J. Pocari, R. Hintermeister, P. Freedson, A. Ward, R. McCarron, J. Ross, and J. Rippe. 1987. Estimation of $\dot{V}O_2$max from a one-mile track walk, gender, age, and body weight. *Medicine and Science in Sports and Exercise* 19:253–259.

Klissouras, V. 1976. Heritability of adaptive variation. *Journal of Applied Physiology* 31:338–344.

Knoops, K., L. deGroot, D. Kromhout, A. Perrin, O. Moreiras-Varela, A. Menotti, and W. vanStaveren. 2004. *Journal of the American Medical Association* 292:1433–1439.

Kobasa, S. 1979. Stressful life events, personality and health: An inquiry into hardiness. *Journal of Personality and Social Psychology* 37:1–11.

Komi, P. 1992. Stretch-shortening cycle. In *Strength and power in sport*, ed. P. Komi. Oxford: Blackwell Scientific.

Komi, P., and E.R. Buskirk. 1972. Effect of eccentric and concentric muscle conditioning on tension and electrical activity of human muscle. *Ergonomics* 15:417–422.

Kong, D. 2004. Aspirin in cardiovascular disorders: What is the optimal dose? *American Journal of Cardiovascular Drugs* 4:151–158.

Kramer, J., M. Stone, H. Obryant, M. Conley, R. Johnson, D. Nieman, D. Honeycutt, and T. Hoke. 1997. Effects of single vs. multiple sets of weight training: Impact of volume, intensity and variation. *Journal of Strength and Conditioning Research* 11:143–147.

Kuh, D., J. Bassey, R. Hardy, A. Sayer, M. Wadsworth, and C. Cooper. 2002. Birth weight, childhood size, and muscle strength in adult life: Evidence from a birth cohort study. *American Journal of Epidemiology* 156(7):627–633.

Kull, M. 2003. Physical activity and mental health: Relationship between depressiveness, psychological disorders and physical activity levels in women. *Biology of Sport* 20:129–138.

Lail, A., J. Marino, A. Russo, R. Serrano, A. Lamonte, J. Wygard, and R. Otto. 2004. The effect of six weeks of balance intervention on trained senior males. *Medicine and Science in Sports and Exercise* 36:S358.

Lakka, T., D. Laaksonen, H. Lakka, N. Mannikko, L. Niskanen, R. Rauramaa, and J. Salonen. 2003. Sedentary lifestyle, poor cardiovascular fitness, and the metabolic syndrome. *Medicine and Science in Sports and Exercise* 35:1279–1286.

Lakka, T., J. Venalainen, R. Rauramaa, R. Salonen, J. Tuomilehto, and J. Salonen. 1994. Relation of leisure-time physical activity and cardiorespiratory fitness to the risk of acute myocardial infarction in men. *New England Journal of Medicine* 330:1549–1554.

Landers, D., and S. Petruzzello. 1994. Physical activity, fitness and anxiety. In *Physical activity, fitness and health*, ed. C. Bouchard, R. Shephard, and T. Stevens. Champaign, IL: Human Kinetics.

Landy, F. 1992. Alternatives to chronological age in determining standards of suitability for public safety jobs, vol. 1. Tech. Rep. Pennsylvania State University.

Larson, E., L. Wang, J. Bowen, W. McCormick, L. Teri, P. Crane, and W. Kukull. 2006. Exercise is associated with reduced risk for incident dementia among persons 65 years of age and older. *Annals of Internal Medicine* 144:73–81.

Leaf, A. 1973. Getting old. *Scientific American* 229:45–55.

Lee, C., A. Jackson, and S. Blair. 1998. U.S. Weight Guidelines: Is it also important to consider cardiorespiratory fitness? *International Journal of Obesity* 22:S2–7.

Lee, I-Min, C. Hsieh, and R. Paffenbarger. 1995. Exercise intensity and longevity in men: The Harvard alumni health study. *Journal of the American Medical Association* 273:1179–1184.

Leibel, R., M. Rosenbaum, and J. Hirsch. 1995. Changes in energy expenditure resulting from altered body weight. *New England Journal of Medicine* 332:621–628.

Leitzmann, M., E. Rimm, W. Willett, D. Spiegelman, F. Grodstein, M. Stampfer, G. Colditz, and E. Giovannucci. 1999. Recreational physical activity and the risk of cholecystectomy in women. *New England Journal of Medicine* 341:777–784.

Lemon, P. 1995. Do athletes need more protein and amino acids? *International Journal of Sports and Nutrition* 5:S39–61.

Leon A., S. Gaskill, C. Bouchard, J. Gagnon, D. Rao, J. Skinner, J. Wilmore, T. Rice, S. Mandel, and J. Bergeron. 2002. Variability in the response of HDL cholesterol to exercise training in the HERITAGE Family Study. *International Journal of Sports Medicine* 23:1–9.

Leonard, J., J. Hofer, and N. Pritikin. 1974. *Live longer now*. Mountain View, CA: World Sports Library.

Librett, J., M. Yore, and T. Schmid. 2003. Local ordinances that promote physical activity: A survey of municipal policies. *American Journal of Public Health* 93:1399–1403.

Lieber, C. 1976. The metabolism of alcohol. *Scientific American* 229:45–55.

Locke, E., and G. Latham. 1985. The application of goal setting to sports. *Journal of Sports Psychology* 7:205–222.

Lopez, S.A., R. Vial, L. Balart, and G. Arroyave. 1974. Effects of exercise and physical fitness on serum lipids and lipoproteins. *Atherosclerosis* 20:1–9.

Lubell, A. 1988. Blacks and exercise. *Physician and Sportsmedicine* 16:162–176.

Macera, C., D. Jones, M. Yore, S. Ham, H. Kohl, C. Kimsey, and D. Buchner. 2003. Prevalence of physical activity, including lifestyle activities among adults—United States, 2000–2001. Centers for Disease Control, *Morbidity and Mortality Weekly Report* 52:764–769.

Mackinnon, L. 1992. *Exercise and immunology*. Champaign, IL: Human Kinetics.

Malina, R., and C. Bouchard. 1991. *Growth, maturation, and physical activity*. Champaign, IL: Human Kinetics.

Malmivaara, A., U. Hakkinen, T. Aro, M. Heinrichs, L. Koskenniemi, E. Kuosma, S. Lappi, R. Paloheimo, C. Servo, V. Vaaranen, and S. Hernberg. 1995. The treatment of acute low back pain: Bed rest, exercises, or ordinary activity? *New England Journal of Medicine* 332:351–355.

Manninen, P., M. Heliovaara, H. Riihimaki, and O. Suomalainen. 2002. Physical workload and the risk or severe osteoarthritis. *Scandinavian Journal of Work Environment and Health* 28:25–32.

Manson, J., F. Hu, J. Rich-Edwards, G. Colditz, M. Stampfer, W. Willet, F. Speizer, and C. Hennekens. 1999. A prospective study of walking as compared with vigorous exercise in the prevention of coronary heart disease in women. *New England Journal of Medicine* 341:650–658.

Manson, J., W. Willett, M. Stampfer, G. Colditz, D. Hunter, S. Hankinson, C. Hennekens, and F. Speizer. 1995. Body weight and mortality among women. *New England Journal of Medicine* 333:677–685.

Marcus, B., and L. Forsyth. 2003. *Motivating people to be physically active.* Champaign, IL: Human Kinetics.

Markoff, R., P. Ryan, and T. Young. 1982. Endorphins and mood changes in long-distance running. *Medicine and Science in Sports and Exercise* 14(1):11–15.

Maslow, A.H. 1954. *Motivation and personality.* New York: Harper.

Massey, B.H., R.C. Nelson, B.J. Sharkey, and T. Comden. 1965. Effects of high-frequency electrical stimulation on the size and strength of skeletal muscle. *Journal of Sports Medicine* 5:136–144.

Matejek, N., E. Weimann, C. Witzel, G. Molenkamp, S. Schwidergall, and H. Bohles. 1999. Hypoleptinaemia in patients with anorexia nervosa and in elite gymnasts with anorexia athletica. *International Journal of Sports Medicine* 20:451–456.

Mayer, J., and B.A. Bullen. 1974. Nutrition, weight control and exercise. In *Science and medicine of exercise and sport*, ed. W.R. Johnson and E.R. Buskirk. New York: Harper and Row.

McArdle, W., F. Katch, and V. Katch. 1994. *Essentials of exercise physiology.* Philadelphia: Lea & Febiger.

McAuley, E., and B. Blissmer. 2000. Self-efficacy determinants and consequences of physical activity. In *Exercise and sports science reviews*, Vol. 28, ed. D. Seals, 85–88. Indianapolis: American College of Sports Medicine.

McCarthy, J., M. Pozniak, and J. Agre. 2002. Neuromuscular adaptations to concurrent strength and endurance training. *Medicine and Science in Sports and Exercise* 34:511–519.

Miller, D., and P. Payne. 1968. Longevity and protein intake. *Experimental Gerontology* 3:231–235.

Miller, E., R. Pastor-Barriuso, D. Dalal, R. Riemersma, L. Appel, and E. Guallar. 2005. Meta-analysis: High dosage of vitamin E supplementation may increase all-cause mortality. *Annals of Internal Medicine* 142:37–46.

Mitchell, J.H., W. Reardon, D.I. McCloskey, and K. Wildnethal. 1977. Possible roles of muscle receptors in the cardiovascular response to exercise. In *The marathon*, ed. P. Milvy, 232–252. New York: New York Academy of Sciences.

Mitchell, T., L. Gibbons, S. Devers, and C. Earnest. 2004. Effects of cardiorespiratory fitness on healthcare utilization. *Medicine and Science in Sports and Exercise* 36:2088–2092.

Mokdad, A., J. Marks, D. Stroup, and J. Gerberding. 2004. Actual causes of death in the United States, 2000. *Journal of the American Medical Association* 291:1238–1245.

Móle, P.A., L.B. Oscai, and J.O. Holloszy. 1971. Adaptation of muscle to exercise: Increase in levels of palmityl CoA synthetase, carnitine palmityl-transferase, and palmityl CoA dehydrogenase, and in the capacity to oxidize fatty acids. *Journal of Clinical Investigation* 50:2323–2329.

Móle, P.A., J. Stern, C. Schultz, E. Bernauer, and B. Holcomb. 1989. Exercise reverses depressed metabolic rate produced by severe caloric restriction. *Medicine and Science in Sports and Exercise* 21:29–33.

Molz, A., B. Heyduck, H. Lill, E. Spanuth, and L. Rocker. 1993. The effect of different exercise intensities on the fibrinolytic system. *European Journal of Applied Physiology and Occupational Physiology* 67:298–304.

Morgan, W.P. 1979. Negative addiction in runners. *Physician and Sportsmedicine* 7:57–70.

Morgan, W.P. 2001. Prescription of physical activity: A paradigm shift. *Quest* 53:366–382.

Morgan, W., P. O'Conner, A. Ellickson, and P. Bradley. 1988. Personality structure, mood states and performance in elite male distance runners. *International Journal of Sport Psychology* 19:247–263.

Morrey, M., and D. Hensrud. 1999. Risk of medical events in a supervised health and fitness facility. *Medicine and Science in Sports and Exercise* 31:1233–1236.

Morris, J., and M. Crawford. 1958. Coronary heart disease and physical activity of work. *Journal of the British Medical Association* 2:1485–1496.

Morris, J.N., and P. Raffle. 1954. Coronary heart disease in transport workers. *British Journal of Industrial Medicine* 11:260–272.

Motl, R., A. Birnbaum, M. Kubik, and R. Dishman. 2004. Naturally occurring changes in physical activity are inversely related to depressive symptoms during early adolescence. *Psychosomatic Medicine* 66:336–342.

Nadel, E.R., ed. 1977. *Problems with temperature regulation during exercise.* New York: Academic Press.

Neary, J., G. Wheeler, I. Maclean, D. Cumming, and H. Quinney. 1994. Urinary free cortisol as an indicator of exercise training stress. *Clinical Journal of Sports Medicine* 4:160–165.

Nelson, M., M. Fiatarone, C. Morganti, I. Trice, R. Greenberg, and W. Evans. 1994. Effects of high-intensity strength training on multiple risk factors for osteoporotic fractures: A randomized controlled trial. *Journal of the American Medical Association* 272:1909–1914.

Nesser T., S. Chen, R. Serfass, and S. Gaskill. 2004. Development of upper body power in junior cross-country skiers. *Journal of Strength and Conditioning Research* 18(1):63–71.

Nevill, A., M. Burrows, R. Holder, S. Bird, and D. Simpson. 2003. Does lower-body BMD develop at the expense of upper-body BMD in female runners? *Medicine and Science in Sports and Exercise* 35:1733–1739.

Newham, D. 1988. The consequences of eccentric contractions and their relationship to delayed onset muscle pain. *European Journal of Applied Physiology* 57:353–359.

Nieman, D. 2003. Current perspectives on exercise immunology. *Current Sports Medicine Reports* 2:239–242.

Nieman, D., D. Henson, and S. McAnulty. 2002. Influence of vitamin C supplementation on oxidative and immune changes following an ultramarathon. *Journal of Applied Physiology* 92:1970–1977.

Nieman, D., D. Henson, S. McAnulty, L. McAnulty, J. Morrow, A. Ahmed, and C. Heward. 2004. Vitamin E and immunity after the Kona Triathlon World Championship. *Medicine and Science in Sports and Exercise* 36:1328–1335.

Nieman, D., and B. Pedersen. 1999. Exercise and immune function: Recent developments. *Sports Medicine* 27:73–80.

Nikkila, E., M. Taskinen, S. Rehunen, and M. Harkonen. 1978. Lipoprotein lipase activity in adipose tissue and skeletal muscle of runners: Relationship to serum lipoproteins. *Metabolism* 27:1661–1667.

Nissen, S., E. Tuzcu, P. Schoenhagen, T. Crowe, W. Sasiela, J. Tsai, J. Orazem, R. Magorien, C. O'Shaughnessy, and P. Ganz. 2005. Statin therapy, LDL cholesterol, C-reactive protein, and coronary artery disease. *New England Journal of Medicine* 352:29–38.

North, T., P. McCullagh, and Z.V. Tran. 1990. Effects of exercise on depression. *Exercise and Sport Science Reviews* 18:379–415.

Nosaka, K., K. Sakamoto, M. Newton, and P. Sacco. 2001. How long does the protective effect on eccentric exercise-induced muscle damage last? *Medicine and Science in Sports and Exercise* 33:1490–1495.

O'Malley, P., D. Jones, I. Feuerstein, and A. Taylor. 2000. Lack of correlation between psychological factors and subclinical coronary artery disease. *New England Journal of Medicine* 343:1298–1304.

Ornish, D. 1993. *Eat more, weigh less*. New York: Harper Collins.

Ornstein, R., and D. Sobel. 1989. *Healthy pleasures*. New York: Addison-Wesley.

Oscai, L.B., and J.O. Holloszy. 1969. Effects of weight changes produced by exercise, food restriction or overeating on body composition. *Journal of Clinical Investigation* 48:2124–2128.

Paffenbarger, R. 1994. Forty years of progress: Physical activity, health and fitness. In *American College of Sports Medicine 40th anniversary lectures*, 93–109. Indianapolis.

Paffenbarger, R., R. Hyde, and A. Wing. 1986. Physical activity, all-cause mortality, and longevity of college alumni. *New England Journal of Medicine* 314:605–613.

Paffenbarger, R., R. Hyde, and A. Wing. 1990. Physical activity and physical fitness as determinants of health and longevity. In *Exercise, fitness, and health*, ed. C. Bouchard, R.J. Shephard, T. Stephens, J.R. Sutton, and B.D. McPherson. Champaign, IL: Human Kinetics.

Panel, E. 1998. Executive summary of the clinical guidelines on the identification, evaluation, and treatment of overweight and obesity in adults. *Archives of Internal Medicine* 158:1855–1867.

Parfitt, G., and C. Gledhill. 2004. The effect of choice of exercise mode on psychological responses. *Psychology of Sport and Exercise* 5:111–117.

Passmore, R., and J. Durnin. 1955. Human energy expenditure. *Physiology Review* 35:801–824.

Pate, R., M. Pratt, S. Blair, W. Haskell, C. Macera, C. Bouchard, D. Buchner, W. Ettinger, G. Heath, A. King, A. Kriska, A. Leon, B. Marcus, J. Morris, R. Paffenbarger, K. Patrick, M. Pollock, J. Rippe, J. Sallis, and J. Wilmore. 1995. Physical activity and public health: A recommendation from the Centers for Disease Control and Prevention and the American College of Sports Medicine. *Journal of the American Medical Association* 273:402–407.

Patel, T., and K. Goldberg. 2004. Use of aspirin and ibuprofen compared with aspirin alone and the risk of myocardial infarction. *Archives of Internal Medicine* 164:852–856.

Pedersen, B., J. Helge, E. Richter, T. Rohde, and B. Kiens. 2000. Training and natural immunity: Effects of diets rich in fat or carbohydrate. *European Journal of Applied Physiology* 82:98–103.

Peeters, A., J. Barendregt, F. Willekens, J. Mackenbach, A. Al Mamum, and L. Bonneux. 2003. Obesity in adulthood and its consequences for life expectancy: A life-table analysis. *Annals of Internal Medicine* 138:24–32.

Pette, D. 1984. Activity induced fast to slow transitions in mammalian muscle. *Medicine and Science in Sports and Exercise* 16:517–528.

Piers, L., M. Soares, L. McCormack, and K. O'Dea. 1998. Is there evidence for an age-related reduction in metabolic rate? *Journal of Applied Physiology* 85:2196–2204.

Pimentel, A., C. Gentile, H. Tanaka, D. Seals, and P. Gates. 2003. Greater rate of decline in maximal aerobic capacity with age in endurance-trained than in sedentary men. *Journal of Applied Physiology* 94:2406–2413.

Plunkett, B., and W. Hopkins. 1995. The cause and treatment of the side pain "stitch." *Medicine and Science in Sports and Exercise* 27:S23.

Pollock, M.L. 1973. The quantification of endurance training programs. In *Exercise and sports sciences reviews*, Vol. 1, ed. J.H. Wilmore. New York: Academic Press.

Pollock, M.L., J. Dimmick, H. Miller, Z. Kendrick, and A. Linnerud. 1975. Effects of mode of training on cardiovascular function and body composition of middle-aged men. *Medicine and Science in Sports and Exercise* 7:139–145.

Powel, K., and R. Paffenbarger. 1985. Workshop on epidemiologic and public health aspects of physical activity and exercise: A summary. *Public Health Reports* 100:118–126.

President's Council on Physical Fitness and Sport. 1975. *An introduction to physical fitness*. Washington, DC: President's Council on Physical Fitness and Sport.

Pritikin, N. 1979. *The Pritikin program for diet and exercise*. New York: Bantam.

Pronk, N. 2003. A sense of urgency to improve employee health: The bottom line and the role of worksite health promotion. *ACSM's Health and Fitness Journal* 7:6–11.

Puchkoff, J., L. Curry, J. Swan, B. Sharkey, and B. Ruby. 1998. The effects of hydration status and blood glucose on mental performance during extended exercise in the heat. *Medicine and Science in Sports and Exercise* 30:S284.

Putman, C., X. Xu, E. Gillies, I. MacLean, G. Bell. 2004. Effects of strength, endurance and combined training on myosin heavy chain content and fiber-type distribution in humans. *European Journal of Applied Physiology* 92:376–384.

Radcliffe, J., and R. Farentinos. 1985. *Plyometrics: Explosive power training*. Champaign, IL: Human Kinetics.

Raebel, M., D. Malone, D. Conner, S. Xu, J. Porter, and F. Lanty. 2004. Health services use and health care costs of obese and nonobese individuals. *Archives of Internal Medicine* 164:2135–2140.

Reis, J., H. Bowles, B. Ainsworth, K. Dubose, S. Smith, and J. Laditka. 2004. Nonoccupational physical activity by degree of urbanization and U.S. geographical region. *Medicine and Science in Sports and Exercise* 36:2093–2098.

Rejeski, W., K. Neal, M. Wurst, P. Brubaker, and W. Ettinger Jr. 1995. Walking, but not weight lifting, acutely reduces systolic blood pressure in older sedentary men and women. *Journal of Aging and Physical Activity* 3:163–177.

Rhea, M., B. Alvar, L. Burkett, and S. Ball. 2003. A meta-analysis to determine the dose response for strength development. *Medicine and Science in Sports and Exercise* 35:456–464.

Ridker, P., C. Hennekens, J. Buring, and N. Rifai. 2000. C-reactive protein and other markers of inflammation in the prediction of cardiovascular disease in women. *New England Journal of Medicine* 342:836–843.

Rising, R., I. Harper, A. Fontvielle, R. Ferraro, M. Spraul, and E. Ravussin. 1994. Determinants of total daily energy expenditure: Variability in physical activity. *American Journal of Clinical Nutrition* 59:800–804.

Robertson, R. 2004. *Perceived exertion for practitioners*. Champaign, IL: Human Kinetics.

Ross, R., H. Pedwell, and J. Rissanen. 1995. Effects of energy restriction and exercise on skeletal muscle and adipose tissue in women as measured by magnetic resonance imaging. *American Journal of Clinical Nutrition* 61:1179–1185.

Roth, D., and D. Holmes. 1985. Influence of physical fitness in determining the impact of stressful life events on physical and psychological health. *Psychosomatic Medicine* 47:164–173.

Roth, E.M., ed. 1968. *Compendium of human responses to the aerospace environment III.* Washington, DC: National Aeronautics and Space Administration.

Ruby, B., and R. Robergs. 1994. Gender differences in substrate utilization during exercise. *Sports Medicine* 17:393–410.

Ruby, B., D. Schoeller, and B. Sharkey. 2001. Evaluation of total energy expenditure (doubly-labeled water) across different measurement periods during arduous work. *Medicine and Science in Sports and Exercise* 33:S274.

Ruby B., G. Leadbetter, D. Armstrong, and S. Gaskill. 2003. Wildland firefighter load carriage: Effects on transit time and physiological responses during simulated escape to safety zone. *International Journal of Wildland Fire* 12:1–6.

Ruby, B., S. Gaskill, D. Heil, B. Sharkey, B. Hansen, and D. Lankford. 2002. Changes in salivary IgA during arduous wildfire suppression relative to work-shift length. *Medicine and Science in Sports and Exercise* 34:S195.

Ruby, B., S. Gaskill, D. Lankford, D. Slivka, D. Heil, and B. Sharkey. 2003. Carbohydrate feedings increase self-selected work rates during arduous wildfire suppression. *Medicine and Science in Sports and Exercise* 35(5):S.

Ryan, A., R. Pratley, D. Elahi, and A. Goldberg. 1995. Resistive training increases fat-free mass and maintains RMR despite weight loss in postmenopausal women. *Journal of Applied Physiology* 79:818–823.

Ryder, H.W., H.J. Carr, and R. Herget. 1976. Future performance in footracing. *Scientific American* 234:109–116.

Sachs, G., D. Weeks, K. Melchers, and D. Scott. 2003. The gastric biology of *Heliobactor pylori*. *Annual Review of Physiology* 65:349–369.

Saelens, B., J. Sallis, J. Black, and D. Chen. 2003. Neighborhood-based differences in physical activity: An environmental scale. *American Journal of Public Health* 93:1552–1558.

Saltin, B. 1977. The interplay between peripheral and central factors in the adaptive response to exercise and training. In *The marathon*, ed. P. Milvy, 224–231. New York: New York Academy of Sciences.

Saltin, B., G. Blomqvist, J.H. Mitchell, R.L. Johnson Jr., K. Wildenthal, and C.B. Chapman. 1968. Response to exercise after bed rest and after training. *Circulation* 38(Suppl. 7):1–78.

Samaha, F., N. Iqbal, P. Seshardi, K. Chicano, D. Daily, J. McGrory. T. Williams, M. Williams, E. Gracely, and L. Stern. 2003. A low-carbohydrate as compared with a low-fat diet in severe obesity. *New England Journal of Medicine* 348:2074–2081.

Sanghavi Goal, M., E. McCarthy, R. Phillips, and C. Wee. 2004. Obesity among U.S. immigrant subgroups by duration of residence. *Journal of the American Medical Association* 292:2860–2867.

Schulze, M., J. Manson, D. Ludwig, G. Colditz, M. Stampfer, W. Willett, and F. Hu. 2004. Sugar-sweetened beverages, weight gain, and incidence of type 2 diabetes in young and middle-aged women. *Journal of the American Medical Association* 292:927–934.

Seals, D. 2003. Habitual exercise and the age-associated decline in large artery compliance. *Exercise and Sport Sciences Reviews* 31:68–72.

Selye, H. 1956. *The stress of life.* New York: McGraw-Hill.

Sharkey, B.J. 1970. Intensity and duration of training and the development of cardiorespiratory endurance. *Medicine and Science in Sports and Exercise* 2:197–202.

Sharkey, B.J. 1974. *Physiological fitness and weight control.* Missoula, MT: Mountain Press.

Sharkey, B.J. 1981. Fitness for wildland firefighting. *Physician and Sportsmedicine* 9:77–83.

Sharkey, B.J. 1984. *Training for cross-country ski racing.* Champaign, IL: Human Kinetics.

Sharkey, B.J. 1986. *Coaches guide to sport physiology.* Champaign, IL: Human Kinetics.

Sharkey, B.J. 1987. Functional vs. chronological age. *Medicine and Science in Sports and Exercise* 19:174–178.

Sharkey, B.J. 1990. *Physiology of fitness.* Champaign, IL: Human Kinetics.

Sharkey, B.J. 1991. *New dimensions in aerobic fitness.* Champaign, IL: Human Kinetics.

Sharkey, B.J. 1997a. *Fitness and health.* 4th ed. Champaign, IL: Human Kinetics.

Sharkey, B.J. 1997b. *Fitness and work capacity.* 2nd ed. Missoula, MT: USDA Forest Service.

Sharkey, B.J., and S. Gaskill. 2006. *Sport physiology for coaches*. Champaign, IL: Human Kinetics.

Sharkey, B.J., and D. Greatzer. 1993. Specificity of exercise, training and testing. In *ACSM's resource manual for guidelines for exercise testing and prescription*, ed. L. Durstine, A. King, P. Painter, and J. Roitman, 82–92. Philadelphia: Lea & Febiger.

Sharkey, B.J., and J.P. Holleman. 1967. Cardiorespiratory adaptations to training at specified intensities. *Research Quarterly* 38:398–404.

Sharkey, B.J., C. Simpson, R. Washburn, and R. Confessore. 1980. HDL cholesterol. *Running* 5:38–41.

Sharkey, B.J., D. Wilson, T. Whiddon, and K. Miller. 1978, September. Fit to work? *Journal of Health, Physical Education and Recreation* 18–21.

Sheehy, G. 1976. *Passages: Predictable crises of adult life*. New York: Bantam.

Simoes, E., T. Byers, R. Coates, M. Serdula, A. Mokdad, and G. Heath. 1995. The association between leisure-time physical activity and dietary fat in American adults. *American Journal of Public Health* 85:240–244.

Siscovick, D., R. LaPorte, and J. Newman. 1985. The disease-specific benefits and risks of physical activity and exercise. *Public Health Reports* 100:180–188.

Siscovick, D., N. Weiss, R. Fletcher, and T. Lasky. 1984. The incidence of primary cardiac arrest during vigorous exercise. *New England Journal of Medicine* 311:874–877.

Slattery, M. 2004. Physical activity and colorectal cancer. *Sports Medicine* 34:239–252.

Sleamaker, R. 1989. *Serious training for serious athletes*. Champaign, IL: Human Kinetics.

Smith, M., and B. Sharkey. 1984. Altitude training: Who benefits? *Physician and Sportsmedicine* 12:48–62.

Smith, R., and O. Rutherford. 1995. The role of metabolites in strength training. 1. A comparison of eccentric and concentric contractions. *European Journal of Applied Physiology and Occupational Physiology* 71:332–336.

Spalding, T., L. Lyon, and B. Hatfield. 2004. Relative efficacy of aerobic training and stress management in lowering cardiovascular activity during psychological stress. *Medicine and Science in Sports and Exercise* 36:S88.

Spiegel, K., E. Tasali, P. Penev, and E. Van Cauter. 2004. Brief communication: Sleep curtailment in healthy young men is associated with decreased leptin levels, elevated ghrelin levels, and increased hunger and appetite. *Annals of Internal Medicine* 141:846–850.

Spirduso, W. 1995. *Physical dimensions of aging*. Champaign, IL: Human Kinetics.

Stampfer, M., F. Hu, J. Manson, E. Rimm, and W. Willett. 2000. Primary prevention of coronary heart disease in women through diet and lifestyle. *New England Journal of Medicine* 343:16–22.

Steed, J., G. Gaesser, and A. Weltman. 1994. Rating of perceived exertion and blood lactate concentration during submaximal running. *Medicine and Science in Sports and Exercise* 26:797–803.

Steinberg, G. 2003. Acute and chronic effects of leptin on skeletal muscle fatty acid metabolism. *Canadian Journal of Applied Physiology* 28:210.

Stephens, T. 1988. Physical activity and mental health in the United States and Canada: Evidence from four population surveys. *Preventive Medicine* 17:35–47.

Stephens, T., D. Jacobs, and C. White. 1985. A descriptive epidemiology of leisure-time physical activity. *Public Health Reports* 100:147–158.

Stone, W., and D. Klein. 2004. Long-term exercisers: What can we learn from them? *ACSM's Health and Fitness Journal* 8:11–14.

Strawbridge, W., S. Deleger, R. Roberts, and G. Kaplan. 2002. Physical activity reduces the risk of subsequent depression for older adults. *American Journal of Epidemiology* 156:328–334.

Stray-Gunderson, J. 1986. The effect of pericardiectomy on maximal oxygen consumption and cardiac output in untrained dogs. *Circulation Research* 58:523–529.

Stubbs, R., D. Hughes, A. Johnstone, G. Horgan, N. King, and J. Blundell. 2004. A decrease in physical activity affects appetite, energy, and nutrient balance in lean men feeding ad libitum. *American Journal of Clinical Nutrition* 79:62–69.

Stunkard, A., T. Foch, and V. Hrubec. 1986. A twin study of human obesity. *Journal of the American Medical Association* 256:51–54.

Sundet, J., P. Magnus, and K. Tambs. 1994. The heritability of maximal aerobic power: A study of Norwegian twins. *Scandinavian Journal of Medical Science in Sports* 4:181–185.

Suzuki, T. 1967. Effects of muscular exercise on adrenal 17-hydroxycorticosteroid secretion in the dog. *Endocrinology* 80:1148–1151.

Swinburn, B., and E. Ravussin. 1993. Energy balance or fat balance? *American Journal of Clinical Nutrition* 57:S766–771.

Takano, T., K. Nakamura, and M. Watanabe. 2003. Urban residential environments and senior citizens' longevity in megacity areas: The importance of walkable green spaces. *Journal of Epidemiology and Community Health* 56:913–918.

Taylor, C., and N. Miller. 1993. Principles of health behavior change. In *ACSM's resource manual for guidelines for exercise testing and prescription*, ed. L. Durstine, A. King, P. Painter, and J. Roitman. Philadelphia: Lea & Febiger.

Tenenbaum, G., and R. Singer. 1992. Physical activity and psychological benefits. Position statement of the International Society of Sport Psychology. *Physician and Sportsmedicine* 20:179–184.

Thacker, S., J. Gilchrist, D. Stroup, and C. Kimsey. 2004. The impact of stretching on sports injury risk: A systematic review of the literature. *Medicine and Science in Sports and Exercise* 36:371–378.

Thompson, D., J. Edelsberg, G. Colditz, A. Bird, and G. Oster. 1999. Lifetime health and economic consequences of obesity. *Archives of Internal Medicine* 159:2177–2183.

Thune, I., T. Brenn, E. Lund, and M. Gaard. 1997. Physical activity and the risk of breast cancer. *New England Journal of Medicine* 336:1269–1275.

Tipton, K., and R. Wolfe. 2004. Protein and amino acids for athletes. *Journal of Sports Sciences* 22:65–79.

Treuth, M., G. Hunter, and T. Kekes-Szabo. 1995. Reduction in intraabdominal adipose tissue after strength training in older women. *Journal of Applied Physiology* 78:1425–1431.

Trichopoulou, A., C. Gnardellis, A. Laagiou, V. Benetou, A. Naska, and D. Trichopoulou. 2001. Physical activity and energy intake selectively predict the waist-to-hip ratio in men but not in women. *American Journal of Clinical Nutrition* 74:574–578.

Tsai, A., and T. Wadden. 2005. Systematic review: An evaluation of major commercial weight loss programs in the United States. *Annals of Internal Medicine* 142:56–66.

Tsang, W., and C. HuiChan. 2004. Effects of exercise on joint sense and balance in elderly men: Tai chi versus golf. *Medicine and Science in Sports and Exercise* 36:658–667.

Tudor-Locke, C., J. Williams, J. Reis, and D. Pluto. 2004. Utility of pedometers for assessing physical activity—construct validity. *Sports Medicine* 34:281–291.

Tutko, T., and U. Tosi. 1976. *Sports psyching*. New York: Hawthorn.

Tuzac, M. 1999. Heart disease prevention must begin in teen years. Paper presented at the annual meeting of the American Heart Association, Dallas, TX.

U.S. Department of Health and Human Services, Public Health Service. 1991. *Healthy People 2000: National health promotion and disease prevention objectives (DHHS #91-50212)*. Washington, DC: U.S. Government Printing Office.

U.S. Department of Health and Human Services (USDHHS), Public Health Service, Centers for Disease Control and Prevention. 1999. *Promoting physical activity: A guide for community action*. Champaign, IL: Human Kinetics.

U.S. Department of Health and Human Services (USDHHS). 1996. *Physical activity and health: A report of the surgeon general*. Washington, DC: U.S. Government Printing Office.

U.S. Department of Health, Education, and Welfare, Public Health Service (USDHEW). 1979. *Smoking and health: A report of the surgeon general. Interaction between smoking and occupational exposure*. Washington, DC: U.S. Government Printing Office.

United States Fire Administration (USFA). 2002. *Firefighter fatality retrospective study*. Federal Emergency Management Agency, National Fire Data Center at www.usfa.fema.gov.

Vaillant, G. 2001. *Aging well*. New York: Little, Brown.

Vailodash, B. 2000. The effects of 22 weeks of cycle training on body weight, heart rate, fitness and diet. Unpublished thesis, The University of Minnesota.

Van Aaken, E. 1976. *Van Aaken method*. Mountain View, CA: World Publications.

Van Linge, B. 1962. The response of muscle to strenuous exercise. *Journal of Bone and Joint Surgery* 44:711–721.

VanderVliet, P., Y. Vanden-Auweele, J. Knapen, R. Rzewnicki, P. Onghena, and H. VanCoppenolle. 2004. The effect of fitness training on clinically depressed patients: An intra-individual approach. *Psychology of Sport and Exercise* 5:153–167.

VanLangendonck, L., J. Lefevre, A. Claessens, M. Thomis, R. Phillippaerts, K. Delvaux, R. Lysens, R. Renson, B. Vanreusel, B. VandenEynde, J. Dequeker, and G. Beunen. 2003. Influence of participation in high-impact sports during adolescence and adulthood on bone mineral density in middle-aged men. *American Journal of Epidemiology* 158:525–533.

VanSchuylenbergh R., B. VandenEynde, P. Hespel. 2004. Effects of air ventilation during stationary exercise testing. *European Journal of Applied Physiology* 92:263–266.

Vasan, R., M. Larson, E. Leip, J. Evans, C. O'Donnell, W. Kannel, and D. Levy. 2001. Impact of high-normal blood pressure on the risk of cardiovascular disease. *New England Journal of Medicine* 345:1291–1297.

Vega deJesus, R., and Siconolfi, S. 1988. Fat mobilization and utilization during exercise at lactates of 2 and 4 mm. *Medicine and Science in Sports and Exercise* 20(Suppl. 71).

Volek, J. 2003. Influence of nutrition on responses to resistance training. *Medicine and Science in Sports and Exercise* 36:689–696.

Votruba, S., R. Atkinson, M. Hirvonen, and D. Schoeller. 2002. Prior exercise increases subsequent utilization of dietary fat. *Medicine and Science in Sports and Exercise* 34:1757–1765.

Walker, J., G. Heigenhauser, E. Hultman, and L. Spriet. 2000. Dietary carbohydrate, muscle glycogen content, and endurance performance in well-trained women. *Journal of Applied Physiology* 88:2151–2158.

Wang, F., T. McDonald, L. Champagne, and D. Edington. 2004. Relationship of body mass index and physical activity to health care costs among employees. *Journal of Occupational and Environmental Medicine* 46:428–436.

Warburton, D., M. Haykowsky, H. Quinney, D. Blackmore, K. Teo, D. Taylor, J. McGavock, and D. Humen. 2004. Blood volume expansion and cardiorespiratory function: Effects of training modality. *Medicine and Science in Sports and Exercise* 36:991–1000.

Washburn, R., B. Sharkey, J. Narum, and M. Smith. 1982. Dryland training for cross-country skiers. *Ski Coach* 5:9–12.

Watson, P., A. Srivastava, and F. Booth. 1983. Cytochrome C synthesis rate is decreased in the 6th hour of hindlimb immobilization in the rat. In *Biochemistry of exercise*, Vol. 13, ed. J. Knutgen, J. Vogel, and J. Poortmans, 378–384. Champaign, IL: Human Kinetics.

Wei, M., J. Kampert, C. Barlow, M. Nichaman, L. Gibbons, R. Paffenbarger, and S. Blair. 1999. Relationship between low cardiorespiratory fitness and mortality in normal weight, overweight, and obese men. *Journal of the American Medical Association* 282:1547–1553.

Weinberg, R., and D. Gould. 2003. *Foundations of sport and exercise psychology*. Champaign, IL: Human Kinetics.

Welle, S. 2002. Cellular and molecular basis of age-related sarcopenia. *Canadian Journal of Applied Physiology* 27:19–41.

Wenger, C. 1988. Human heat acclimatization. In *Human performance physiology and environmental medicine at terrestrial extremes*, ed. K. Pandolf, M. Sawka, and R. Gonzalez. Indianapolis: Benchmark.

Wenger, H., and G. Bell. 1986. The interaction of intensity, duration and frequency of exercise training in altering cardiorespiratory fitness. *Sports Medicine* 3:346–356.

Weuve, J., J. Kang, J. Manson, M. Breteler, J. Ware, and F. Grodstein. 2004. Physical activity, including walking, and cognitive function in older women. *Journal of the American Medical Association* 292:1454–1461.

Whaley, M., J. Kampert, H. Kohl, and S. Blair. 1999. Physical fitness and clustering of risk factors associated with the metabolic syndrome. *Medicine and Science in Sports and Exercise* 31:287–293.

Whiddon, T.R., B.J. Sharkey, and R.J. Steadman. 1969. Exercise, stress and blood clotting in men. *Research Quarterly* 40:431–434.

Willett, W. 2001. *Eat, drink and be healthy*. New York: Simon and Schuster.

Williams, P. 1974. *Low back and neck pain*. Springfield, IL: Charles C Thomas.

Willis, J., and L. Campbell. 1992. *Exercise psychology*. Champaign, IL: Human Kinetics.

Wilmore, J.H. 1983. *Athletic training and physical fitness.* Boston: Allyn & Bacon.

Wilson, P.K., W. Castelli, and W. Kannel. 1987. Coronary risk prediction in adults (the Framingham Study). *American Journal of Cardiology* 59:91–94.

Witvrouw, E., N. Mahieu, L. Danneels, and P. McNair. 2004. Stretching and injury prevention: An obscure relationship. *Sports Medicine* 34:443–449.

Womack, C., P. Nagelkirk, and A. Coughlin. 2003. Exercise-induced changes in coagulation and fibrinolysis in healthy populations and patients with cardiovascular disease. *Sports Medicine* 33:795–807.

Wood, P. 1975. Middle-aged joggers show healthy lipoprotein pattern. *Medical Tribune* 38:27.

Wood, R., R. Reyes, M. Welsch, J. Favaloro Sabatier, M. Sabatier, C. Lee, L. Johnson, and P. Hooper. 2001. Concurrent cardiovascular and resistance training in healthy older adults. *Medicine and Science in Sports and Exercise* 33:1751–1758.

Wright, J., J. Kennedy-Stephenson, C. Wang, M. McDowell, and C. Johnson. 2004. Trends in intake of energy and macronutrients—United States, 1971–2000. Centers for Disease Control and Prevention, *Morbidity and Mortality Weekly Report* 53:80–82, at www.cdc.gov/mmwr.

Young, A. 1988. Human adaptation to cold. In *Human performance physiology and environmental medicine at terrestrial extremes,* ed. K. Pandolf, M. Sawka, and R. Gonzalez. Indianapolis: Benchmark.

Zauner, C.W., J.J. Burt, and D.F. Mapes. 1968. The effect of strenuous and mild premeal exercise on postprandial lipemia. *Research Quarterly* 39:395–401.

Zhang, K., M. Sun, A. Kovera, J. Albu, F. PiSunyer, and C. Boozer. 2002. Sleeping metabolic rate in relation to body mass index and body composition. *International Journal of Obesity* 26:376–383.

Zuti, W.B., and L. Golding. 1976. Comparing diet and exercise as weight reduction tools. *Physician and Sportsmedicine* 4:59–62.

Index

Note: The italicized *f* and *t* following page numbers refer to figures and tables, respectively.